THE MOTOR SYSTEM:
NEUROPHYSIOLOGY AND MUSCLE MECHANISMS

THE MOTOR SYSTEM: NEUROPHYSIOLOGY AND MUSCLE MECHANISMS

PROCEEDINGS OF A SATELLITE SYMPOSIUM TO THE XXVIth
INTERNATIONAL CONGRESS OF PHYSIOLOGY, HELD IN INDIA
1974

Edited by

Professor MANIK SHAHANI

*E.C.I. Institute of Electrophysiology for
Fundamental and Applied Research,
Parel, Bombay 400 012, India*

ELSEVIER SCIENTIFIC PUBLISHING COMPANY
Amsterdam — Oxford — New York   1976

ELSEVIER SCIENTIFIC PUBLISHING COMPANY
335 Jan van Galenstraat
P.O. Box 211, Amsterdam, The Netherlands

AMERICAN ELSEVIER PUBLISHING COMPANY, INC.
52 Vanderbilt Avenue
New York, New York 10017

ISBN: 0-444-41374-x

Printed in The Netherlands

Preface

This book is a record of some of the papers presented at a meeting on The Motor System — Neurophysiology and Muscle Mechanisms, that was organised by Professor Manik Shahani as a Satellite Symposium in connection with the XXVIth International Congress of Physiology, held in New Delhi in October, 1974. The meeting achieved everything that a satellite meeting should: it took the opportunity created by the presence of a large gathering of physiologists in India to bring together a group of specialists from all over the world to exchange information and opinions in a particular field of physiology; at the same time, the prospect of coming to this meeting in Bombay was an additional stimulus to physiologists from other countries to make the journey to India for the Congress.

Like the Congress itself, this meeting was greatly appreciated and enjoyed by the participants. The scientific interest of the meetings was combined with the excitement of what was for most of us the first visit to India, and we were experiencing for ourselves a little of the variety, the contrasts, the problems and the opportunities of that great country. We all feel a deep debt of gratitude to Professor Shahani, to the civic authorities of Bombay, and to all the others who contributed to the organisation of the meeting and to the hospitality that we received.

The scientific sessions covered all physiological aspects of the motor system of mammals — central and peripheral, sensory and motor, nervous and muscular. Every one of us benefited both from meeting colleagues from all parts of the world, and from being brought into contact with lines of work related to our own. We shall all return to our own specialities with a greater realisation of how our own work can benefit from neighbouring branches of physiology, and of ways in which we can contribute to them.

Department of Physiology,
University College London,
London WCIE 6BT, U.K.

Andrew Huxley

Royal Society Research Professor

Acknowledgements

It is indeed my great privilege to thank my friends amongst the many fellow scientists whose advice helped me to plan the meeting on the Motor System—Neurophysiology and Muscle Mechanisms: Sir Andrew Huxley (London), Sir John Eccles (Buffalo), Prof. Maurice Hugon (Marseille), Prof. E. Gutmann (Prague), Dr. Pavel Hnik (Prague), Prof. Jozef Zachar (Bratislava), Prof. Albrecht Struppler (Munich), Prof. Karleric Hagbarth (Uppsala) and Prof. Plato Kostyuk (Kiev), are a few of the names which I am taking the liberty to mention. The success of the meeting was assured by the support I received from Mr. M.W. Desai, Dr. E.P. Bharucha, Dr. T.H. Rindani, Dr. C.K. Deshpande, Dr. V.N. Acharya and Miss D.H. Dastoor, besides many others.

Mr. Avinash Khopkar typed almost all the manuscripts that have gone to form this volume. Miss Gospi Capadia gave her assistance in the preparation of the index etc. I am grateful to all the authors who have contributed to this volume; without their prompt response, it would not have been possible to keep to the time schedule. Finally, I cannot forget all the encouragement and understanding which was given by my wife, Professor Mira Shahani, and my children, Uma and Sanjay.

Manik Shahani

List of contributors

Adrian, R.H.	Physiological Laboratory, University of Cambridge, Downing Street, Cambridge, U.K.
Agarwal, G.C.	Department of Biomedical Engineering, Rush-Presbyterian—St. Luke's Medical Centre, Chicago, Illin is, U.S.A.
Beaubaton, D.	Département de Neurophysiologie générale, Institute de Neurophysiologie et Psychophysiologie, C.N.R.S., Marseille, France.
Blair, S.M.	Department of Physiology-Anatomy, University of California, Berkeley, California 94720, USA.
Bratzlavsky, M.	Department of Neurology, University of Ghent, B-9000 Ghent, Belgium.
Burg, D.	Neurological Clinic of the Technical University of Munich, Munich, G.F.R.
Delwaide, P.J.	Section of Neurology, Institute of Medicine, Hôpital de Bavière, Liège, Belgium.
Dessalle, M.	Section of Neurology, Institute of Medicine, Hôpital de Bavière, Liège, Belgium.
Ellaway, P.H.	Department of Physiology, University College London, London, U.K.
Gottlieb, G.L.	Department of Biomedical Engineering, Rush-Presbyterian—St. Luke's Medical Centre, Chicago, Illinois, U.S.A.
Gutmann, E.	Institute of Physiology, Czechoslovak Academy of Sciences, Prague, Czechoslovakia.
Gydikov, A.	Institute of Physiology, Bulgarian Academy of Sciences, Sofia 13, Bulgaria.
Henneman, E.	Harvard Medical School, Boston Massachusetts 02114, U.S.A.
Juprelle, M.	Section of Neurology, Institute of Medicine, Hôpital de Bavière, Liège, Belgium.
Kirkwood, P.A.	Sobell Department of Neurophysiology, Institute of

Neurology, Queen Square, London W.C.1, U.K.

Kojima, S.   Department of Neurophysiology, Primate Research In-
                    stitute, Kyoto University, Inuyama, Japan.

Kostyuk, P.G.   A. Bogomoletz Institute of Physiology, Kiev, U.S.S.R.

Kubota, K.   Department of Neurophysiology, Primate Research In-
                    stitute, Kyoto University, Inuyama, Japan.

Lange, W.   Physiological Institute, University of Munich, D-8000
                    Munich 2, G.F.R.

Mai, J.   Department of Neurology, Aarhus Kommunehospital,
                    Aarhus, Denmark.

Massion, J.   Département de Neurophysiologie générale, Institute de
                    Neurophysiologie et Psychophysiologie, C.N.R.S., Mar-
                    seille, France.

Paillard, J.   Département de Neurophysiologie générale, Institute de
                    Neurophysiologie et Psychophysiologie, C.N.R.S., Mar-
                    seille, France.

Partridge, L.D.   Department of Physiology and Biophysics, University of
                    Tennessee, Centre for the Health Sciences, Memphis,
                    Tennessee, U.S.A.

Peachey, L.D.   Department of Biology, University of Pennsylvania,
                    Philadelphia, Pennsylvania 19174, U.S.A.

Pedersen, E.   Department of Neurology, Aarhus Kommunehospital,
                    Aarhus, Denmark.

Regis, H.   Département de Neurophysiologie générale, Institute de
                    Neurophysiologie et Psychophysiologie, C.N.R.S., Mar-
                    seille, France.

Rubia, F.J.   Physiological Institute, University of Munich, D-8000,
                    Munich 2, G.F.R.

Sears, T.A.   Sobell Department of Neurophysiology, Institute of
                    Neurology, Queen Square, London W.C.1, U.K.

Shahani, B.T.   Massachusetts General Hospital, Boston, Massachusetts
                    02114, U.S.A.

Shahani, M.   E.C.I. Institute of Electrophysiology for Fundamental
                    and Applied Research, Parel, Bombay-400 012, India.

Stålberg, E.   Department of Clinical Neurophysiology, University
                    Hospital, Uppsala, Sweden.

Stephens, J.A.   The Sherrington School of Physiology, St. Thomas's
                    Hospital Medical School, London S.E.1, U.K.

Struppler, A.   Neurological Clinic of the Technical University of
                    Munich, Munich, G.F.R.

Stuart, D.G.   Department of Physiology, College of Medicine, Univer-
                    sity of Arizona, Tucson, Arizona 85724, U.S.A.

Szumski, A.J.   Department of Physiology, Medical College of Virginia,
                    Richmond, Virginia 23298, U.S.A.

Trouche, E.   Département de Neurophysiologie générale, Institute de Neurophysiologie et Psychophysiologie, C.N.R.S., Marseille, France.

Velho, F.   Neurological Clinic of the Technical University of Munich, Munich, G.F.R.

Westheimer, G.   Department of Physiology-Anatomy, University of California, Berkeley, California 94720, U.S.A.

Young, R.R.   Massachusetts General Hospital, Boston, Massachusetts 02114, U.S.A.

Contents

Preface   v
Acknowledgements   vii
List of contributors   ix
Contents   xiii
Introduction   1

Section I. MUSCLE
1. The multiple regulation of contractile and histochemical properties of cross-
   striated muscle
   by E. Gutmann   5
2. The propagation of excitation in striated muscle
   by R.H. Adrian   15
3. Structure and function of the T-system in skeletal muscle cells
   by L.D. Peachey   25

Section II. THE MOTOR UNIT
1. The recruitment order of motor units and its significance for the behaviour of
   tendon organs during normal muscle activity
   by D.G. Stuart and J.A. Stephens   37
2. The potential of the motor unit
   by A. Gydikov   49
3. The extent of voluntary control of human motor units
   by E. Henneman, B.T. Shahani and R.R. Young   73
4. Single fibre electromyography for motor unit study in man
   by E. Stålberg   79

Section III. AFFERENTS, MUSCLE SPINDLES AND CENTRAL EXCITATION
1. Influence of a voluntary innervation on human muscle spindle sensitivity
   by D. Burg, A.J. Szumski, A. Struppler and F. Velho   95
2. Pharmacological blocking of the human fusimotor system
   by J. Mai and E. Pedersen   111
3. Monosynaptic excitation of thoracic motoneurones from both primary and
   secondary spindle afferents in the anaesthetised cat
   by P.A. Kirkwood and T.A. Sears   117
4. Recurrent inhibition of gamma motoneurones
   by P.H. Ellaway   119

5. Afferent inflow from the human bladder in relation to filling and voiding
by E. Pedersen and J. Mai   127

Section IV. REFLEX PHYSIOLOGY
1. Human brainstem reflexes
by M. Bratzlavsky   135
2. Behaviour of human brainstem reflexes in muscles with antagonistic function
by M. Bratzlavsky   155
3. The effects of caloric vestibular stimulation on the tonic vibration reflex in
man
by P.J. Delwaide, M. Dessalle and M. Juprelle   163
4. Reflex physiology in man
by P.J. Delwaide   169
5. Effects of vibration on human spinal reflexes
by G.C. Agarwal and G.L. Gottlieb   181
6. Effect of vibration on the F response
by B.T. Shahani and R.R. Young   189
7. Single muscle spindle afferent recordings in human flexor reflex
by A. Struppler and F. Velho   197

Section V. CENTRAL CONTROL OF MOVEMENT
1. Supraspinal mechanisms on a spinal level
by P.G. Kostyuk   211
2. Functional organization of the primate oculomotor system
by G. Westheimer and S.M. Blair   237
3. The spatial distribution of climbing fibre suppression of Purkinje cell activity
by F.J. Rubia and W. Lange   247
4. Visual input and its influence on motor and sensory systems in man
by M. Shahani   261
5. The effects of tonic, isometric contraction on the evoked EMG
by G.C. Agarwal and G.L. Gottlieb   283
6. The EMG analysis of certain negative symptoms caused by lesions of the central nervous system
by B.T. Shahani and R.R. Young   293
7. Asterixis — a disorder of the neural mechanisms underlying sustained muscle
contraction
by B.T. Shahani and R.R. Young   301
8. A review of physiological and pharmacological studies of human tremor
by B.T. Shahani and R.R. Young   307

Section VI. ORGANIZATION OF LEARNT MOVEMENTS
1. Prefrontal unit activity of under-trained monkeys in delayed-response tasks
by K. Kubota and S. Kojima   317
2. Triggered and guided components of visual reaching. Their dissociation in
split-brain studies
by J. Paillard and D. Beaubaton   333
3. Movement and associated postural adjustment
by H. Regis, E. Trouche and J. Massion   349
4. A proposal for study of a state description of the motor control system
by L.D. Partridge   363

Subject index   371
Author index   383

Introduction

The last twenty-five years have registered tremendous advances in the knowledge of the motor system in man, pursued on an experimental basis. This has been possible, no doubt, due to the availability of sophisticated electronic equipment and computer technology. Animal experiments, which have been the backbone of physiology, can now be performed with great ease, with the result that there has been almost a flood of papers in the different branches of neurophysiology. Yet, looking at the diary of international meetings and symposia, one finds hardly any devoted to the motor system. It was with this background and a consciousness of the need to bring scientists both from human and animal physiology together, that a meeting on 'The Motor System — Neurophysiology and Muscle Mechanisms' was organized in Bombay on October 29th, 30th and 31st, 1974, immediately after the XXVIth International Congress of Physiological Sciences held in Delhi.

The meeting took about two years to organise, and an attempt was made to cover the entire motor system, from cortex to a single muscle fibre, incorporating as far as possible all that lies between — cerebellum, central control through descending tracts, reflex physiology, and various sensory inputs. Geographically as well, almost the whole world of science was covered, as the scientists who participated came from eminent universities and institutes from many different countries including Belgium, Bulgaria, Czechoslovakia, Denmark, France, Germany, Japan, Sweden, U.K., U.S.A. and U.S.S.R. There were young as well as old workers in the field, and there were scientists dedicated to fundamental research as well as applied work related to pathophysiology. This volume, therefore, is a unique book which may find its place on the shelf of a pure physiologist, clinical neurophysiologist, psychophysiologist, neurologist, physiotherapist, and all those who are concerned with the motor system in one way or another including the ergonomist, engineer and orthopaedic surgeon.

Muscle

1. The multiple regulation of contractile and histochemical properties of cross-striated muscle
   by E. Gutmann   5

2. The propagation of excitation in striated muscle
   by R.H. Adrian   15

3. Structure and function of the T-system in skeletal muscle cells
   by L.D. Peachey   25

The multiple regulation of contractile and histochemical properties of cross-striated muscle

E. GUTMANN

Recent studies have shown the remarkable capacity of skeletal muscle and muscle fibres to respond to new functional demands, especially with respect to dynamic properties and histochemical muscle fibre pattern (for reviews see Close, 1972; Gutmann, 1973). The high degree of this adaptational capacity is revealed by the great diversity of muscles and muscle fibres adapted to different functional demands, the considerable changes in muscle during ontogenetic development (Nyström, 1968; Close, 1972; Gutmann et al., 1974) and observations on transformation of speed, metabolism and muscle fibre pattern produced by a change of nerve supply (Buller et al., 1960; Drahota and Gutmann, 1963; Guth et al., 1968). The basic conditions of such studies were the recognition of (a) the histochemically distinct groups of muscle fibres with respect to oxidative and glycolytic activities (Dubowitz and Pearse, 1960; Stein and Padykula, 1962) and of ATPase (Engel, 1962); (b) the close correlation between speed of contraction and enzymic properties of the muscle (Bárány, 1967; Close, 1972) and (c) the close correlation between the properties of neurone and muscle fibres in slow and fast mammalian motor units (Henneman and Olson, 1965; Edström and Kugelberg, 1968, and others).

The classification of muscle fibres into two types may be an oversimplification, especially with respect to the existence of a group of 'intermediate' fibres (see Barnard et al., 1971). It must also be remembered that the identification of fast—white and slow—red muscles and muscle fibres, introduced by Ranvier (1874) is not at all a general one. Fast muscle fibres may be 'red' or 'white', i.e. fast contracting types may differ in oxidative enzyme activity and fatigue resistance (Hall-Cragg, 1968; Schiaffino et al., 1970; Burke et al., 1971; Gutmann and Syrový, 1971). For instance, the differentiation in speed of contraction is similar in the fast extensor digitorum longus and in the slow soleus muscle of both the rabbit and the hare. However, both extensor digitorum longus and soleus muscle of the hare are 'red' due to the general adaptation response to 'endurance' in the wild living hare (Bass et al., 1974).

The classification of fast and slow muscles remains, however, a useful tool in studies of the basic mechanisms of adaptation.

The regulatory influence of the neurone was revealed by observations on transformation of contraction time and properties of the contractile proteins during development and after cross-innervation. Since, in slow and fast mammalian motor units, properties of the neurone are closely matched to properties of the muscle fibres, it is understandable that the mechanisms responsible for plasticity of muscle were primarily studied and looked for with respect to neuronal function. There is, however, increasing evidence for a multiple regulation of contractile and histochemical (the muscle fibre pattern) properties of muscle, including neural (i.e. impulse and non-impulse), myogenic, hormonal, vascular and peripheral influences. The main questions concerning this regulation appear to be the characterisation of the neural mechanisms and the differentiation of the different components of regulation.

NEURAL INFLUENCES

Transformation of contraction time and myosin properties (ATPase activity and low molecular weight protein — light chains of myosin) is observed after cross-union of nerves (Buller et al., 1960, 1969; Bárány and Close, 1971; Samaha et al., 1970, and others) and cross-transplantation of muscles (Gutmann and Carlson, 1975; Hanzlíková and Gutmann, 1974). The transformation concerns also non-contractile structures, such as glycogen content and intracellular ionic composition (Drahota and Gutmann, 1963) and the contractural response to caffeine, related to a change in Ca^{2+} transport (Gutmann and Hanzlíková, 1967; Miledi and Stefani, 1969), however the initiating signal for the transformation is a presynaptic one, related to a change in end-plate structure (Hník et al., 1967). The latter signal apparently also changes membrane characteristics such as the sensitivity to acetylcholine (ACh) (Elul et al., 1970). The spread of ACh sensitivity after denervation was thought to be due to the absence of a 'neurotrophic' factor (Miledi, 1960). Stimulation experiments of muscle (Jones and Vrbová, 1971; Lomo and Rosenthal, 1972) suggested, however, that regulation was achieved by nerve impulse; blocking experiments (Albuquerque et al., 1972), on the contrary, suggested regulation by non-impulse ('neurotrophic') activities. The neuronal influence on contraction properties could be related to impulse (frequency pattern or degree of activity) or to non-impulse activity of the neurone. Long-term electrical stimulation of a fast muscle results in slowing of contraction time (Salmons and Vrbová, 1969) and in a change of ATPase activity and myosin light chains corresponding to those of a slow muscle (Sreter et al., 1973). The frequency of stimulation in these experiments was low, suggesting the importance of the frequency pattern of stimulation on regulation of contractile properties. However, stimulation of a fast denervated muscle results in shortening of contraction time, both in vivo (Brown, 1973; Melichna and Gutmann, 1974) and in vitro (Gutmann et al., 1969). Both frequency pattern and total activity apparently affect contractile properties. Denervation experiments provide evidence for the assumption that regulation of contraction properties is primarily related to neuronal impulse and not to non-impulse activities. After nerve section, progressive prolongation of contraction time is observed in a fast muscle (Gutmann et al., 1972). If contraction time were regulated by impulse activity no difference should be observed in a denervated muscle, irrespective of whether the nerve was sectioned close to or distally from the muscle, since impulse activity is abolished simultaneously on both sides. This has been shown to be the case in 'long–short' nerve stump experiments (Gutmann et al., 1975). On the other hand this type of experiment shows conclusively that 'neurotrophic' activities also affect muscle properties. For instance, onset of degeneration of end plates and decrease of glycogen synthesis (Gutmann et al., 1955), fibrillation potentials (Luco and Eyzaguirre, 1955), neuromuscular transmission (Slater, 1966) and other membrane and intracellular denervation changes occur earlier in a muscle denervated close to nerve entry (Gutmann, 1973). These properties are apparently due to neurotrophic influences, mediated by the axoplasmic flow which is exhausted sooner after denervation of a muscle with a short nerve stump. It thus appears that the primary contention, that contraction properties are regulated by a trophic factor released from the nerve (Buller et al., 1960) can no longer be maintained.

A developmental study may serve as an example of the mechanism by which the neuronal impulse activity changes speed and muscle fibre pattern. Slow and fast muscles exhibit a differential behaviour during development. Slow muscles show a prolongation, fast muscles a progressive shortening of contraction time. This is best seen in the slow soleus muscle of the guinea pig, which is fast at birth and slow in the adult animal and this is apparently related to the increasing response of the 'tonic' muscle to antigravity forces. Correspondingly the muscle fibre pattern changes from a mixed muscle fibre pattern according to ATPase activity to a uniform pattern with fibres of low ATPase activity. The light chain pattern of myosin also changes from a 3-band ('fast') pattern of the soleus muscle at birth to a 2-band ('slow') pattern in the adult animal (Gutmann et al., 1974). Developmental transformation takes place apparently due to a decrease of ATPase activity in originally fast muscle fibres.

Collateral sprouting of axons was suggested as a mechanism resulting in transformation of muscle (Guth, 1974). Normally innervated muscle will not receive a new nerve supply but sprouts have been shown to take over territories and functions of denervated axons (Weddell et al., 1941; Edds, 1953) and a denervated muscle may become innervated at any place on the muscle membrane (Gutmann and Young, 1944). The skeletal muscle fibre may accept additional innervation from a foreign nerve if the original nerve is temporarily interrupted (Gutmann and Hanzlíková, 1967) or blocked (Jansen et al., 1973). It was thus possible to produce muscle fibres with two end plates and, correspondingly, a change in contraction properties of the 'hyper-neurotized' muscle (Gutmann and Hanzlíková, 1967). A mechanism of selective enlargement of slow motor units during development with the corresponding changes in speed of contraction and fibre pattern (see Gutmann et al., 1974) may thus be possible. The significance of this mechanism has still to be shown.

MYOGENIC INFLUENCES

It is well known that the first stages of muscle development proceed independently of neural influences (see Fishman, 1972). Moreover, differentiation of some fast and slow muscles may be evident already at very early stages of development (Sréter et al., 1972). These observations point to myogenic factors in the process of differentiation.

The importance of myogenic properties is shown in experiments in which a slow muscle is transplanted into the place of the androgen-sensitive (fast) levator ani muscle of the rat. According to the 'fast' nerve supply of the pudendal nerve, now re-innervating the slow muscle, contraction time of the slow soleus muscle is changed to a fast one. However, the grafted skeletal muscle does not acquire hormone sensitivity to androgens, i.e. no change of contraction time or weight is observed after castration or testosterone administration, as it is the case in the androgen-sensitive ('target') muscle (Hanzlíková and Gutmann, 1974). Thus, the neuronal impulse activity transforms the muscle with respect to contraction time and muscle fibre pattern, but hormone sensitivity is not changed, being primarily of myogenic origin.

HORMONAL INFLUENCES

The experiments quoted suggest the importance of hormonal influences on muscle properties. The effects of hormones differ, however, in target (highly sensitive) and non-target muscles. Castration, i.e. lack of androgens, results in prolongation of the contraction time, while administration of testosterone causes a shortening of contraction time (Burešová and Gutmann, 1971). Moreover, testosterone administration results in a change of muscle fibre pattern especially with respect to glycolytic enzymes. The 'female' red temporalis muscle is transformed into a 'male' white one after administration of testosterone to female guinea pigs (Gutmann et al., 1970). The effects of testosterone on non-target muscles are relatively small and may be due to changes in motor activity related to the hormone administration (Hanzlikova and Gutmann, 1974).

VASCULAR INFLUENCES

Increased blood supply in muscles adapted especially for endurance work results in an increase of oxidative enzyme activities and density of capillaries. Bearing this in mind the differences between slow 'red' and fast 'white' muscles (see Hudlická, 1973) may be understood as being due to a differential adaptation to endurance and phasic motor activities. Endurance and speed of contraction may be independently controlled. Accordingly, fast—white and fast—red muscle fibres will be found (see Barnard et al., 1970; Bass et al., 1973; Burke and Tsairis, 1974, and others).

PERIPHERAL FACTORS

Peripheral factors also affect contraction time and muscle fibre pattern. Compensatory hypertrophy of a muscle induced by tenotomy of the synergistic muscles is accompanied by prolongation of contraction time and decrease of tension output and is apparently due to the stretching of the muscle (Gutmann et al., 1971; Hník et al., 1974). The relation between length and tension is well known (Ramsey and Street, 1940) and depends apparently on the degree of overlap between the two sets of filaments (Gordon et al., 1966). Some of the effects of change of length of muscle can be reproduced also in vitro or in denervated muscle. Stretching of a muscle increases protein synthesis (Burešová et al., 1969) and the number of sarcomeres (Goldspink et al., 1974). Immobilisation and denervation of the limb (by plaster casts) in an extended position results in relative prolongation of contraction time and increase in weight; immobilisation in a flexed position, on the other hand, causes a relative shortening of contraction time and a decrease of weight in the denervated muscle (Melichna and Gutmann, 1974). The denervated muscle immobilized in a lengthened position does also produce 25% more sarcomeres in series, whilst that immobilized in a shortened position loses 35% (Goldspink et al., 1974).

It will be remembered that conflicting data are reported with respect to the effect of immobilization on contraction properties. Decrease of contraction time after immobilization has been described in the slow soleus (Fischbach and Robbins, 1969; Mann and Salafsky, 1970; Booth and Kelso, 1973) but not in fast muscle (Booth and Kelso, 1973). Peripheral factors have to be taken into consideration and could affect the results reported.

The following conclusions are possible:

(1) A multiple regulation, i.e. neural, vascular, hormonal and peripheral factors affect contractile and histochemical properties of muscle.

(2) Changes in contraction time and muscle fibre pattern are primarily due to nerve-impulse activities, the 'neurotrophic', non-impulse activities being primarily related to maintenance and growth processes of the neurone affecting the muscle.

(3) Tranformation of contractile and histochemical properties is affected by changeability of muscle fibre types; collateral innervation may take part in this process.

REFERENCES

ALBUQUERQUE, E.X., WARNICK, J.E., ROSSE, J.R. and SANSONE, F.M. (1972) Effects of Vinblastine and Colchicine on neural regulation of fast and slow skeletal muscles of the rat: an electrophysiological and ultrastructural study. Exp. Neurol., 37, 607—634.

BÁRÁNY, M. (1967) ATPase activity of myosin correlated with speed of muscle shortening. J. Gen. Physiol., 50, 197—218.

BÁRÁNY, M. and CLOSE, R.I. (1971) The transformation of myosin in cross-innervated rat muscle. J. Physiol. 213, 455—474.

BARNARD, R.J., EDGERTON, V.R. and PETER, J.B. (1970) Effect of exercise on skeletal muscle. I. Biochemical and histochemical properties. J. Appl. Physiol., 28, 762—766.

BARNARD, R.J., EDGERTON, V.R., FURUKAWA, T. and PETER, J.B. (1971) Histochemical, biochemical and contractile properties of red, white and intermediate fibers. Am. J. Physiol., 220, 410—414.

BASS, A., GUTMANN, E., MELICHNA, J. and SYROVÝ, I. (1973) Contraction, histochemical and enzyme properties of fast and slow muscles of the rabbit and the hare. Physiol. Bohemoslov., 22, 477—486.

BOOTH, F.W. and KELSO, J.R. (1973) Effect of hind limb immobilization on contractile and histochemical properties of skeletal muscle. Pflügers Arch., 342, 231—238.

BROWN, M.D. (1973) Role of activity in the differentiation of slow and fast muscles. Nature, 244, 178—179.

BULLER, A.J., ECCLES, J.C. and ECCLES, R.M. (1960) Interactions between motoneurones and muscles in respect to the characteristic speeds of their responses. J. Physiol., 150, 417—439.

BULLER, A.J., MOMMAERTS, W.H.F. and SERAYDARIAN, K. (1969) Enzymic properties of myosin in fast and slow twitch muscles of the cat following cross-innervation. J. Physiol., 205, 581—597.

BUREŠOVÁ, M. and GUTMANN, E. (1971) Effect of testosterone on protein synthesis and contractility of the levator ani muscle of the rat. J. Endocrinol., 50, 643—651.

BUREŠOVÁ, M., GUTMANN, E. and KLICPERA, M. (1969) Effect of tension upon rate of incorporation of amino acids into proteins of cross-striated muscle. Experientia, 25, 144—145.

BURKE, R.E., LEVINE, D.M., ZAJAC, F.E., TSAIRIS, P. and ENGEL, W.K. (1971) Mammalian motor units. Physiological-histochemical correlation in 3 types in cat gastrocnemius. Science, 174, 709—712.

BURKE, R.E. and TSAIRIS, P. (1974) The correlation of physiological properties with histochemical characteristics in single muscle units. In: Trophic functions of the neuron. Ann. N.Y. Acad. Sci., 228, 145—159.

CLOSE, R.I. (1972) Dynamic properties of mammalian skeletal muscles. Physiol. Rev., 52, 129—197.

DRAHOTA, Z. and GUTMANN, E. (1963) Long-term regulatory influence of the nervous system on some metabolic differences in muscle of different function. Physiol. Bohemoslov., 12, 339—348.

DUBOWITZ, V. and PEARSE, A.G. (1960) A comparative histochemical study of oxidative enzyme and phosphorylase activity in skeletal muscle. Histochemie, 2, 105—117.

EDDS, M.V. (1950) Collateral nerve regeneration. Rev. Biol. 28, 260—276.

EDSTRÖM, L. and KUGELBERG, E. (1968) Histochemical composition, distribution of fibers and fatiguability of single motor units. J. Neurol. Neurosurg. Psychiat., 31, 424—433.

ELUL, R., MILEDI, R. and STEFANI, E. (1970) Neural control of contracture in slow muscle fibres of the frog. Acta Physiol. Lattinoam., 20, 194—226.

ENGEL, W.K. (1962) The essentiality of histo- and cytochemical studies of skeletal muscle in the investigation of neuromuscular disease. Neurology, 12, 778—794.

FISCHBACH, G.D. and ROBBINS, N. (1969) Changes in contractile properties of disused soleus muscles. J. Physiol. (Lond.), 201, 305—320.

FISCHMAN, D.A. (1972) Development of striated muscle. In: The Structure and Function of Muscle, Vol. 1, Academic Press, New York, pp. 75—148.

GOLDSPINK, G., TABARY, C., TABARY, J.C., TARDIEU, C. and TARDIEU, G. (1974) Effect of denervation on the adaptation of sarcomere number and muscle extensibility of the functional length of the muscle. J. Physiol., 236, 733—742.

GORDON, A.M., HUXLEY, A.F. and JULIAN, F.J. (1966) Tension development in highly stretched vertebrate muscle fibres. J. Physiol. (Lond.), 184, 143—169.

GUTH, L. (1974) Trophic interactions between nerve and muscle. Int. Congr. Ser. 334, Excerpta Medica, Amsterdam, p. 1.

GUTH, L., WATSON, P.K. and BROWN, W.C. (1968) Effects of cross-reinnervation on some chemical properties of red and white muscles of rat and cat. Exp. Neurol., 20, 52—69.

GUTMANN, E. (1973) Critical evaluation and implications of denervation and reinnervation studies of cross striated muscle. In: Methods of Neurochemistry, Vol. 5, M. Dekker, Inc., New York, pp. 189—254.

GUTMANN, E. (1973) The multiple regulation of muscle fibre pattern in cross striated muscle. Nova Acta Leopoldina, 38, 193—218.

GUTMANN, E. and CARLSON, M.B. (1975) Contractile and histochemical properties of regenerating cross-transplanted fast and slow muscles in the rat. Pflügers Arch., 353, 227—239.

GUTMANN, E., HÁJEK, I. and HOSRKÝ, P. (1969) Effect of excessive use on contraction and metabolic properties of cross-striated muscle. J. Physiol., 203, 46—47P.

GUTMANN, E. and HANZLÍKOVÁ, V. (1967) Effects of accessory nerve supply to muscle achieved by implantation into muscle during regeneration of its nerve. Physiol. Bohemoslov., 16, 244—250.

GUTMANN, E., HANZLÍKOVÁ, V. and LOJDA, Z. (1970) Effects of androgens on histochemical fibre type. Differentiation in the temporal muscle of the guinea pig. Histochemie, 24, 287—291.

GUTMANN, E., MELICHNA, J. and SYROVÝ, I. (1972) Contraction properties and ATPase activity in fast and slow muscle of the rat during denervation. Exp. Neurol., 36, 488—497.

GUTMANN, E., MELICHNA, J. and SYROVÝ, I. (1974) Developmental changes in contraction time, myosin properties and fibre pattern of fast and slow skeletal muscles. Physiol. Bohemoslov., 23, 19—27.

GUTMANN, E., MELICHNA, J. and SYROVÝ, I. (1975) Lack of effect of length of nerve stump on contraction properties of denervated muscle. Physiol. Bohemoslov., (in press).

GUTMANN, E., SCHIAFFINO, S. and HANZLÍKOVÁ, V. (1971) Mechanism of compensatory hypertrophy in the skeletal muscle of the rat. Exp. Neurol., 31, 451—464.

GUTMANN, E. and SYROVÝ, I. (1971) Contractile behaviour and ATPase activity of the semitendinosus muscle of the rat. Physiol. Bohemoslov., 20, 1—9.

GUTMANN, E., VODIČKA, Z. and ZELENÁ, J. (1955) Changes in striated muscle after section of nerve, as a function of the length of the peripheral segment. Physiol. Bohemoslov., 4, 200—204.

GUTMANN, E. and YOUNG, J.Z. (1944) The reinnervation of muscle after various periods of atrophy. J. Anat., 78, 15—42.

HALL-CRAGGS, E.C.B. (1968) The contraction times and enzyme activity of two laryngeal muscles. J. Anat., 102, 241—255.

HANZLÍKOVÁ, V. and GUTMANN, E. (1974) The absence of androgen-sensitivity in the grafted soleus muscle innervated by the pudendal nerve. Cell. Tiss. Res., 145, 121—129.

HENNEMAN, E. and OLSON, C.B. (1965) Relations between structure and function in the design of skeletal muscle. J. Neurophysiol., 28, 581—598.

HNÍK, P., JIRMANOVÁ, I., VYKLICKÝ, L. and ZELENÁ, J. (1967) Fast and slow muscles of the chick after nerve cross-union. J. Physiol., 193, 309—325.

HNÍK, P., MACKOVÁ, E., SYROVÝ, I., HOLAS, M. and KRISHNA-REDDY, V. (1974) Contractile properties of muscle undergoing 'compensatory' hypertrophy and its increased susceptibility to denervation and reflex atrophy. Pflügers Arch., 349, 171—181.

HUDLICKÁ, O. (1973) Circulation in Skeletal Muscle. Elsevier, Amsterdam.

JANSEN, J.K.S., LOMO, T., NICOLAYSEN, K. and WESTGAARD, R.H. (1973) Hyperinnervation of skeletal muscle fibres: dependence on muscle activity. Science, 181, 559—561.

JONES, R. and VRBOVÁ, G. (1971) Can denervation hypersensitivity be prevented? J. Physiol., 217, 67—75.

LOMO, T. and ROSENTHAL, J. (1972) Control of ACh sensitivity by muscle in the rat. J. Physiol., 221, 493—513.

LUCO, J.V. and EYZAGUIRRE, C. (1955) Fibrillation and hypersensitivity to ACh in denervated muscle: effects of length of degenerating nerve fibers. J. Neurophysiol., 18, 65—73.

MANN, W.S. and SALAFSKY, B. (1970) Enzymic and physiological studies on normal and diseased developing fast and slow cat muscles. J. Physiol., 208, 33—47.

MELICHNA, J. and GUTMANN, E. (1974) Stimulation and immobilization effects on contractile and histochemical properties of denervated muscle. Pflügers Arch., 348, 165—178.

MILEDI, R. (1960) Properties of regenerating neuromuscular synapses in the frog. J. Physiol., 154, 190—205.

MILEDI, R. and STEFANI, E. (1969) Non-selective reinnervation of slow and fast muscle fibres in the rat. Nature, 222, 569—571.

NYSTRÖM, B. (1968) Histochemistry of developing cat muscles. Acta Neurol. Scand., 44, 405—439.

RAMSEY, R.W. and STREET, S.F. (1940) The isometric length-tension diagram of isolated skeletal muscle fibres of the frog. J. Cell. Comp. Physiol., 15, 11—34.

SALMONS, S. and VRBOVÁ, G. (1969) The influence of activity on some contractile characteristics of mammalian fast and slow muscles. J. Physiol. (Lond.), 201, 535—549.

SAMAHA, F.J., GUTH, L. and ALBERS, R.W. (1970) The neural regulation of gene expression in the muscle cell. Exp. Neurol., 27, 276—282.

SCHIAFFINO, S., HANZLÍKOVÁ, V. and PIEROBON, S. (1970) Relations between structure and function in rat skeletal muscle fibers. J. Cell. Biol., 47, 107—119.

SLATER, C.R. (1966) Time course of failure of neuromuscular transmission after motor nerve section. Nature, 209, 305—306.

SRÉTER, F.A., GERGELY, J., SALMONS, S. and ROMANUL, F. (1973) Synthesis by fast myosin light chains characteristic of slow muscle in response to long-term stimulation. Nature New Biol., 241, 17—19.

SRÉTER, F.A., HOLTZER, S., GERGELY, J. and HOLTZER, H. (1972) Some properties of embryonic myosin. J. Cell. Biol., 58, 586—594.

STEIN, J.M. and PADYKULA, H.A. (1962) Histochemical classification of individual skeletal muscle fibers of the rat. Am. J. Anat., 110, 103—124.

WEDDEL, G., GUTMANN, L. and GUTMANN, E. (1941) The extension of nerve fibres into denervated areas of skin. J. Neurol. Psychiat., 4, 206—225.

2

The propagation of excitation in striated muscle

R.H. ADRIAN

The electrical activity of a nerve fibre results in transmitter release at discrete sites in the nerve; elsewhere the nerve is specialized for the rapid longitudinal propagation of the signal. The electrical activity of a vertebrate muscle fibre produces a contraction throughout the substance of the fibre. In such a muscle fibre not only does the action potential propagate along the fibre, but an electrical signal spreads radially in the transverse tubular system so that superficial and axial myofibrils contract within about 1 msec of each other (Gonzalez-Serratos, 1971). A.V. Hill (1948) first stated the problems raised by the very rapid activation of contraction throughout the cross-section of a muscle fibre.

Recently, L.D. Peachey and I (Adrian and Peachey, 1973) have tried to calculate how an action potential might spread along a sartorius muscle fibre and in the transverse tubular system. We have tried, as far as possible, to take into account what is known about the ionic currents of frog muscle (Adrian et al., 1970), the morphology of the transverse tubular system (Porter and Palade, 1957; Peachey, 1965) and the characteristics of the capacity of muscle fibre (Falk and Fatt, 1964; Schneider, 1970; Hodgkin and Nakajima, 1972a,b). In the context of the possible presence in the membrane of gating charges for activation (Schneider and Chandler, 1973) for sodium current (Armstrong and Bezanilla, 1973; Keynes and Rojas, 1973) and any other possible mechanisms, it is as well to state explicitly that we have made no provision for the sort of non-linear capacitance which such charge movements would imply.

Conventional cable theory assumptions are used to describe longitudinal and radial current spread in the fibre and the tubular system (Adrian et al., 1969). The Hodgkin–Huxley equations, suitably modified, describe the behaviour of the non-linear sodium and potassium currents in the surface membrane of the muscle fibre and in the membrane of the transverse tubules. Following Hodgkin and Huxley (1952) we have calculated the solution for a wave propagating at a uniform velocity along the longitudinal cable, by converting the partial differential equation describing the longitudinal spread into an ordinary differential equation with time as the independent variable. Radial propagation in the transverse tubular system is described by dividing the cross-section of the fibre into a central disc and fifteen concentric annuli, writing for each annulus the differential equation for the voltage change across the tubular wall capacity and tubular ionic conductances. In this way the tubular system is represented by a non-linear cable made up of sixteen elements, each of which is made up of the following current pathways in parallel; a leak conductance, a linear capacity, an activatable sodium current, and an activatable potassium current. Each of these elements is joined to neighbouring cable elements by resistances representing the radial resistances of the tubular lumen. The complete set of differential equations describing currents and voltage in each of the sixteen tubular elements and the fibre surface were solved simultaneously by a fourth order Runge—Kutta method using both an Atlas 2 computer (Titan) in Cambridge and a PDP 6 in the Medical Computer Centre of the University of Pennsylvania.

In a system of such relative complexity there is considerable scope for arbitrary choice of parameters. As far as possible we have tried to use experimentally determined values. For the morphology of the transverse tubular system we have used values derived from Peachey's electron microscopy (Peachey, 1965): we have assumed that there is no systematic radial variation in this morphology. Values for the activatable ionic currents in the surface of the muscle fibre follow closely the results of voltage clamp experiments by Adrian et al. (1970). These experiments are probably a reasonable guide to the surface currents but could not have measured activatable tubular currents (Adrian and Peachey, 1973). For this reason our estimates of tubular sodium and potassium conductances and, a fortiori, the kinetic characteristics of those tubular currents are no better than guesses. We have chosen to suppose that the rate-constant equations, and the equations describing changes in m, h and n are the same in fibre surface and tubular membrane: we have no evidence for or against such a choice.

The distribution of the capacity between the surface and the tubular system is not as straightforward as it might at first sight appear. The area of tubular wall associated with one square centimetre of surface depends on the fibre radius; it increases linearly with the fibre radius. Likewise, as one might expect, the membrane capacity increases with increasing fibre radius (Hodgkin and Nakajima, 1972a,b). Frog sartorius fibres of average diameter (80 μ; *Rana temporaria*) have a capacity measured with constant current pulses of about 8 μF/cm^2 of fibre surface and morphological measurements suggest that the area of the tubular wall is about seven times the surface area in fibres of that diameter. In calculating the action potential we have assumed a capacity of 0.9 μF/cm^2 for both the fibre surface and for the wall of the transverse tubule. This would be consistent with the constant current measurements and also with the observation that fibres with the tubular system functionally disconnected from the surface by treatment with glycerol (Eisenberg and Gage, 1967) have a membrane capacity of 1.0 μF/cm^2 when this is measured by means of the propagation velocity and the rate of rise of the foot of the action potential (Tasaki and Hagiwara, 1957; Hodgkin and Nakajima, 1972a).

To predict the electrical behaviour of the fibre and tubular systems one must know how to represent the electrical connection between the extracellular fluid and the tubular lumen. We have supposed that there is an access resistance (R_s) at the circumference of the tubular system which must be crossed by any current passing between the extracellular fluid and the tubular lumen. If the value of R_s is substantially greater than the effective radial resistance of the tubular lumen (R_R) the equivalent circuit of the surface membrane and tubular system for small voltage displacements will approximate to the circuit shown in Fig. 1. This equivalent circuit was proposed by Falk and Fatt (1964) from a.c. impedance measurements with intracellular micro-electrodes. Their results were fitted best by assuming that C_M and C_T in Fig. 1 had values of 2.6 μF/cm^2 and 4.1 μF/cm^2. In the model for calculating the action potentials making R_s much greater than R_R would produce values for C_M and C_T of 0.9 μF/cm^2 and 6.3 μF/cm^2 respectively. Others have made a.c. impedance studies of muscle fibres. Schneider (1970) concludes that a radial resistance of about 300 Ω cm^2 is distributed in the tubular lumen and that there is no special access resistance. Eisenberg (personal communication) feels that there may be some access resistance but that it cannot be much greater than 50 Ω cm^2. It is probably true to say, therefore, that the model which we have used for calculating action potentials is not, in detail, compatible with any equivalent circuits derived from a.c. impedance studies, and for that reason, if for no other, must be cautiously interpreted. It remains to be seen whether non-ideal behaviour of the capacity of the kind produced by mobile changes or dipoles in the membrane can account for these discrepancies. Like the action potential calculations the impedance analyses assume that the capacities in the equivalent circuit behave in a linear manner.

Fig. 2 compares experimentally recorded action potentials with calculated

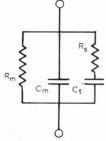

Fig. 1. Two time-constant equivalent circuits for surface membrane (R_m and C_m) and for the tubular system (R_s and C_T) of a muscle fibre.

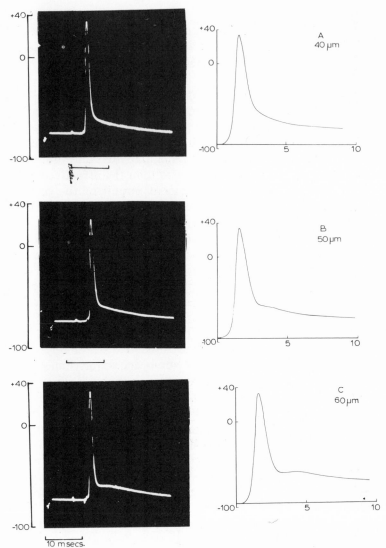

Fig. 2. Experimentally recorded action potentials from three fibres in the same muscle. Radii: 46 μm, 38 μm and 53 μm (from above down). Below each record the time represents 10 msec. On the right, action potentials for fibres with three radii are calculated assuming that the sodium channels in the tubular wall have a twentieth of the density of sodium channels in the surface membrane. For details of the assumptions made in the calculations see text and Adrian and Peachey (1973). Ordinate in each case is potential (mV). Abscissa for the calculated action potentials is time (msec).

action potentials for fibres of three different diameters. The recorded potentials are all from the same muscle and illustrate the considerable variation in the after-potential configuration. For the calculated action potentials, which are for fibres of different diameters, the total available sodium conductance ($\bar{g}_{Na}$) in the fibre surface is about three times that in the tubules. If the ratio of tubular to surface area is seven, the density of sodium channels in the surface is about twenty times the density in the tubular walls. The calculated longitudinal propagation velocity for the fibre with radius 50 μm is 200 cm/sec; the time constant for the exponentially rising foot of this action potential is 200 μsec. These figures produce a capacity from the foot of the action potential of 1.81 μF/cm^2. The corresponding average experimental figures from Hodgkin and Nakajima (1972b) are 209 cm/sec, 127 μsec, and 2.59 μF/cm^2. The agreement is reasonably satisfactory. Nevertheless, to achieve an adequate propagation velocity we have had to make the apparent high frequency capacity (1.81 μF/cm^2) less than that measured experimentally either by the action potential foot (2.59 μF/cm^2) or by a.c. methods ($\sim$2.5 μF). If we assume a value for the capacity of the surface membrane which is suggested by the impedance measurements (2.0–2.5 μF/cm^2) and change no other assumptions the calculated propagation velocity would be reduced. Increasing either α_m or $\bar{g}_{Na}$ for the surface could compensate for this reduction, but the propagation velocity is relatively insensitive to $\bar{g}_{Na}$ and the increases would have to be large.

The calculated action potentials of Fig. 2 assume that the surface and tubular membranes have the same specific capacitance (0.9 μF/cm^2) and that an access resistance of 150 Ω cm^2 separates the extracellular fluid from the tubular lumen. Fig. 3 compares action potentials calculated with and without access resistance to show the consequences of this assumption. Each part of Fig. 3 plots a series of action potentials shown side by side. Each of the action potentials is what would be recorded between an electrode in sarcoplasm and an electrode in either the extracellular fluid or the tubular lumen. At the front and back of each stack is the action potential which would be recorded between an intracellular electrode and a conventional extracellular electrode; this action potential is what would be recorded in a real experimental situation. In between are the action potentials which would be recorded if it were possible to introduce an electrode into the tubular lumen and record as one pushed this hypothetical electrode through the tubular lumen from one side of the fibre to the other.

Figs. 3A and 2B are derived from the same calculation. Fig. 3A differs from 2B in that the access resistance is set to 0 Ω cm^2 rather than to 150 Ω cm^2. The most obvious difference between the two patterns of potential changes is the greater simultaneity of the potential changes in the fibre without access resistance. Though both calculations show a negative after-potential, the characteristic step appears only in the fibre with access resistance, reflecting somewhat delayed tubular potential changes. Absence of access resistance increases the effect of the tubular capacity on the action potential in the fibre surface. Currents generated in the fibre surface play a greater part in the tubular potential changes in Fig. 3B than in Fig. 3A. This

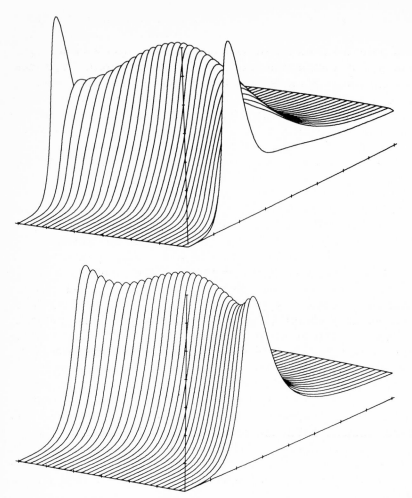

Fig. 3. Calculated action potentials for a fibre with a radius of 50 μm, activatable sodium currents as in Fig. 2 and (A) with an access resistance (R_s) of 150 Ω cm² and (B) without an access resistance. In (A) the longitudinal propagation velocity is 200 cm/sec, in (B) 109 cm/sec. The vertical coordinate is potential, such that each division represents 20 mV. The horizontal receding coordinate is time such that each division represents 1 msec. The second horizontal coordinate is the fibre diameter divided into six equal divisions, each division represents 8.33 μm.

is reflected in the calculated conduction velocity for the two cases. Removing the access resistance reduces the longitudinal velocity from 200 cm/sec to 109 cm/sec. Likewise, the capacity calculated from the exponential foot of the action potential is increased from 1.81 μF/cm² to 3.98 μF/cm².

In general one can say from these calculations that a high longitudinal propagation velocity requires that only a small part of the charge on the tubular capacity be provided by currents in the fibre surface. An access resistance provides a means of uncoupling the surface and tubular systems to some extent; the larger the access resistance the less is the passive electrotonic spread of potential from the surface, and the more necessary are regenerative currents in the tubular system to amplify the signal from the surface. If rapid longitudinal propagation is important, it can be achieved by reducing the electrotonic interaction of the tubular and surface membranes, to the level required to initiate a self-propagating signal in the tubular system. The actual numbers used in the calculations of Fig. 3 are guesses in several important respects. Until we have independent experimental information these calculations can only be used to examine the consequences of particular assumptions.

There is one important consequence of a tubular action potential which is independent of the particular numerical assumptions made in these calculations. If the tubular potential change is generated by conductance changes in the tubular wall, rather than by electrotonic spread of surface action potential, the ionic concentrations within the tubule will be changed as a result of the electrical activity. The surface volume ratio of the tubules (10^6 cm^2/cm^3) is much larger than for even very small nerve fibres so that a single action potential can give rise to appreciable changes in concentration. There is good experimental evidence (Costantin, 1970) that tubular potential changes are altered by tetrodotoxin, so we can safely assume that a movement of sodium ions takes place from tubular lumen to sarcoplasm in the rising phase of the tubular action potential. In the absence of any replenishment from the extracellular fluid the tubular content of sodium ions is equivalent to the sodium movement for between 100 and 200 action potentials. Radial diffusion times for ions in the tubular system (Hodgkin and Horowicz, 1959; Almers, 1972) are of the order of 1 second, so that one would expect to see the effects of sodium depletion at high, and possibly unphysiological rates of firing. Bezanilla et al., (1972) have described failure of contraction during tetanic stimulation which they attribute to tubular sodium depletion.

If the changes of tubular sodium concentration seem unlikely to have physiological effects, the same cannot be said of the changes in tubular potassium concentration. If a movement of sodium depolarizes and a movement of potassium repolarizes the tubular membrane a single action potential will raise the tubular potassium concentration by about 0.5 mM. This concentration increase will decay over about a second. A train of impulses could easily produce a substantial rise in the tubular potassium concentration. A raised tubular potassium would depolarize the tubular membrane, and by electrotonic spread also depolarize the surface, though in general the tubular depolarization would be greater than the surface depolarization. The surface depolarization would be detectable as a slowly decaying after-potential which increased in size with the number of action potentials in a train. Freygang et al., (1964) have described such an after-potential in the frog and they attributed it to potassium accumulation in the tubular system. The relative size of tubular and surface depolarization will depend on the relative conductances of the fibre surface and tubular wall. A high conductance in the fibre surface will reduce the after-potential due to tubular potassium accumulation. It is possible that the chloride conductance of vertebrate skeletal muscle serves this purpose.

In some recent experiments with S.H. Bryant (Adrian and Bryant, 1974) on muscle fibres from normal goats and goats with congenital myotonia (Brown and Harvey, 1939), we have recorded trains of action potentials set up by long-lasting constant currents delivered by an internal micro-electrode. In muscle fibres from myotonic animals a train of 10—15 impulses usually results in a discharge of impulses which outlasts the stimulating current, and the 'spontaneous' impulses arise from a long-lasting after depolarization which builds up during the initiating train of impulses. This behaviour is shown in Fig. 4, which shows two trains of impulses in a myotonic fibre, one of seven impulses which does not give rise to a continued discharge and one of ten driven impulses which just does. The same behaviour can be seen in normal muscle fibres if the chloride in the extracellular solution is replaced

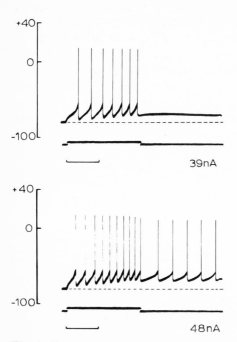

Fig. 4. Trains of action potentials in a muscle fibre from a myotonic goat. A constant current of 39 nA lasting just over 200 msec produced seven action potentials and a long-lasting, depolarizing, after potential. 48 nA produced ten action potentials and firing continued after the current stopped. This firing lasted for 2—3 sec. The horizontal line represents 100 msec. The vertical scale is potential in mV.

by sulphate, an impermeant anion. If the connection between the surface membrane and tubular system is disrupted by glycerol treatment of myotonic fibres, a constant current produces a train of impulses for as long as the current lasts, but this impulse train is not followed by a long-lasting after depolarization and a discharge of impulses does not continue beyond the end of the current. It is known that myotonic muscle fibres lack the high chloride permeability of normal muscle fibres (Bryant, 1969). We suggest that there is potassium accumulation in the tubular system of both normal and myotonic fibres, but that, in the former, surface depolarization is small because the conductance of the fibre surface is high. Moreover, the presence of chloride current in the surface membrane will shift the threshold for initiating an action potential to a more positive potential. If the steady state activation of the sodium system (proportional to $m_\infty^3 h_\infty$) is low at that potential the fibre may not be able to maintain a repetitive discharge in response to a constant depolarizing stimulus.

Radial propagation of excitation in the transverse tubular system complicates the action potential of striated muscle in two distinct ways. First the large capacity of the tubular system would act to slow longitudinal propagation: the longitudinal propagation velocity could be made to some extent independent of the tubular capacity by a resistance concentrated at the tubular mouths, in reality perhaps achieved by having a small number of tubular openings. Such an access resistance, by reducing the electrotonic interactions of surface and tubules, makes regenerative ionic currents in the tubular wall necessary for an adequate electrical signal at the centre of the fibre. The second complication arises because the very small volume of the tubules makes significant ionic concentration changes follow even a single tubular excitation. The consequences of these concentration changes which may be the cause of myotonic discharges, are prevented in normally functioning muscle by the high chloride conductance of the fibre surface.

REFERENCES

ADRIAN, R.H. and BRYANT, S.H. (1974) On the repetitive discharge in myotonic muscle fibres. J. Physiol., (in preparation).
ADRIAN, R.H., CHANDLER, W.K. and HODGKIN, A.L. (1969) The kinetics of mechanical activation in frog muscle. J. Physiol., 204, 207—230.
ADRIAN, R.H., CHANDLER, W.K. and HODGKIN, A.L. (1970) Voltage clamp experiments in striated muscle fibres. J. Physiol., 208, 607—644.
ADRIAN, R.H. and PEACHEY, L.D. (1973) Reconstruction of the action potential of frog sartorius muscle. J. Physiol., 235, 103—131.
ALMERS, W. (1972) Potassium conductance changes in skeletal muscle and the potassium concentration in the transverse tubules. J. Physiol., 225, 33—56.
ARMSTRONG, C.M. and BEZANILLA, F. (1973) Currents related to movement of the gating particles of the sodium channels. Nature, 242, 459—461.

BEZANILLA, F., CAPUTO, C., GONZALES-SERRATOS, H. and VENOSA, R.A. (1972) Sodium dependence of the inward spread of activation in isolated twitch muscle fibres in the frog. J. Physiol., 223, 507—523.

BROWN, G.L. and HARVEY, A.M. (1939) Congenital myotonia in the goat. Brain, 62, 343—363.

BRYANT, S.H. (1969) Cable properties of external intercostal muscle fibres from myotonic and non-myotonic goats. J. Physiol., 204, 539—550.

COSTANTIN, L.L. (1970) The role of sodium current in the radial spread of contraction in frog muscle fibres. J. Gen. Physiol., 55, 703—715.

EISENBERG, R.S. and GAGE, P.W. (1967) Changes in the electrical properties of frog skeletal muscle fibres after disruption of the transverse tubular system. Science, 158, 1700—1707.

FALK, G. and FATT, P. (1964) Linear electrical properties of striated muscle fibres observed with intracellular electrodes. Proc. Roy. Soc. B, 160, 69—123.

FREYGANG, W.H., GOLDSTEIN, D.A. and HELLAM, D.C. (1964) The after potential that follows a train of impulses in frog muscle fibres. J. Gen. Physiol., 47, 929—952.

GONZALEZ-SERRATOS, H. (1971) Inward spread of activation in vertebrate muscle fibres. J. Physiol., 212, 777—799.

HILL, A.V. (1948) On the time required for diffusion and its relation to processes in muscle. Proc. Roy. Soc. B., 135, 446—453.

HODGKIN, A.L. and HOROWICZ, P. (1959) The influence of potassium and chloride ions on the membrane potential of single muscle fibres. J. Physiol., 148, 127—160.

HODGKIN, A.L. and HUXLEY, A.F. (1952) A quantitative description of membrane current and its application to conduction and excitation in nerve. J. Physiol., 117, 500—544.

HODGKIN, A.L. and NAKAJIMA, S. (1972a) The effect of diameter on the electrical constants of frog skeletal muscle fibres. J. Physiol., 221, 105—120.

HODGKIN, A.L. and NAKAJIMA, S. (1972b) Analysis of the membrane capacity in frog muscle. J. Physiol., 221, 121—136.

KEYNES, R.D. and ROJAS, E. (1973) Characteristics of the sodium gating current in the squid giant axon. J. Physiol., 233, 28—30P.

PEACHEY, L.D. (1965) The sarcoplasmic reticulum and transverse tubules of the frog's sartorius. J. Cell. Biol., 25, 209—231.

PORTER, K.R. and PALADE, G.E. (1957) Studies on the endoplasmic reticulum III. Its form and distribution in striated muscle cells. J. Biophys. Biochem. Cytol., 3, 269—300.

SCHNEIDER, M.F. (1970) Linear electrical properties of the transverse tubules and surface membrane of skeletal muscle fibres. J. Gen. Physiol., 56, 640—671.

SCHNEIDER, M.F. and CHANDLER, W.K. (1973) Voltage-dependent charge movement in skeletal muscle: a possible step in excitation-contraction coupling. Nature, 242, 224—246.

TASAKI, I. and HAGIWARA, S. (1957) Capacity of muscle fibre membrane. Am. J. Physiol., 188, 423—429.

3

Structure and function of the T-system in skeletal muscle cells

Lee D. PEACHEY

Just as a reminder, and to put the present subject into the right context, let me briefly review the nature of the structure and function of a vertebrate motor unit. A motor unit can be looked at morphologically as a series of structures, and functionally as a sequence of events taking place in association with these structures (Fig. 1). The motor nerve impulse starts in the central nervous system and travels along the motor axon as a propagated action potential. The mechanism of such nerve action potentials is based on sodium

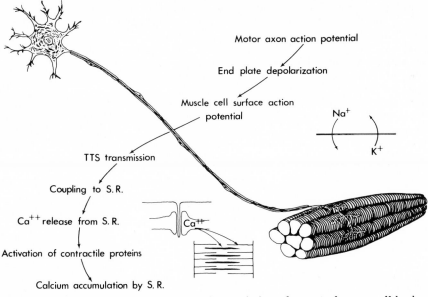

Motor axon action potential

End plate depolarization

Muscle cell surface action potential

Na^+

K^+

TTS transmission

Coupling to S.R.

Ca^{++} release from S.R.

Ca^{++}

Activation of contractile proteins

Calcium accumulation by S.R.

Fig. 1. Diagram of a typical motor unit consisting of a central nerve cell body and motor axon innervating a group of muscle cells. The events in the sequence of activation and relaxation of this unit are connected by arrows, and the inserts present details of certain of these events.

ion entry and delayed potassium ion exit from the nerve fiber, and has been described in the well-known experimental and theoretical analysis of Hodgkin and Huxley. Upon arrival at the motor nerve ending, or myoneural junction, the nerve cell action potential, through a chemical transmitter, initiates a propagated action potential that spreads over the whole surface of the muscle fiber in a few milliseconds. The mechanism of this muscle cell surface action potential is very similar to that of the nerve cell action potential, and recently has been described by Adrian et al. (1970). The next step involves the inward spread of an electrical signal along the membranes of the T-system tubules in the muscle cell, and it is the structural basis of this that will be the focus of my presentation. The electrical events in the T-system have already been discussed in the preceding chapter by Dr. Adrian. Next in the sequence of events in motor unit activity is a coupling of the T-system depolarization to some event in the sarcoplasmic reticulum that results in release of calcium ions from the latter structures. This calcium diffuses to the myofibrils, where it causes activation of contraction by binding to specific sites on the contractile myofilaments. The resulting twitch ends when the calcium ions are re-accumulated by the sarcoplasmic reticulum, and the motor unit returns to its resting state.

I would like now to review briefly the structure of the internal membrane systems in skeletal muscle cells. There has been microscopic evidence for a reticular network in striated muscle cells for almost 100 years, though this morphological evidence has not always been integrated into physiological thinking about muscle contraction. One of the early microscopic papers was published in 1902 by the Italian histologist Emilio Veratti (1902). Using a heavy metal impregnation method, Veratti described reticula in a variety of muscle cells, pointing out that these reticula were periodic in structure, and that they were intimately associated with the striations of the myofibrils. While Veratti's staining method was very capricious, and the variability of his results left some uncertainty about the real nature of the reticula, these early studies literally provided a framework for an interesting story of a specific cellular structure and function.

Most of this story has been written in the last 20 years, since the 'rediscovery' of the sarcoplasmic reticulum (SR) and transverse tubules (T-system) in the electron microscope by Bennett, Porter, Palade and others in the early 1950s (Bennett and Porter, 1953; Porter and Palade, 1957). What has come out of these and subsequent studies of thin sections by electron microscopy has been a picture of the typical appearance of these membrane systems in a variety of muscle cells. Fig. 2 shows a typical electron micrograph of the SR and T-system from the ever-popular frog sartorius muscle. Fig. 3 is a three-dimensional drawing of the structure of these membrane systems as deduced from such micrographs (Peachey, 1965). It depicts the SR and T-system disposed in a very regular way around a little more than one sarcomere length of a few fibrils in a frog muscle.

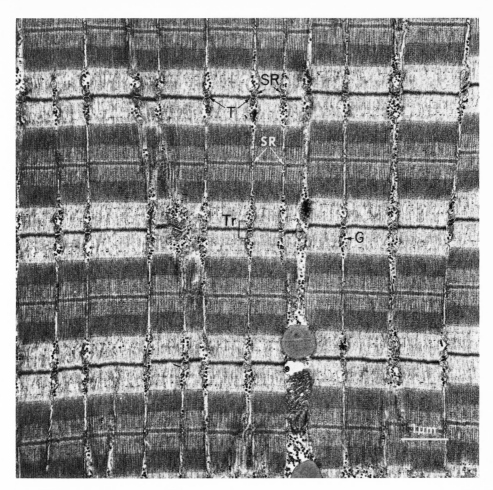

Fig. 2. Electron micrograph of a longitudinal thin section of frog skeletal muscle fiber. The SR and T-system (T) lie between the striated myofibrils, with triads (Tr) located adjacent to the Z-lines of the myofibrils. Bar indicates 1 μm.

It is important, in considering the function of the T-system (or transverse tubular system), to note that it is structurally an inward continuation or invagination of the surface plasma membrane of the muscle cell. Ezerman and Ishikawa (1967) have demonstrated that the T-system forms during cellular differentiation in myoblasts by successive caveolation of the cell surface. Also, studies using ferritin or peroxidase as an extracellular marker for electron microscopy (Huxley, 1964; Page, 1964; Eisenberg and Eisenberg, 1968; Peachey and Schild, 1968) show entry of these large molecules into the T-system of mature fibers, confirming the T-system's surface connection and the extracellular nature of its content. More recently, a tannic

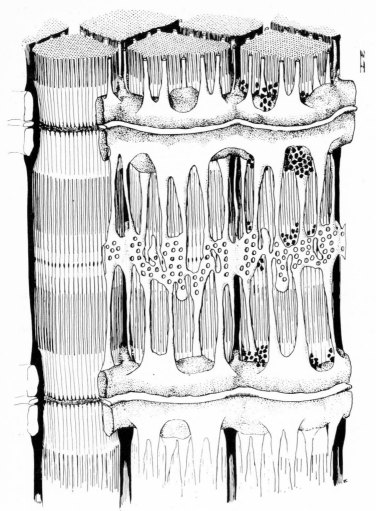

Fig. 3. Three-dimensional drawing of the SR and T-system associated with a few myofibrils in a frog skeletal muscle, as deduced from electron micrographs of thin sections.
(Reproduced from Peachey, 1965).

acid fixation (Rodewald and Karnovsky, 1974) and bismuth subnitrate staining method has been used by Dr. Richard Rodewald and myself to visualize
directly the openings of the T-system at the fiber surface in adult frog
skeletal muscle.

Summarizing up to this point, the SR is an intracellular membrane system
of some complexity, intimately associated with the myofibrils. The SR also
associates closely with the membranes of the T-system network. The tubules

of the T-system network are inward extensions of the cell surface membrane. For the rest of this talk, I will focus my attention on the T-system.

An early clue to the possible function of the T-system in excitation-contraction coupling came from the local experiments of A.F. Huxley and collaborators, also in the 1950s (Huxley and Straub, 1958; Huxley and Taylor, 1958; Huxley and Peachey, 1964). In frog twitch muscles, where the T-system is precisely localized at the Z-lines of the fibrillar striations, activation of contraction was obtained only when the spot locally depolarized was over the Z-lines (Huxley and Taylor, 1958). In some other muscles, including those of a crab, local depolarization gave rise to contraction only near the ends of the A-bands (Huxley and Peachey, 1964), and electron microscopy (Peachey, 1967) showed this to be the location of the transverse tubules in these muscles.

Thus, we early were led to suspect that the function of the transverse tubules is to convey a signal, probably an electrical depolarization of the tubular membranes, into the depths of the fiber as one step in the coupling of excitation to contraction (Huxley and Taylor, 1958; Peachey and Porter, 1959).

The next phase in the development of this story was an effort to determine the exact nature of the signal carried by the transverse tubules, and I think it is fair to say that we know the general form of the answer, though some detail remains to be worked out.

The morphological studies I have already discussed formed a sort of starting point for the analysis of the T-system by Adrian et al. (1969a) as an electric cable, as had been done earlier for the nerve fiber. Fig. 4 indicates why the analysis was different from that used for an essentially one-dimensional nerve fiber: the T-system was considered to be a two-dimensional network, lying roughly in a plane transverse to the fiber axis: there being many such T-systems in the length of the muscle fiber.

Without going into detail, I would just say at this point that initially the T-system was treated as if it were a passive cable, with linear electrical properties. This led to the prediction of a sag of a few millivolts in depolarization toward the center of the fiber, in experimental situations in which the surface was held by voltage-clamp techniques at a fixed level of depolarization near the contraction threshold (Adrian et al., 1969a,b).

Experiments to check this were done by Adrian et al. (1969b). They seemed to confirm the predicted passive behavior of the T-system in that the distance the contraction spread inward toward the fiber axis was graded with the size of the depolarization of the surface membrane. These experiments, however, were done in the presence of tetrodotoxin, which blocks sodium activation in nerve and muscle cell membranes. When Costantin (1970) later repeated these experiments without tetrodotoxin, he found a different behavior. His results strongly suggested that the T-system was not a passive cable network, but that it propagated an action potential. This action poten-

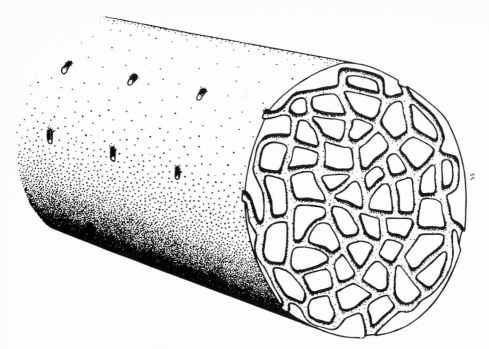

Fig. 4. Somewhat idealized representation of T-systems as irregular, planar networks of branched tubules lying transverse to the fiber axis. One T-system network is cut through to show its tubules. Other T-system networks are seen only as openings at the surface of the fiber. The size of the network mesh is exaggerated compared to the fiber diameter for clarity of presentation: in reality the tubules are smaller and closer together than shown.

tial depended on the presence of external sodium ions and could be blocked with tetrodotoxin. Thus, it looked as if the T-system had at least some similarity in its electrical properties to the surface membrane of the muscle fiber, from which it was derived and to which it remained connected. Specifically, this similarity was in the ability to propagate a sodium-dependent action potential. Dr. Adrian has already discussed this in greater depth.

I would now like to return to morphology for a moment and discuss some recent results on the structure of the T-system obtained with high-voltage electron microscopy. Dr. Brenda Eisenberg and I have been using the exogenous peroxidase method for the study of the T-system network in thick slices. It is necessary to selectively stain the T-system if it is to be visualized in slices of the order of 1 μm in thickness, since the T-system tubules are so small, and this method seems to give us the selectivity of staining that we need. Fig. 5 shows a portion of the T-system in a transverse slice about 0.7 μm thick, as seen in a transmission electron microscope with an accelerating potential of 1000 kV. This figure shows how well this staining method

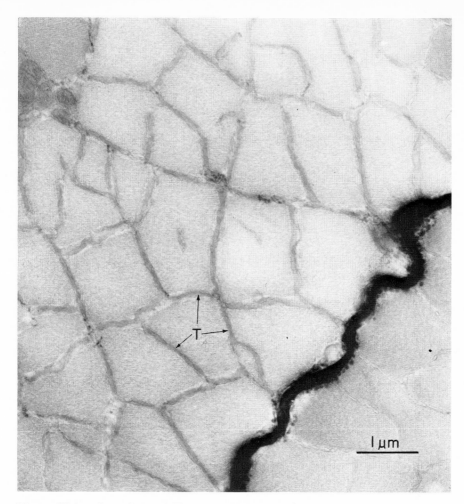

Fig. 5. High voltage (1000 kV) electron micrograph of a transverse slice of frog skeletal muscle treated with peroxidase and stained with diaminobenzidine—H_2O_2—osmium tetroxide to increase the contrast of the T-system. The very dark line is the extracellular space between two fibers. The less dense network in the fiber above is the T-system surrounding the myofibrils, and in some cases ending within a fibril or between two incompletely separated fibrils. Thickness 0.7 μm. Micrograph taken at the University of Colorado.

delineates the T-system and shows its form over relatively large areas in such thick slices.

Using low-magnification micrographs, covering the whole transverse area of a fiber, and in following the T-system through successive serial slices, we have not only been able to reconstruct the T-system completely across the

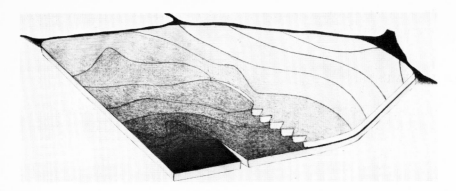

Fig. 6. Drawing intended to show the helical arrangement of bands and T-system network in a frog muscle fiber, as recently deduced from examination of serial transverse thick slices by high-voltage electron microscopy. The lines represent boundaries where the T-system network passes from one slice into the next. The upper turn of the helix is cut off (zig-zag edge) to show the face of the lower turn. A dislocation in the T-system network is seen near the center of the fiber, and another is seen at the front near the left.

fiber, but we also have come upon an interesting point about T-system structure. In brief, the result is that we have found that the T-system takes a helical course in the fiber, so that we can trace the T-system network continuously through several sarcomeres along the length of the fiber. Fig. 6 shows diagramatically how this result appears in a series of consecutive slices.

There are two interesting implications of this helical form of the T-system. First, since the T-system is precisely localized at the level of the Z-lines of the fibrillar striations in amphibian muscle, then if the T-system is helical, the striations must also be helical. Second, if the striations are helical, there must be places where the striations are shifted longitudinally in adjacent myofibrils. These shifts seem to correspond to the vernier formations commonly observed in living fibers as well as in longitudinal sections of fixed or frozen tissue.

Finally, I should like to point out that the observation of helical bands in skeletal muscle fibers has been made before, though apparently forgotten. Tiegs reported finding helical Krause's membranes (Z-lines) in a variety of muscle fibers in 1922–24, and reviewed his observations in 1955. Tiegs also mentions that helical bands were reported by van Leeuwenhoek in 1718, a few years after he made the very first observation of the bands themselves.

The physiological implications of the helical bands and T-system are not entirely clear. I do not think we need to change drastically our views of the electrical behavior of the intact fiber, since adjacent T-systems along the length of fiber are activated approximately at the same time as the action potential travels along the fiber at about 200 cm/sec. It may, however, provide an explanation for the slow contractile waves observed in skinned fibers by

Natori (1965) and by Costantin and Podolsky (1967), if these are propagated along the helical T-system.

ACKNOWLEDGEMENTS

This work was supported by grants from the N.I.H. (RR-592 and HL-15835) and from the Muscular Dystrophy Associations of America.

REFERENCES

ADRIAN, R.H., CHANDLER, W.K. and HODGKIN, A.L. (1970) Voltage clamp experiments in striated muscle fibers. J. Physiol., 208, 607—644.
ADRIAN, R.H., CHANDLER, W.K. and HODGKIN, A.L. (1969a) The kinetics of mechanical activation in frog muscle. J. Physiol., 204, 207—230.
ADRIAN, R.H., COSTANTIN, L.L. and PEACHEY, L.D. (1969b) Radial spread of contraction in frog muscle fibres. J. Physiol., 204, 231—267.
BENNETT, H.S. and PORTER, K.R. (1953) An electron microscope study of sectioned breast muscle of the domestic fowl. Am. J. Anat., 93, 61—105.
COSTANTIN, L.L. (1970) The role of sodium current in the radial spread of contraction in frog muscle fibers. J. Gen. Physiol., 55, 703—715.
COSTANTIN, L.L. and PODOLSKY, R.J. (1967) Depolarization of the internal membrane system in the activation of frog skeletal muscle. J. Gen. Physiol., 50, 1101—1124.
EISENBERG, B. and EISENBERG, R.S. (1968) Selective disruption of the sarcotubular system in frog sartorius muscle, J. Cell Biol., 39, 451—467.
EZERMAN, E.B. and ISHIKAWA, H. (1967) Differentiation of the sarcoplasmic reticulum and T-system in developing chick skeletal muscle in vitro. J. Cell Biol., 35, 405—420.
HUXLEY, A.F. and STRAUB, R.W. (1958) Local activation and interfibrillar structures in striated muscle. J. Physiol., 143, 40—41P.
HUXLEY, A.F. and TAYLOR, R.E. (1958) Local activation of striated muscle fibres. J. Physiol., 144, 426—441.
HUXLEY, A.F. and PEACHEY, L.D. (1964) Local activation of crab muscle. J. Cell Biol., 23, 107A.
HUXLEY, H.E. (1964) Evidence for continuity between the central elements of the triads and extracellular space in frog sartorius muscle. Nature, 202, 1067—1071.
NATORI, R. (1965) Propagated contractions in isolated sarcolemma-free bundles of myofibrils. Jikei Med. J., 12, 214—221.
PAGE, S. (1964) The organization of the sarcoplasmic reticulum in frog muscle. J. Physiol., 175, 10—11P.
PEACHEY, L.D. (1965) The structure of the sarcoplasmic reticulum and transverse tubules of the frog's sartorius. J. Cell Biol., 25, 209—231.
PEACHEY, L.D. and SCHILD, R.F. (1968) The distribution of the T-system along the sarcomeres of frog and toad sartorius muscles. J. Physiol., 194, 249—258.
PEACHEY, L.D. (1967) Membrane systems of crab fibers. Am. Zool., 7, 505—513.
PEACHEY, L.D. and PORTER, K.R. (1959) Intracellular impulses conduction in muscle cells. Science, 129, 721—722.

PORTER, K.R. and PALADE, G.E. (1957) Studies on the endoplasmic reticulum. III. Its form and distribution in striated muscle cells. J. Biophys. Biochem. Cytol., 3, 269—300.

RODEWALD, R. and KARNOVSKY, M.J. (1974) Porous substructure of the glomerular slit diaphragm in the rat and mouse. J. Cell Biol., 60, 423—433.

TIEGS, O.W. (1955) The flight muscles of insects — their anatomy and histology: with some observations on the structure of striated muscle in general. Phil. Trans. R. Soc. (Lond.), B238, 221—348.

VERATTI, E. (1902) Richerche sulla fine struttura della fibra muscolare striata. Mem. Inst. Lombardo Sci. Lett., 19, 87—133. (Reprinted and translated in J. Biophys. Biochem. Cytol. 10, suppl. pp. 1—59, 1961.)

The motor unit

1. The recruitment order of motor units and its significance for the
   behaviour of tendon organs during normal muscle activity
   by D.G. Stuart and J.A. Stephens   37

2. The potential of the motor unit
   by A. Gydikov   49

3. The extent of voluntary control of human motor units
   by E. Henneman, B.T. Shahani and R.R. Young   73

4. Single fibre electromyography for motor unit study in man
   by E. Stålberg   79

The recruitment order of motor units and its significance for the behaviour of tendon organs during normal muscle activity

Douglas G. STUART and John A. STEPHENS

The behaviour of Golgi tendon organs during single motor unit contractions is discussed in relation to motor unit recruitment and the type of information these receptors might supply to the central nervous system. It is concluded that while the responses of a single Ib afferent are not related to the forces generated at the tendon by different motor units acting on the receptor, the collective response of many tendon organs during normal muscle activity would be expected to be related to the total force developed by the muscle. The behaviour of individual receptors during normal muscle activity is shown to depend on the details of motor unit recruitment, and in particular on the relationship between the order of motor unit recruitment and changes in their firing rate at various levels of contraction strength.

For many years tendon organs have been regarded as high-threshold force detectors serving a protective function via the spinal Ib inhibitory pathway. More recently, however, these receptors have been shown in fact to be exquisitely sensitive to in-series force development, capable of responding to the contraction of even the smallest motor unit (Houk and Henneman, 1967; Stuart et al., 1970, 1972a,b). This new information demands that the functional role of tendon organs and the type of information these receptors supply to the central nervous system be reassessed.

In our laboratory we have recently completed a study of the tendon organs of medial gastrocnemius and the mechanical properties of motor units found to excite them (Stephens et al., 1973; Stephens and Stuart, 1974a,b; Reinking et al., 1975a,b; Stephens et al., 1975a,b; Stephens and Stuart, 1975a,b). Before discussing these findings, however, it is essential to understand the anatomical arrangement of these receptors and their surrounding muscle fibres.

Golgi tendon organs are located primarily at the musculo-tendinous junctions of skeletal muscle (See Fig. 1A). In each receptor the Ib afferent endings are enclosed within a fusiform capsule surrounding bundles of col-

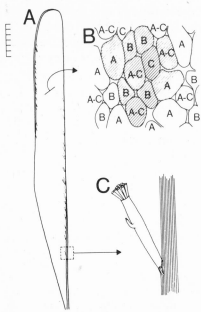

Fig. 1. The arrangement between muscle fibres and tendon organs in cat medial gastrocnemius. For full details see Reinking et al., 1975b. (A) is modified from Swett and Eldred
(1960) and shows a lateral or imaginary sagittal view of the left medial gastrocnemius
muscle in a 1 Kg kitten. The scale is 1 mm per division. Tendon organs beneath the
superficial aponeurosis of origin are shown with solid lines and those lining the deep distal
aponeurosis with broken line. There are 44 tendon organs; 25 proximal and 19 distal. Not
included are receptors within the tendon proper which usually comprise about 7% of the
total number (Barker, 1974). (B) shows a cross section of adult cat medial gastrocnemius
redrawn from a slide prepared by V.R. Edgerton. Fibres are labelled A, B and C on the
basis of their myosin ATPase and DPNH—diapharase activity (for review of nomenclature
see Close, 1972). Some fibres are labelled A-C to indicate high myosin ATPase activity
and intermediate DPHN activity. Ten adjacent fibres are shaded, this number being the
near average number of muscle fibres associated with a single tendon organ (Barker,
1974). (C) is modified from Schoultz and Swett (1972) and shows the way in which the
capsule of a single tendon organ merges with the aponeurosis of insertion (or origin) at
one end while enclosing the collagenous terminations of a number of muscle fibres at the
other end. The length of a tendon organ capsule ranges from 500 to 1200 μ and the
diameter at mid-section from 100 to 120 μ (see Stuart et al., 1972a).

lagen which connect a number of striated muscle fibres (typically 10—11 in
cat hind limb muscles) with the aponeurosis of origin or insertion (Schoultz
and Swett, 1974; Barker, 1974). Active contraction or stretch of any of
these muscle fibres is thought to provide the significant input to the receptor
(Houk and Henneman, 1967; Stuart et al., 1972a,b; Fig. 1C). In view of the
wide distribution of the muscle fibres of a single motor unit amongst those
of other units, with few fibres from the same unit adjacent to one another
(Brandstater and Lambert, 1973; Burke and Tsairis, 1973), we may calculate

that, in general, each of the muscle fibres associated with a tendon organ form part of a different motor unit (Reinking et al., 1975b). Furthermore, because of the intermingling of muscle fibres of different histochemical type as shown in Fig. 1B, we would expect the tendon organs of a heterogeneous muscle such as cat medial gastrocnemius to be responsive to contractions of motor units with a wide range of mechanical properties.

Fig. 2 shows results from our experiments which demonstrate this arrangement. Notice that each receptor was found to respond to contraction of a representative sample of motor unit types present in cat medial gastrocnemius. Both slow and fast twitch units with a broad range of fatigue resistance were found to excite each receptor.

Another important feature of tendon organ physiology is that there is no correlation between the Ib firing rate attained and the forces developed at the muscle tendon when the responses of a single afferent to the contraction of several motor units are compared (Houk and Henneman, 1967; Reinking

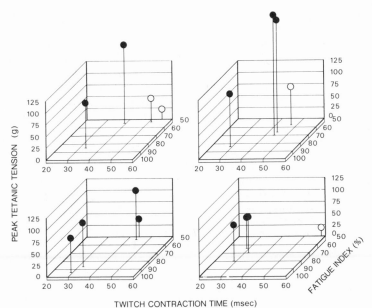

Fig. 2. The mechanical properties of motor units whose contraction excited the same tendon organ. Notice that all 4 afferents responded to motor units with a wide range of mechanical properties. Fast twitch units (twitch contraction time $\leqslant 45$ msec) have filled circle tops and slow twitch units open circle tops. Peak tetanic tension for each unit was measured at optimum length (stimulation rate 200 pps for fast twitch and 100 pps for slow twitch units). Twitch contraction time was measured at the optimum length for twitch of each unit after potentiation. Fatigue index is that percentage of the cumulative force developed after 2 minutes of a 4 minute fatigue test (Stimulation rate at 40 pps for 330 msec of every second). Non-fatigable units have an index close to 50% and highly fatigable units near 100%. For further details see Reinking et al., 1975a,b.

TABLE 1

Lack of correlation between Ib firing rate and force of motor unit contraction when the responses of the same afferent to contraction of different motor units are compared.

Afferent 1		Afferent 2		Afferent 3	
Δf[a] (g)	Δr[b] (pps)	Δf (g)	Δr (pps)	Δf (g)	Δr (pps)
18	78	45	33	16	55
48	70	103	18	17	27
71	71	198	108	71	98
149	45	209	15	75	40

[a] Force of motor unit contraction recorded at muscle tendon.
[b] Increase in Ib afferent firing during motor unit contraction.

et al., 1975b). In Table 1, for example, the changes in Ib firing rate (Δr) associated with contraction of 4 different motor units are shown for each of 3 afferents. In each case the motor units are ranked in order of increasing contraction strength. Notice that the corresponding Δr values do not rank accordingly. This result emphasizes that during a motor unit contraction it is the force exerted in series with the receptor by one of its muscle fibres which provides the significant input to the receptor, not the total force exerted at the tendon by all the fibres of the unit.

During normal muscle activity the total force developed at the tendon is determined by the sum of the forces developed by each active motor unit. A single tendon organ can be regarded as taking a sample of those forces. While such individual samples based on the force of contraction of only one muscle fibre of each motor unit are unrepresentative of the forces exerted at the tendon, we may suppose that the sum of many such samples from many receptors might faithfully follow changes in the total force developed at the tendon.

In order to test this hypothesis we have examined the summed responses of 12 Ib afferents to contractions of 27 motor units (Reinking et al., 1975b). In Fig. 3A the motor units were first ranked in order of increasing tetanic tension. These tensions were then summed progressively and plotted against the fraction of the sample used to form each sum. Notice that the resulting curve is convex to the X axis because the distribution of tetanic tension for this set of motor units was essentially rectangular. The 45° line would be expected if all the units developed the same tetanic tension. In Fig. 3B the corresponding Ib firing rates associated with contraction of each of these motor units have also been summed progressively. This cumulative curve lies very close to the 45° line as would be expected if there were no relationship

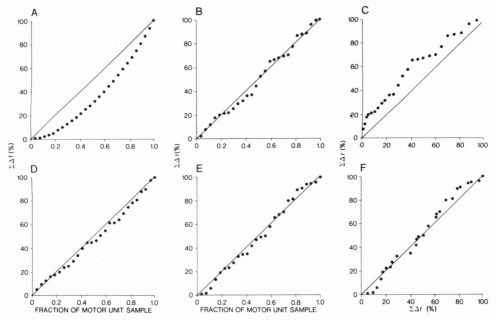

Fig. 3. The summed response of tendon organs. Data taken from the responses of 12 Ib afferents during contraction of 27 motor units in 5 experiments. Muscle length was set at —4mm relative to the optimum length for tetanus of the parent whole muscle in each case. For A, B and C motor units were first ordered according to contraction strength. For D, E and F motor units were taken in random order. For full report see Reinking et al., 1975b.

between tetanic tension developed and Ib firing rate. In Fig. 3C the curves of Fig. 3A and B have been combined with the cumulative force shown on the X axis and the cumulative Ib firing rate on the Y axis. The 45° line would be expected if the cumulative firing rates attained were proportional to the cumulative force. Notice that the curve in Fig. 3C is concave to the X axis indicating that at low cumulative force levels the summed Ib response is relatively more powerful than at high force levels. This plot simply reflects the fact that in general small motor units can excite Ib afferents as strongly as larger motor units.

To illustrate the importance of the order of motor unit recruitment on the relationship between total cumulative Ib response and muscle force, we have repeated the process shown in Fig. 3A, B and C in Fig. 3D, E and F except that in this case the motor units were first ranked in random order. Notice that in contrast to Fig. 3C the curve relating cumulative force and Ib response in Fig. 3F now lies close to a 45° line.

It is clear from Fig. 3 that despite the lack of correlation between Ib firing rate of a single receptor and the forces developed by its exciting motor units at the tendon, the summed response of many Ib afferents may well be related to the total force developed during normal muscle activity. The exact form of this relationship will depend, however, on the nature of motor unit recruitment as shown in Fig. 3. There is now direct experimental evidence, at least during graded voluntary contractions of the 1st dorsal interosseous muscle in man, that motor units are recruited in order of increasing contraction strength (Milner-Brown et al., 1973a). Indirect support for this mode of recruitment can be found by an analysis of the association of motor unit

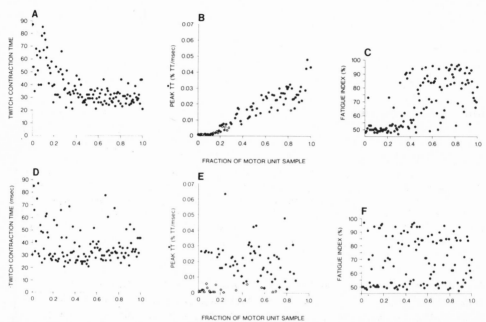

Fig. 4. The ordering and association of motor unit mechanical properties in medial gastrocnemius. Sample of 126 motor units studied in 12 adult cats (3.0 to 5.1 Kg). In A, B and C units are ordered according to tetanic tension and in D, E and F according to axonal conduction velocity. In A and D twitch contraction times were measured at the optimum length for twitch for each unit after potentiation. In B and C peak rate of rise of tetanic tension (TT) is expressed in units of percentage parent whole muscle tetanic tension developed per msec. Fast twitch units (twitch contraction time ≤ 45 msec) stimulated at 200 pps are shown with closed circles and slow twitch units stimulated at 100 pps with open circles. Closed diamonds indicate those fast twitch units stimulated at 100 pps and open diamonds those slow twitch units stimulated at 200 pps. In C and F fatigue index is that percentage of cumulative force developed at 2 minutes in a 4 minute fatigue test (stimulation rate 40 pps for 330 msec every second). Non-fatigable units have an index near 50% and highly fatigable units near 100%. In each part of figure, after initial ordering, the properties of each unit are plotted against the fraction of the motor unit sample so far considered. Thus, for example, motor unit number 63 in the order is plotted on the X axis at 0.5 and number 126 at 1.0. Modified from Stephens and Stuart, 1975a.

mechanical properties in cat medial gastrocnemius (Reinking et al., 1975a; Stephens and Stuart, 1975a) which emphasizes certain useful functional consequences.

Figs 4A, B and C show that ordering motor units according to their tetanic tension results in the selection of units with progressively increasing contraction times and rates of rise of tetanic tension. Small units are non-fatigable while larger faster contracting units have a broad range of fatigue resistance (Stephens et al., 1973; Stephens and Stuart, 1974a; Reinking et al., 1975a; Stephens and Stuart, 1975a). It is significant that this mode of recruitment would permit the gastrocnemius to act both as a low contraction strength, slow fatigue-resistant muscle and at high contraction strength as a fast contracting but less fatigue-resistant muscle. Such an arrangement ideally suits the gastrocnemius for its varied tasks from quiet standing, where it develops small forces (Grillner, 1972), to galloping and jumping, which require powerful and rapid contractions. The increased fatigability that would result from the recruitment of larger, faster motor units is perhaps of little functional consequence because of the phasic rather than sustained nature of these contractions. If on the other hand, units are ordered according to their axonal conduction velocities, as shown in Figs 4D, E and F, no sequencing of speed or fatigability results. Indeed the relationship between axonal conduction velocity and motor unit mechanical properties in medial gastrocnemius is obscure (Stephens and Stuart, 1975a) as is shown in Fig. 5.

Returning to the significance of motor unit recruitment for the behaviour of tendon organs, it remains uncertain to what extent, during a graded voluntary muscle contraction, the discharge rate of a single receptor depends on changes in the number of active muscle fibres in series with the receptor due to motor unit recruitment, or to changes in the force of contraction of those already active due to changes in motor unit firing rate.

Recently, Vallbo (1974) has observed the behaviour of tendon organs during isometric contractions of the long finger flexors of the hand in man. A striking feature of his results was that while the force of contraction increased smoothly, Ib afferent firing changed in discrete steps with little increase in firing between each step (5—8, 9—12 and 20—25 pps; see Fig. 1 in Vallbo, 1974). Presumably these step-like changes in Ib firing were due to changes in the number of active motor units contributing force to the receptor capsule and the small changes in firing between each step reflected relatively minor changes in the force contributed by each unit. This situation may not be representative at higher contraction strengths, however, because once all the fibres associated with each receptor are active, changes in Ib afferent firing can only result from changes in the force exerted by each motor unit. Certainly changes in Ib firing rate can be demonstrated during the graded contraction of single motor units either by using the force — length property of muscle or during fatiguing contractions (Stephens et al., 1975b).

Fig. 6 shows the changes in Ib firing rate of two Ib afferents during

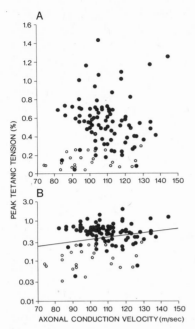

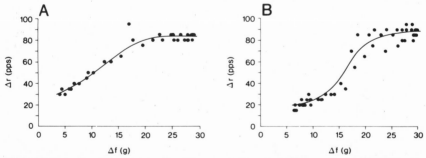

Fig. 5. Peak tetanic tension plotted against axonal conduction velocity for a sample of 177 medial gastrocnemius motor units (12 experiments). For full details see Stephens and Stuart (1975a). Peak tetanic tension (TT) expressed as a percentage of whole muscle TT. (B) has the same data as (A) but with TT shown on a logarithmic scale. In (A) the coefficient of linear correlation between TT and CV was not significantly different from zero ($P > 0.1$) when either taking all the data together or the fast (contraction time ⩽ 45 msec) and slow populations alone. In B the coefficient of correlation between log TT and CV for the total data did reach significance at the 5% level although it was small ($r = 0.21$). The corresponding best fit line has been drawn in (B). However, when the fast and slow populations were considered alone, in neither case was the correlation significant.

Fig. 6. The responses of two Ib afferents during fatiguing motor unit contractions (stimulation rate 40 pps for 330 msec each second). Changes in Ib firing rate (Δr) associated with each contraction are plotted against the force recorded at the tendon (Δf). Modified from Stephens et al., 1975b.

fatiguing motor unit contractions. Notice that in each case the Ib firing rate reaches a maximum before the maximum contraction strength of the units is reached. In other words, the excitatory effect of a single motor unit appears to be limited. A similar conclusion can be drawn from the behaviour of tendon organs during motor unit contractions at different muscle lengths (Stephens et al., 1975b). On this basis it appears that at high contraction strengths, where all the muscle fibres associated with each tendon organ are active, the Ib firing rate may change little, despite further increases in their force of contraction. At intermediate contraction strengths, however, changes in Ib firing rate with changes in motor unit firing rate might be more important, as the force exerted increases along the steep part of the force firing rate curve shown in Fig. 6.

In their recent study of the changes in firing rate of human motor units during linearly changing voluntary contractions, Milner-Brown et al. (1973b) concluded that at low levels of contraction strength motor unit recruitment is the major mechanism for increasing the force of contraction but that increased firing rate becomes the more important mechanism at intermediate to high force levels (see, however, Hannertz, 1974). Certainly the relative importance of recruitment and increasing firing rate as mechanisms for increasing the force of voluntary contraction will be reflected in the behaviour of tendon organs.

There is now obviously need for a systematic study of the behaviour of tendon organs during normal muscle activity. Such experiments would provide a unique opportunity not only to study the behaviour of the receptors themselves but also, like the nervous system with which they communicate, to follow the process of motor unit recruitment.

ACKNOWLEDGEMENTS

This work was supported in part by USPHS grant NS 07888 and the General Research Support Fund of the University of Arizona, College of Medicine. We would like to thank Ms. Rebecca L. Gerlach, Ms. Mary Ellen Burrows and Mr. Edward K. Stauffer, who assisted at various stages in our study.

REFERENCES

BARKER, E. (1974) Morphology of muscle receptors: In (C.C. Hunt, Ed.) Handbook of Sensory Physiology, Vol. III/2, Springer Verlag, New York, pp. 1—190.
BRANDSTATER, M.E. and LAMBERT, E.H. (1973) Motor unit anatomy. Type and spatial arrangement of muscle fibers. In (J.E. Desmedt, Ed.) New Developments in Electromyography and Clinical Neurophysiology, Vol. 1, Karger, Basel, pp. 14—22.

BURKE, R.E. and TSAIRIS, P. (1973) Anatomy and innervation ratios in motor units of cat gastrocnemius. J. Physiol., 234, 749—765.

CLOSE, R.I. (1972) Dynamic properties of mammalian skeletal muscles. Physiol. Rev., 52, 129—197.

GRILLNER, S. (1972) The role of muscle stiffness in meeting the changing postural and locomotor requirements for force development by the ankle extensors. Acta Physiol. Scand., 86, 92—108.

HANNERTZ, J. (1974) Discharge properties of motor units in relation to recruitment order in voluntary contraction. Acta Physiol. Scand., 91, 374—384.

HOUK, J.C. and HENNEMAN, E. (1967) Responses of Golgi tendon organs to active contractions of the soleus muscle of the cat. J. Neurophysiol., 30, 466—481.

MILNER-BROWN, H.S., STEIN, R.B. and YEMM, R. (1973a) The orderly recruitment of human units during voluntary isometric contractions. J. Physiol., 230, 359—370.

MILNER-BROWN, H.S., STEIN, R.B. and YEMM, R. (1973b) Changes in firing rate of human motor units during linearly changing voluntary contractions. J. Physiol., 230, 371—390.

REINKING, R.M., STEPHENS, J.A. and STUART, D.G. (1975a) The motor units of cat medial gastrocnemius: problem of their classification on the basis of mechanical properties. Exp. Brain Res. (In press).

REINKING, R.M., STEPHENS, J.A. and STUART, D.G. (1975b) The tendon organs of cat medial gastrocnemius: Significance of motor unit type and size for the activation of Ib afferents. J. Physiol. (In press).

SCHOULTZ, T.W. and SWETT, J.E. (1972) The fine structure of the Golgi tendon organ. J. Neurocytol., 1, 1—26.

SCHOULTZ, T.W. and SWETT, J.E. (1974) Ultrastructural organization of sensory fibers innervating the Golgi tendon organ. Anat. Rec., 179, 147—162.

STEPHENS, J.A., GERLACH, R.L., REINKING, R.M. and STUART, D.G. (1973) Fatigability of medial gastrocnemius motor units in the cat. In (R.B. Stein, K.S. Pearson, R.S. Smith and J.B. Redford, Eds) Control of Posture and Locomotion, Plenum Press, New York, pp. 179—185.

STEPHENS, J.A., REINKING, R.M. and STUART, D.G. (1975a) The motor units of cat medial gastrocnemius: electrical and mechanical properties as a function of muscle length. J. Morphol. (In press).

STEPHENS, J.A., REINKING, R.M. and STUART, D.G. (1975b) The tendon organs of cat medial gastrocnemius: responses to active and passive forces as a function of muscle length. J. Neurophysiol. (In press).

STEPHENS, J.A. and STUART, D.G. (1974a) The classification of motor units in cat medial gastrocnemius muscle. J. Physiol., 240, 43—44 p.

STEPHENS, J.A. and STUART, D.G. (1974b) The responses of Golgi tendon organs to contraction of single motor units in a mixed mammalian muscle. J. Physiol., 242, 62—63 p.

STEPHENS, J.A. and STUART, D.G. (1975a) The motor units of cat medial gastrocnemius: speed-size relations and their significance for the recruitment order of motor units. Brain Res., 91, 177—195.

STEPHENS, J.A. and STUART, D.G. (1975b) The motor units of cat medial gastrocnemius: twitch potentiation and twitch-tetanus ratio. Pflug. Arch., 356, 359—372.

STUART, D.G., GOSLOW, G.E., MOSHER, C.G. and REINKING, R.M. (1970). Stretch responsiveness of Golgi tendon organs. Exp. Brain Res., 10, 463—476.

STUART, D.G., MOSHER, C.S. and GERLACH, R.L. (1972a) Properties and central connections of Golgi tendon organs with special reference to locomotion. In (B. Banker, R.J. Pryzbylsky, J. Van Der Meulen and M. Victor, Eds) Research in Muscle Development and the Muscle Spindle, Excerpta Medica, Amsterdam, pp. 437—462.

STUART, D.G., MOSHER, C.G., GERLACH, R.L. and REINKING, R.M. (1972b) Mechanical arrangement and transducing properties of Golgi tendon organs. Exp. Brain Res., 14, 274—292.

SWETT, J.E. and ELDRED, E. (1960) Distribution and numbers of stretch receptors in medial gastrocnemius and soleus muscles. Anat. Rec., 137, 453—460.

VALLBO, A.B. (1974) Afferent discharge from human muscle spindles in non-contracting muscles. Steady state impulse frequency as a function of joint angle. Acta Physiol. Scand., 90, 303—318.

2

The potential of the motor unit

A. GYDIKOV

The concept of the motor unit was proposed by Liddel and Sherrington in 1925 to describe the structure consisting of one alpha motoneurone and the group of muscle fibres innervated by it. In the case of mammals, each muscle fibre is innervated by only one axon (Brown and Mathews, 1960). The neuromuscular synapses are usually situated along the middle of the muscle fibres, which lie parallel from one tendon to another. In man it is only m. gracilis and m. sartorius that have fibres running in series. The muscle fibres in the remaining muscles are approximately as long as the muscle itself, or shorter if they are situated obliquely, as is the case with the pinnate muscles. The neuromuscular synapses are usually situated in a strip 1 to 2 mm wide which lies along a straight or a curved line specified by the mutual positions of the tendons (Cöers and Wolf, 1957).

The motor units possess a variable number of muscle fibres—from several to several thousand. On average, they are bigger in the bigger muscles. In a cross-section of the muscle, the fibres of the different motor units are inter-mixed, those belonging to a particular motor unit being situated in a definite and approximately oval territory whose area is between 10 and 30 times bigger than the sum of the cross-sections of the fibres belonging to that motor unit (Buchthal et al., 1957b, 1959; Brandstater and Lambert, 1973). The separate fibres lie individually, and it is only rarely that groups of two or more fibres from the same motor unit can be found. The frequency of such grouping corresponds to that which is to be expected if we assume that it is of a random character (Brandstater and Lambert, 1973). The diameter of the territory of the separate motor unit is different. For human muscles it is about 5 mm in the upper extremities and about 10 mm in the lower ones (Buchthal et al., 1957b, 1959).

In a normal state, each impulse of the alpha motoneurone causes excitation in all muscle fibres of the motor unit. When the depolarization of the subsynaptic membrane reaches a certain threshold level, this leads to the appearance of spreading depolarization. The forefront of the depolarization spreads from the synapse towards the two ends of the muscle fibre at a particular velocity, v. The depolarization at each point of the membrane increases over a particular period of time (DT) and, after that, repolarization is to be observed, which also lasts a certain time (RT). If we exclude the after-potentials, the total time for the rapid changes of the trans-membrane potential, DRT, becomes the sum of these two times:

$$DRT = DT + RT \tag{1}$$

As a result of the spreading of the depolarization toward the two ends of the fibre and of the repolarization processes taking place, a depolarized zone appears around the synapse. This zone increases in length, then it divides into two depolarized zones which move toward the two ends of the fibre and, having reached these ends, they decrease in length until their complete disappearance. If we assume that, at each point of the membrane, DRT and v are constant quantities, then the length of each one of the two depolarized zones (b) after their division and before reaching the end of the fibre is equal to:

$$b = v\text{DRT} \tag{2}$$

The duration of the rapid electric changes at the excitation of the muscle fibre (T) is determined from the following equation:

$$T = \frac{L + b}{v} = \frac{L}{v} + \text{DRT} \tag{3}$$

where L is the distance from the motor end plate to the longer end of the muscle fibre.

At each impulse of the alpha monoteurone all muscle fibres of the motor unit are excited almost synchronously. Nevertheless, there exists a certain degree of desynchronization determined by a number of causes, namely: (a) the terminal ramifications of the axon are different in length and they conduct at different velocities, on account of which the impulse does not arrive absolutely simultaneously in the different synapses; (b) the synaptic delay is not a strictly constant quantity; (c) the motor end plates do not lie strictly on one line and (d) the velocity of conduction along the individual muscle fibres may not be the same. Due to this last factor the desynchronization can change, depending on the distance to the motor end plates.

Due to the desynchronization, equations (1), (2) and (3) in the motor unit remain valid if the participating quantities are defined in the following manner: DT_s — time from the beginning to the maximum of the summated depolarization in a given cross-section of a motor unit; RT_s — time from the beginning to the end of repolarization in a given cross-section of a motor unit (the after-potentials excluded); DRT_s — time from the beginning to the end of the rapid changes of the transmembrane potentials in a given cross section of a motor unit; b_s — the length of the summated depolarization zone, i.e. the distance from the beginning of the depolarization in the fibre in which it had moved closest to its end, to the end of the repolarization in the fibre in which it is the farthest from its end; v_s — velocity of spreading of the forefront of the summated depolarized zone; L_s — the greatest distance from a motor end plate to one of the ends of the respective muscle fibre in the motor unit; and T_s — duration of the rapid electric changes at the excitation of the motor unit.

The potential of the motor unit upon placing the leads in the muscle or on its surface is the sum of the extracellular potentials of the muscle fibres, potentials occurring as a result of the volume conduction in the muscle. It depends on several groups of factors: (a) on the parameters of the excitation of the separate muscle fibres (DT, RT, DRT, v, b and L); (b) on the number of the muscle fibres in the motor unit, on its territory, on the distribution of the fibres within the territory and on the desynchronization; (c) on the properties of the volume conductor: resistance, homogeneity, anisotropy, and presence and configuration of the dielectric walls and (d) on the place and manner of leading-off the potential.

The object of the present paper is to examine the dependence of the potential of the motor unit on these factors.

DEPENDENCE OF THE MOTOR UNIT POTENTIAL ON THE PLACE AND MANNER OF RECORDING

The potentials of the motor unit can be led off in a monopolar or in a bipolar manner, using different areas of the electrodes. The latter can be situated at different radial distances, r, to the particular motor unit (the precise definition of r will be given further on) and at different axial distances to the line approximating the position of the motor end plates (l). Bipolar leads are usually employed in electromyographic studies. In this case the potential constitutes the difference of the potentials recorded by the two poles of the electrode. That is why we shall first examine the potentials led off in a monopolar manner and later on we shall examine on that basis the potentials recorded in a bipolar manner. The potentials existing in numerous neighbouring points are 'averaged' on the surface of the leads. The closer the two points, the smaller is the difference of the potentials between them, provided all other conditions are the same. That is why we shall examine first recordings with electrodes which have a small area and give potentials that are approximately characteristic of a given point.

The point from which a particular recording is made can be situated within the territory of the motor unit or outside this territory. Intra-territorial recordings are usually employed in the course of electromyographic studies. The potentials in this case are of complex and varying shapes depending on the distances between the electrode and the closest muscle fibres. Upon extra-territorial recording the potentials are relatively uniform and in this manner it is easier to study the influences of various other factors. That is why we shall first examine the monopolar extra-territorial recordings with electrodes having a small surface.

The potentials thus led off at distances from the motor area smaller than L_s can have not more than four phases (Gydikov and Kosarov, 1972a,b)—Fig. 1A. The dependence of the amplitude of the separate phases on l and r is shown in Fig. 1B, C, D and E. In the motor area the potential starts with a negative phase, followed by a low-amplitude positive phase, and ending with a terminal positive phase. With the increase of l the potential changes from a three-phase to a four-phase one, beginning with a positive phase. The negative maximum draws increasingly farther away from the beginning of the potential, while the second positive phase draws nearer to it. The terminal positive phase does not shift. At distances close to L_s the second positive phase coincides with the terminal positive phase and the

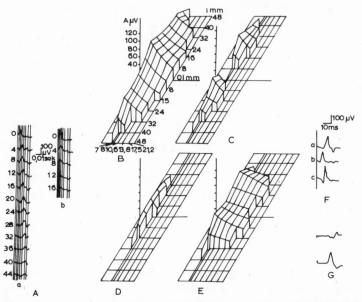

Fig. 1. Volume conduction of the potentials. (A) Potentials from a motor unit in m. biceps br. at different axial (a) and radial (b) distances; (B, C, D and E) dependences of the amplitude of the different phases on the axial and the radial distance; (B) negative phase; (C) first positive phase; (D) second positive phase; (E) terminal positive phase; (F) Potentials having a terminal positive phase recorded by different needle monopolar electrodes; (a) with small leading-off area; (b) with larger leading-off area; (c) with needle multi-electrode; (G) Potentials from a motor unit in m. opponens pol. at axial distances $l > L$ and $l = 0$ (after Bergmans).

potential becomes a three-phase one. The negative and the terminal positive phases are summated at the end of the motor unit. The potential is of the biphasic type at distances greater than L_s, with initial positive phase and a negative phase coinciding in time with the terminal positive phase upon recording from distances considerably smaller than L_s (Fig. 1Aa). The amplitude of the separate phases decreases with the increase of r. The slowest is the decrease of the amplitude of the terminal positive phase (Fig. 1Ab,E).

The phases of the potential are not symmetric. For instance, the ascending part of the negative phase lasts less than the descending part. The ratio between the two parts, K_s, is always smaller than 1 . K_s grows with the increase of r, i.e. the potentials become more symmetric.

The negative phase is conditioned by the depolarized zone moving under the electrode. The positive phases before and after the negative one are conditioned by the volume conduction, just as in the case of potentials from nerve fibres (Lorente de No, 1947). The terminal positive phase described by us (Gydikov and Kosarov, 1972a) is characteristic of the monopolarly recorded potentials in the muscle (Fig. 1F). Some records from the publications by Jasper and Balem (1949), Petersen and Kugelberg (1949) and Lundervold and Li (1953) show that the terminal positive phase can be observed at any monopolar recording. According to results obtained from studies of ours, these phases are not to be observed in about 20% of the motor units. Some records from publications by Katz and Miledi (1965) and Bergmans (1970) show the terminal negative phase of the potential upon recording from a point for which $l > L$ (Fig. 1G).

DEPENDENCE OF EXTRA-TERRITORIAL MONOPOLARY RECORDED MOTOR UNIT POTENTIALS ON PARAMETERS OF EXCITATION AND DESYNCHRON-IZATION

Significance of L

In investigating the excitation in the nerve fibres and in the nerve, the fibres are considered as being infinitely long. This is not possible in the case of the muscle fibres and of the motor units, since L and L_s are relatively small.

L and L_s can be varied in the experiment by investigating the potentials of one and the same motor unit upon passively expanded or contracted muscle (Gydikov and Kosarov, 1973). Besides that they are different for the different muscles and are approximately familiar from anatomical studies. L_s can easily be measured experimentally by determining the distance $l_k = L_s$ up to which a shift of the negative phase of the extracellular monopolar potentials from the beginning of the impulse still exists (on Fig. 1A, $L_s = 40$ mm).

Fig. 2A shows motor unit potentials from muscles of different lengths,

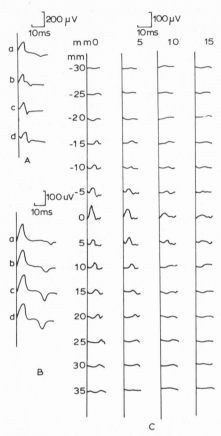

Fig. 2. The influence of L on the extra-territorial motor unit potential. (A) Motor units from muscles with different lengths: (a) m. biceps br.; (b) m. pronator ter.; (c) m. opponens pol.; (d) m. interosseus dors., I. (B) Potentials from a motor unit in m. biceps br. at different muscle lengths; (a, b, c and d) increasing passive shortening; (C) from m. flexor carpii rad. with two terminal positive phases. Potentials recorded at different axial and radial distances shown in the figure.

while Fig. 2B shows potentials from different lengths of one and the same muscle. The change in the length of the muscle does not affect v_s, but as shown by the figures it changes the duration of the potentials. This duration upon monopolar recording, on physical considerations, is equal to T_s. The dependence between T_s and L_s is directly proportional and, consequently, according to (1) the change of L_s affects neither b_s nor TDR_s.

Therefore the terminal positive phase of the potentials of a motor unit occurs when the depolarization zone reaches the end of the motor unit. If the motor end plates are not in the middle of the muscle fibres then we must expect two terminal positive phases. This is precisely what is observed in the experiment (Fig. 2C; Gydikov and Kosarov, 1972b).

The change in L_s does not affect DT_s and RT_s, and the assymmetry of the negative phase at the different radial distances is therefore preserved. Since b_s undergoes no change, the change in L_s does not lead to a change in the desynchronization. This in its turn signifies that the extracellular potentials of the individual muscle fibres must change with the change of L_s, as is the case with the extra-territorial potentials.

In the course of investigations of individual muscle fibres (Håkansson, 1957), biphasic potentials have been recorded with the initial positive phase having an amplitude almost equal to that of the negative phase. However, the measurements were taken at rather close distances to the muscle fibre (less than 1 mm). The extra-territorial potential of a motor unit is the sum of the extracellular potentials of the separate muscle fibres at big radial distances. At such distances, with the existing recording amplifiers and on account of the small amplitude, it is not possible to record potentials from individual fibres. That is why a mathematical model of an excitable fibre was worked out in our laboratory (Dimitrova, 1973, 1974; Dimitrova and Dimitrov, 1974; Dimitrov and Dimitrova, 1974a,b,c). In actual fact this model is a concrete form of the model of the solid angle of Woodbury (1965) and Plonsey (1965, 1969). The model of the solid angle determines the extracellular potential $\varphi(l,r)$ at a given point of the volume conductor in the following manner:

$$\varphi(l,r) = \frac{\sigma_a}{4\,\pi\sigma_0} \int_s V d\Omega \tag{4}$$

wherein σ_a is the conductivity of the axoplasm, σ_o is the conductivity of the surrounding medium, V is the intracellular potential, and Ω is the solid angle subtended at a point with coordinates l and r by a surface element, d_S.

If we assume that the muscle fibre is a cylinder and that the intracellular potential may be approximated with rectangular wave forms, as shown on Fig. 3A, the following expression is obtained for $\varphi(l,t)$ ensuing from (4):

$$\varphi(l,r) = \frac{V\sigma_a}{4\,\pi\sigma_0 N} \sum_{i=1}^{N} (\Omega_{1i} + \Omega_{2i} + \Omega_{3i} + \Omega_{4i}) \tag{5}$$

where Ω_{1i} and Ω_{2i} are the solid angles subtended at a point with coordinates l,r by the cross-sections of the muscle fibre which determine the ith rectangular component of one depolarized zone, Ω_{3i} and Ω_{4i} being analogous to the other depolarized zone (Fig. 3B).

By definition, the solid angle is directly proportional to the section of the fibre S which is perpendicular to the radius-vector R and is inversely proportional to the square of this radius-vector (Fig. 3C). On that account (3) can

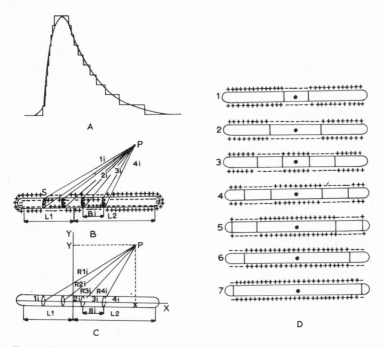

Fig. 3. Model of a single muscle fibre. (A) The intracellular potential and the approximation with rectangular waveform. (B) The solid angles subtended by one rectangular waveform composing the two depolarized zones. (C) Computing the extracellular potentials
according to the model of Dimitrova; (D) Seven consecutive stages of the depolarisation.

be transformed into:

$$\varphi(l,r) = \frac{V\sigma_a}{4\,\pi\sigma_0 N} \sum_{i=1}^{N} \left(\frac{S_{1i}\cos\alpha_{1i}}{R_{1i}^2} + \frac{S_{2i}\cos\alpha_{2i}}{R_{2i}^2} + \frac{S_{3i}\cos\alpha_{3i}}{R_{3i}^2} + \frac{S_{4i}\cos\alpha_{4i}}{R_{4i}^2} \right) \quad (6)$$

wherein S_{1i} and S_{2i} are the areas of the fibre sections determining the ith
rectangular wave for one depolarized zone, S_{3i} and S_{4i} being for the other
depolarized zone; R_i are the distances to the centre of the corresponding
sections, while α_i are angles between R_i and the normal of the corresponding
section.

It is assumed in the model that S_i are constant along the entire length of
the fibre ($S_i = \pi a_1^2$, wherein a_1 is the radius of the fibre), and that they
decrease to zero only at the end. It is likewise assumed that at the initial
moments after activation of the fibre the two depolarized zones have one
real part (at the forefront) and one non-operative part (at the rear), the real
part gradually growing until it becomes equal to the entire zone. After that
each one of the zones moves at a constant speed towards the ends of the

fibre, and at the very end we again have one real (at the rear) and one non-operative (at the forefront) part of the depolarized zone, the real part decreasing until it disappears completely. The rate of increase and decrease in the length of the real parts is equal to the velocity of spreading of the zone along the fibre.

Using a computer and upon approximation of the intracellular potential with 200 rectangular wave forms, the extracellular potentials were calculated at different points of the volume conductor. The results of the modelling showed that the extracellular potential of a separate fibre has the same four phases as the extra-territorial potentials of the motor unit. In particular, there exists a terminal positive phase which appears when the depolarized zone reaches the end of the fibre. Two terminal positive zones are to be observed when the position of the synapse is asymmetric in relation to the two ends of the fibre. The amplitude of each one of the phases changes upon an increase of l analogous to the extra-territorial potentials. The same holds true of the change in the amplitude of the separate phases with the growth of r. The model calculations embrace quantities of r from zero to the maximum ones at which the extra-territorial potentials were observed in the experiment. Near the fibre the initial positive phase has an amplitude which is almost equal to the amplitude of the negative phase, while the second positive phase and the terminal positive phase have very small amplitudes. With the increase of r the amplitude of the first positive phase drops most quickly, the decline in the amplitude of the negative phase being slower, that of the amplitude of the second positive phase being still slower, and the slowest decline being that of the amplitude of the terminal positive phase. Close to the fibre — provided we have used the amplifications at which the first two phases are to be observed — the second two phases are rather small and the potential looks like being a two-phase one. The ratio between the amplitudes changes upon increasing the distance from the fibre, and the potential looks like being a four-phase one. The absence of a terminal positive phase in some motor units may be explained by a possible turning of the ends of the muscle fibres, by their unequal lengths, or by some other factors.

In the model we obtain the dependence (3) and, particularly, the directly proportional dependence between T and L, b and v being constant.

Significance of the remaining parameters of excitation and desynchronization

It has not been possible as yet to influence v_s, b_s, DRT_s, DT_s, RT_s and desynchronization in an isolated manner in the course of experiments. All these parameters undergo changes under effects such as temperature changes, fatigue and hypoxia. However, the separate effects do not alter these parameters to the same degree. For instance, we know the dependence of v_s on the temperature: v_s increases with the rise of the temperature in the muscle.

It was established, however, that the temperature influences DRT_s as well (Gydikov et al., 1974c). DRT_s decreases with the warming of the muscle and increases upon cooling. The influence on v_s is stronger than the influence on DRT_s, and in this manner b_s is prolonged with the rise in temperature and is shortened upon cooling. The method of measuring b_s is based on dependence (3), L_s being determined by the manner described (Gydikov and Kosarov, 1974). Following the determination of b_s it is easy to find DRT_s using dependence (2).

The changes of v_s, DRT_s, and b_s have an influence on T_s. The changes in the extracellular potentials with temperature variations are shown on Fig. 4A. Changes in the amplitude of the potentials also occur parallel with the changes in T_s.

Fatigue and hypoxia prolong b_s (Kosarov and Gydikov, 1973; Gydikov

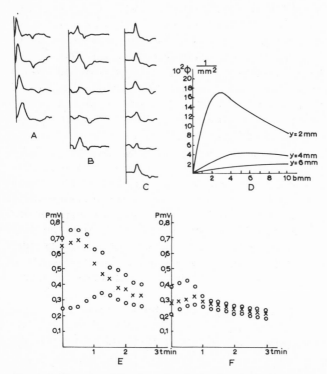

Fig. 4. Influence of the length of the depolarized zone on the motor unit potentials. (A) Potentials of a motor unit from m. biceps br. at different temperature; (B) Potentials of a motor unit from m. opponens pol. upon long lasting high-frequency stimulation and after switching off the stimulation; (C) Potentials from a motor unit in m. biceps br. after interruption of the blood supply and restoration of the blood circulation; (D) Dependence of the negative phase amplitude of the extracellular potential of a muscle fibre at different radial distances (y) on the length of the depolarized zone (model); (E) and (F) Negative phase amplitude of the potentials of two motor units during fatigue at different radial distances.

and Kosarov, 1974). There is a decrease of v_s in the case of hypoxia. After stimulation leading to fatigue the same trend is to be observed in the changes of v_s. In these two cases, however, the influence on DRT_s is much stronger and the final result is prolongation of b_s (Gydikov et al., 1974c). This leads to an increase of T_s (Fig. 4B).

Upon modelling the potentials of a separate muscle fibre the changes of v and b are shown to influence T in much the same manner. The changes of b account for changes in the amplitude of the negative phase which are different at different radial distances (Fig. 4C). Fig. 4C shows that with the prolongation of b the amplitude of the negative phase increases, this being followed by a decrease, the maximum for greater distances being reached at a higher b (Dimitrova, 1973). Consequently, it is possible upon the prolongation of b for the amplitude of the potentials to decrease at small radial distances and to increase at big distances. This conclusion obtained from the model was experimentally confirmed (Gydikov et al., 1974b).

Use was made of Bergmans' method (1970, 1973) for isolated electric stimulation of a separate axon, as modified in the course of our work. Upon continuous high-frequency stimulation changes occur in the potentials under the effect of fatigue (Fig. 4Ba), amplitude changes in particular. It can be seen from Fig. 4D that the amplitude changes show different dynamics at different radial distances. Such non-simultaneous changes at different radial distances cannot be due to changes in the desynchronization or in the membrane resting potential.

The model data indicate that the prolongation of b influences also the amplitudes of the other phases of the extracellular potentials.

As already mentioned, the extra-territorial monopolarly recorded potentials are asymmetric. This asymmetry is conditioned by the asymmetry of the intracellular potentials, but in view of the specificities of volume conduction it is different at different radial distances. Another factor which may influence asymmetry is desynchronization. Since desynchronization is due to numerous random factors it may be expected that the distribution of the forefronts of the depolarized zones along the length of the motor unit will be symmetric. Growing desynchronization will not only prolong b_s but it will also make the extra-territorial potentials more symmetric.

On recording from the same radial distance, cooling makes the potentials more symmetric, while warming makes them more asymmetric. The changes are mainly at the expense of the ascending phase of the potentials. There exists a close inverse correlation between that phase and v_s. The potentials become more asymmetric during continuous high-frequency stimulation, on account of a considerable prolongation of the duration of the descending phase, although the duration of the ascending phase shows an increase as well, be it a small one. After discontinuing the stimulation b_s promptly becomes shorter, but the potentials become more symmetrical compared with those prior to stimulation. This result could be explained by the assumption that upon high-frequency stimulation there occurs a prolongation of the DRT_s at the expense partly of the increased desynchronization and mainly on account of prolonged repolarization. It may be assumed that, upon discontinuing the stimulation, RT_s returns to the initial values before the growth of the desynchronization has disappeared (Gydikov et al., 1974c).

On modelling the extracellular potentials of a separate muscle fibre it was found that the asymmetry of the intracellular potentials is of great significance. It determines the asymmetry of the extracellular potentials which decreases with the increase of the radial distance. The increase in the asymmetry of the intracellular potentials increases the amplitude of the negative phase at small radial distances and reduces that amplitude at large radial distances.

The data from the model indicated that asymmetry is the cause of the non-simultaneous occurrence of the maximum of the negative phase at different radial distances. At large distances the maximum shows a delay in time, compared with the maximum at short distances. This effect in the vicinity of the motor end plate is highly influenced also by the summation of the potential fields conditioned by the two zones of depolarization. As a result of the effect of the two factors, with v remaining constant, the velocity of spreading of the negative maximum in the volume conductor along the length of the muscle fibre is irregular (Fig. 5A), and it approximates the genuine velocity only when l is quite large. The velocity measured in the volume conductor changes differently at different radial distances (Dimitrov and Dimitrova, 1974a). This conclusion from the model was confirmed experimentally (Dimitrov et al., 1974). Fig. 5B shows the changes in the velocity of spreading — measured in the volume conductor — of the negative maximum of the potential of a motor unit at various radial distances. In view of this dependence, v_s was measured in the course of our studies by two leads situated at considerable distances from the motor end plates.

On Fig. 5C and D we see potentials from a separate muscle fibre measured experimentally at different radial distances, as taken from the works of Håkansson (1957) and Stålberg (1966). We can see the model-predicted shifts of the maximum of the negative phase and a decrease in the asymmetry of the extracellular potentials with the increase in the radial distance.

The methods described of measuring T_s, L_s and v_s by the extra-territorial monopolar potentials provide for the experimental determination of b_s and DRT_s. The determination of the b_s changes is easier since, if we ensue from (3) that

$$b_s = b_{s1} - b_{s2} = T_{s1}v_{s1} - L_s - T_{s2}v_{s2} + L_s = T_{s1}v_{s1} - T_{s2}v_{s4} , \qquad (7)$$

there is no need to measure L_s. Experimentally, it is easy to follow the change in the asymmetry at a particular radial distance and to judge indirect-

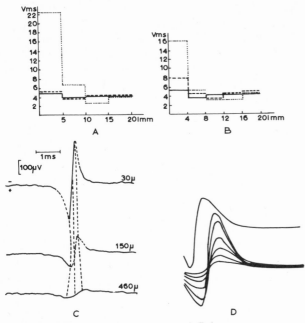

Fig. 5. Velocity of propagation of muscle potentials and single muscle fibre potentials at different *r*. (A) Velocity of propagation of single muscle fibre potentials in a volume conductor at different *r* (the different lines); (B) Propagation velocity of extra-territorial motor units potentials at different *r* (the different lines); (C) and (D) Single muscle fibre potentials at different *r* (experimentally); (C) after Håkensson, 1957; (D) after Stålberg, 1966.

ly the changes of DT_s and RT_s, and also the extent to which they are conditioned mainly by changes in the desynchronization or by DT and RT.

DEPENDENCE OF THE EXTRA-TERRITORIAL MONOPOLARY RECORDED MOTOR UNIT POTENTIALS ON THE NUMBER OF MUSCLE FIBRES AND ON THE SIZE OF THE UNIT'S TERRITORY

The number of muscle fibres is a rather important factor which determines the amplitude of the summated potentials of a motor unit. We have found out that the amplitude of the separate phase of the extra-territorial potentials is highly dependent on *l* and *r*. At given values of *l* and *r*, however, its size is directly proportional to the number of fibres contained in the motor unit and to their diameter. The extra-territorial monopolar leads can be used for location of the motor units and for determining their size. Different variants of the method have been worked out to this end (Kosarov et al., 1971; Gydikov et al., 1972; Gydikov and Kosarov, 1972b; Kosarov et al., 1974). The greatest advantages are obtained upon using four surface

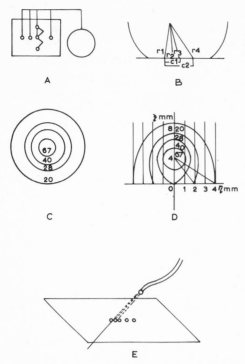

Fig. 6. Location of motor units and extra-territorial potential field. (A) Multi-electrode for location; (B) Cross-section of a muscle—the principle of location of a motor unit; (C) extra-territorial potential field of a motor unit in an infinite volume conductor (cross-section); (D) Extra-territoral potential field of a motor unit in an infinite volume conductor (cross-section); (D) Extra-territorial potential field of a motor unit in a volume conductor limited by a dielectric wall (cross-section); (E) Multi-electrode for location and studying the extra-territorial potential field of the motor units.

monopolar leads arranged in the manner shown in Fig. 6A. The electrodes lie in one line and are placed perpendicular to the direction of the muscle fibres. Measurements are taken of the average amplitude of the negative phase of the potentials upon recording with each one of the electrodes (P_i). On the basis of these measurements it is possible, with a certain degree of precision, to determine the place of the electric axis of the motor unit in the cross-section of the muscle corresponding to the position of the electrodes. By the term 'electric axis' is meant the imaginary line along which it is possible to place a generator equivalent to all muscle fibres of the motor unit in such a manner that the same potentials shall be obtained from it at the respective distances. P_i depends on r_i in the following manner:

$$P_i = \frac{a}{r_i^{n_i}} \qquad (i = 1 \div 4) \tag{8}$$

All values of r in the present paper are related precisely to the distance between the electrode and the electric axis of the motor unit; a is the potential which would have been measured at a distance of 1 mm from the electric axis provided the muscle fibres had been substituted by an equivalent generator; and n_i is a quantity different for each point, which is dependent on a variety of factors and in a complex manner. The closer two points are to one another the smaller is the difference between their corresponding values of n_i. It may be assumed in a first approximation that $n_1 = n_2 = n_3 = n_4$ in the case of the four leads used for the purpose of location. Besides that, as can be seen in Fig. 6B, r_2 is a median of the triangle made up of r_1, r_3 and c_1, while r_3 is a median of the triangle made up of r_1, r_4 and c_2. We can therefore work out the following system of equations:

$$P_1 = \frac{a}{r_1^{n_1}}$$

$$P_2 = \frac{a}{r_2^{n_2}}$$

$$P_3 = \frac{a}{r_3^{n_3}}$$

$$P_4 = \frac{a}{r_4^{n_4}}$$

$$r_2^2 = \frac{1}{2} r_1^2 + \frac{1}{2} r_3^2 - c_1^2$$

$$r_3^2 = \frac{1}{2} r_1^2 + \frac{1}{2} r_4^2 - c_2^2 \qquad (9)$$

By solving this system we find the place of the electric axis of the motor unit in the cross-section of the muscle and the quantity a which, provided all other conditions are equal, is indicative of the size of the motor unit. In the course of the studies carried out, a showed variations within very broad limits—from 0.10 to about 10.00 mV; a is a relative indicator of the size of the motor unit. Besides depending on the number and diameter of the muscle fibres, a is dependent on a number of other factors as well, such as the amplitude of the intracellular potentials, b, the asymmetry of the intracellular potentials, the desynchronization among the muscle fibres, and certain parameters of the volume conductor. However, it is obvious that the most significant factor is the number of the muscle fibres of the motor unit. It is only the variations within this number that can account for the broad limits of the variation of a.

The data obtained in the modelling, which indicate that on account of asymmetry of the intracellular potentials and the summation of the effect of the two depolarized zones the maximum of the negative phase does not occur simultaneously at different radial distances, warrant the logical conclusion that the increase in the diameter of the territory of the motor unit is analogous to an increase of desynchronization and will consequently lead to a decrease of a.

The parameter n_i indicates the rate of decrease of the amplitude of the negative phase of potentials with the increase of the radial distance. The data obtained from the modelling indicated that a variety of factors tend to influence this rate: it decreases with the prolongation of b and increases with the increase in the asymmetry of the intracellular potentials. The summation of the effect from the two depolarized zones has a considerable influence around the motor end plate area.

DEPENDENCE OF THE EXTRA-TERRITORIAL MONOPOLARY RECORDED MOTOR UNIT POTENTIALS ON THE PROPERTIES OF THE VOLUME CONDUCTOR

The inhomogeneity of the muscle as a volume conductor is not very large and can be neglected. Conductivity in the direction of the muscle fibres, according to data obtained by various authors and for different muscles, is between 2 and 14 times higher than the conductivity in a transverse direction (Galeotti, 1902; Sapengo, 1930; Burger and van Dongen, 1960—1961; Ruch et al., 1963; Geddes and Baker, 1967). Practically, the resistance of the muscle is purely resistive (Plonsey, 1969; Rosenfalck, 1969; Pattle, 1971) and is determined by the resistance and configuration of the space in which the extracellular fluid is to be found and consequently by the orientation of the muscle fibres.

The model data have shown that the extracellular potentials of the muscle fibres essentially depend on anisotropy. The amplitude of the negative phase increases at close distances and decreases at larger distances; thereby there is a growth in the values of n_i. Anisotropy leads to an increase in the delay of the occurrence of the negative maximum at large radial distances, and this influences the velocity of its spreading in the volume conductor in an axial direction.

The potential of the motor unit depends essentially on the existence and configuration of the dielectric walls. The dielectric walls increase the potentials in comparison with the amplitude they would have had in an infinite volume conductor. The closer the dielectric walls are to the motor unit, the greater this increase. The influence of the dielectric walls depends on their configuration. A flat dielectric wall causes a two-fold rise in the amplitude of the potentials measured at its surface. In the depth of the muscle the changes in amplitude decrease with the increase in the distance of a given point from the wall. Fig. 6C shows the equipotential lines of the extra-territorial potential field of a motor unit in a cross-section of the muscle in an infinite volume conductor. In Fig. 6Db there is a volume conductor limited by a flat wall. At each point of the volume conductor the amplitude of the potentials is equal to the amplitude which would have been obtained in an infinite volume conductor under conditions of simultaneous excitation of two equal motor units situated at equal distances on either side of the line crossing the dielectric wall (Fig. 6D; Dimitrov, 1974).

The skin surface is a dielectric wall. A flat wall of this kind is formed upon pressing a multi-electrode to the skin. The potentials of the motor units which are close to this wall are essentially influenced by it. The distant curved dielectric walls have no such essential influence and it may be expected that the extra-territorial potential field around the motor unit will not differ very much from that shown on Fig. 6D. When a tubule (Fig. 6E) is placed in the multi-electrode, through which it is possible to drive a needle electrode in the muscle, the amplitudes of the potentials at different points of the volume conductor actually do not differ essentially from those predicted on the basis of the location of the motor unit with surface electrodes. In addition it turned out that, as can be seen from Fig. 6D, it is possible for the electrode to move farther away from the motor unit and nevertheless for the amplitude of the potential to increase, if the electrode draws closer to a dielectric wall. This is to be observed when the electrode is to the side of the electric centre of the motor unit (Gydikov et al., 1974a).

THE MOTOR UNIT POTENTIAL AS RECORDED BY INTRA-TERRITORIAL MONOPOLAR LEADS

The differences between the distances from the electrode to the separate muscle fibres of the motor unit are small when it is placed extra-territorially, and the contribution of the potentials of the individual fibres in the formation of the summated potential is approximately of the same order. However, upon intra-territorial location these differences are critical. That is why the potentials from the closest muscle fibres are of fundamental significance to the summated potential. Since the muscle fibres in the closest vicinity of the electrode can be at various distances and the depolarized zones may be differently displaced in time upon excitation, the intra-territorial potential of the motor unit may have various forms at the different points of the territory. It may show various types of unevenness and even several phases. The unevenness and polyphasic nature are due to the non-coincidence in time of the negative maxima (spikes) determined by two or more muscle fibres. This in turn may be due to the desynchronization and unequal radial distance from the electrode to these fibres. Unevenness is to be observed upon a slight displacement of the two spikes. Polyphasic behaviour is obtained with a bigger shift, on account of the large amplitude of the initial positive phase at small radial distances.

When one or more muscle fibres are very near to the lead, the amplitude of the potential is so large that, when a corresponding amplification is used, the terminal positive phase is not to be seen. It can be seen, however, with proper amplification. The duration of the potential T_s, recorded until the end of the terminal positive phase, depends in the same manner on v_s, L_s and b_s, as in the case of extra-territorial leads, but the experimental follow-up of the changes of DT_s and RT_s with needle-type intra-territorial electrodes is a difficult proposition. Their changes may be observed in the manner described by simultaneous extra-territorial surface recordings. By examining the changes in the asymmetry of the separate spikes at a constant radial distance, it is possible to gauge the changes in DT and RT of individual muscle fibres -- this being impossible in the case of extra-territorial leads. It is likewise possible to determine the v of separate fibres (Stålberg, 1966). Equation (2) is also valid.

It should be pointed out that recording with the multi-electrode of Buchthal et al. (1957a), using one of the terminal electrodes as reference, is not pure monopolar recording. For instance, upon using a reference electrode situated at a large distance (50—60 mm) we obtain larger amplitudes of the potentials, smaller values for n_i, and longer duration of the negative phase when moving farther away from the electric centre of the motor unit (Kosarov and Gydikov, 1974).

THE MOTOR UNIT POTENTIAL USING BIPOLAR RECORDING

As already pointed out, the potential of the motor unit using bipolar recording represents the difference of the potentials recorded by the two poles. When both poles of the bipolar electrode are placed at $l < L$, one essential result is the disappearance or the sharp reduction of the amplitude of the terminal positive phase (Fig. 7A). Depending on the position of the two poles, the 'remainder' from the terminal positive phase may also be of the opposite sign. When one of the poles is at a distance $l < L$, and the other pole is at a distance $l > L$, the terminal positive phase has a much higher amplitude, which may also have an opposite sign depending on which one of the electrodes is at a distance $l > L$ (Fig. 7B).

It is of essential significance to the bipolar recordings whether one or both poles are situated extra-territorially, or intra-territorially, respectively, and whether they are situated along the length of or transversely to the muscle fibres. Of great significance also is the inter-electrode distance, and in some cases the area of the recording electrodes as well.

When both poles are situated extra-territorially and transversely to the muscle fibres, the potential obtained in the motor area is an almost monophasic one, whereas outside the motor area it is an almost biphasic potential with an initial positive phase (Fig. 7C). The zero-to-maximum or peak-to-peak amplitude of these potentials depends on the inter-electrode distance

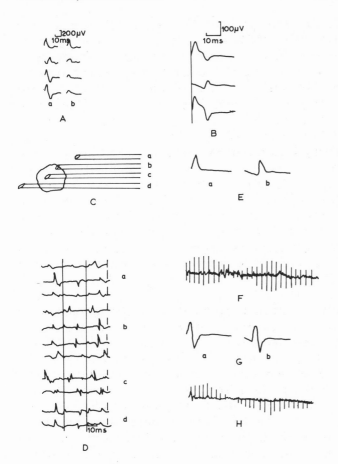

Fig. 7. Bipolar records of motor unit potentials; (A) from top to bottom (a) monopolar records from two points at different l, the bipolar record from the same points and the calculated difference between the two monopolar records; (b) monopolar records from two points at different r, the bipolar record from the same points and the calculated difference between the two monopolar records; (B) from top to bottom—monopolar records at $l = 0$ and $l > L$ and the bipolar record from the same two points; (C) Four different possible positions of the concectric needle electrode with respect to the motor unit territory; (D) Records of motor unit potentials by a concentric needle electrode (centre) simultaneously with monopolar records from the cannulae (left) and from the different electrode (right) corresponding to the four positions in Fig. 7C; (E) Bipolar records of motor unit potentials at $l = 0$ (a) and $l < L$ (b). The two poles of the electrode at equal axial distance; (F) Changes of the amplitude of the potentials of a motor unit upon moving a bipolar electrode across the end plate area. The two poles of the electrode are on a line parallel to the muscle fibres; (G) Bipolar records of motor unit potentials; (a) one pole of the electrode at $l = 0$, the other pole at $l < L$; (b) one pole of the electrode at $l_1 > L$, the other pole at $l_2 < L$ ($l_2 > l_1$); (H) Changes of the amplitude of the potentials of a motor unit upon moving a bipolar electrode transverse to the muscle fibres. The two poles of the electrode at equal axial distance.

and on the difference in the radial distances of the two poles. It is larger on a greater difference in the two radial distances, which may be obtained with a greater inter-electrode distance. However, even in the case of a large inter-electrode difference, the two radial distances could be the same if the electrode is situated symmetrically on either side of the electric axis of the motor unit (Fig. 7D). The amplitude depends not only on the difference in the radial distances but on their absolute values as well: with the growth of the absolute values the amplitude decreases (Fig. 7D).

When both poles are located extra-territorially and longitudinally to the muscle fibres, with one of them in the motor area, the bipolarly recorded potential is almost a biphasic one, while if both poles are outside the motor end plate area it is a triphasic potential (Fig. 7E). The peak-to-peak amplitude increases with the increase in the inter-electrode distance and upon drawing closer to the motor area. However, if the two poles are on either side of the motor area, the amplitude decreases and may become equal to zero — upon a symmetric location of the two poles in relation to the area (Fig. 7F). The increase in the radial distance leads to a decrease of the amplitude.

The duration of the extra-territorially and bipolarly recorded potentials is always shorter than T_s because the terminal positive phase is lost. It does not depend on L_s, according to dependence (3). With a transverse location of the electrodes it increases with the increase of DRT_s. It also increases with the prolongation of b_s and upon the decrease of v_s. A precise quantitative dependence cannot be worked out for the following reason: theoretically, the duration of the potential recorded under these conditions should be equal to T_s. Due to the dropping of the terminal positive phase, the end of the potential is measured to the end of the positive phase that follows after the negative one. However, it has a small amplitude which becomes still smaller upon subtraction, and estimation becomes practically impossible.

An analogous situation is found upon measuring the duration in the case of a longitudinally located bipolar electrode. In this instance too, due to uncertainty in recording the end of the potential initiated with the pole that is farther away from the motor area, it is not possible to work out a quantitative expression for the duration of the potential. Here the duration increases with the increase in the inter-electrode distance. DRT_s, b_s and v_s have an analogous influence on the recordings as in a transverse line.

The area of the recording electrodes when extra-territorial leads are used has no essential effect on the amplitude of the potentials.

The area of the electrodes is a factor of essential significance in the case of intra-territorial bipolar recording. What has been said about the influence of the orientation of the electrodes is valid in relation to the parameters of the separate spikes. When there is more than one spike, the position of the poles of the electrode toward their generators is different, and their dislocation affects each spike in a different manner. There exist analogous dependences on the DRT, *b* and *v* of the amplitude and duration of the spikes, but they are difficult to observe on account of the summation of the potentials from different muscle fibres. Whereas the amplitude of the potential in such a recording depends on the amplitude of the largest spike, the duration largely depends on the desynchronization of the excitation of the individual muscle fibres.

Essentially, in the case of standard recording with concentric electrodes, there are four possible positions of the electrode in relation to the territory of the motor unit (Fig. 7G), namely: (a) the cannula and the electrode can lie extra-territorially; (b) the electrodes can be located intra-territorially and the cannula mainly extra-territorially; (c) the electrode can lie intra-territorially and the cannula mainly intra-territorially also; and (d) the electrode can lie extra-territorially and the cannula mainly intra-territorially. The above four combinations are obtained upon monopolar recording from the electrode and from the cannula (Fig. 7E). In certain cases also the potential recorded in a standard manner can show unevenness or even 'phases' which are determined by the non-simultaneous peaks of the potential upon recording from both poles.

CONCLUSION

On account of the lower noise level and of certain other factors of convenience, bipolar or concentric electrodes, introduced intra-territorially, are usually employed in the electromyographic investigations of potentials from individual motor units. Nevertheless, monopolar recordings, extra-territorial in particular, convey considerably more information about the functional state of the motor units. As a result of physiological investigations carried out, a more extensive use of such recordings in clinical electromyography is recommended.

REFERENCES

BERGMANS, I. (1970) The Physiology of Single Human Nerve Fibres. Vander, Louvain.

BERGMANS, I. (1973) Physiological observations on single human nerve fibres. In: (J.E. Desmedt, Ed.) New Developments in Electromyography and Clinical Neurophysiology, Vol. 2, Karger, Basel, pp. 89–127.

BRANDSTATER, M.E. and LAMBERT, E.H. (1973) Motor unit anatomy. In: (J.E. Desmedt, Ed.) New Developments in Electromyography and Clinical Neurophysiology, Vol. 1, Karger, Basel, pp. 14–22.

BROWN, M.C. and MATTHEWS, P.B.C. (1960) An investigation into the possible existence of polyneuronal innervation of individual skeletal muscle fibres in certain hindlimb muscles of the cat. J. Physiol., 151, 436–457.

BUCHTHAL, F., ERMINIO, F. and ROSENFALCK, P. (1959) Motor unit territory in different human muscles. Acta Physiol. Scand., 45, 72–87.

BUCHTHAL, F., GULD, C. and ROSENFALCK, P. (1957a) Volume conduction of the spike of the motor unit potential investigated with a new type of multi-electrode. Acta Physiol. Scand., 38, ·33—354.

BUCHTHAL, F., GULD, C. and ROSENFALCK, P. (1957b) Multi-electrode study of the territory of a motor unit. Acta Physiol. Scand., 39, 83—104.

BURGER, H.C. and VAN DONGEN, R. (1960—1) Specific electric resistance of body tissues. Phys. Med. Biol., 5, 431—447.

CÖERS, C. and WOLF, A.L. (1957) The Innervation of Muscle. Blackwell, Oxford, pp. 14—20.

DIMITROV, G. (1974) Extracellular potential field of a single striated muscle fiber, immersed in anisotropic volume conductor, limited by infinite dielectric wall. C.R. Acad. Bulg. Sci., 27, 1133—1136.

DIMITROV, G. and DIMITROVA, N. (1974a) Influence of the distribution asymmetry of the depolarization on the extracellular potential field generated by an excitable fibre. Electromyogr. Clin. Neurophysiol, 14, 255—275.

DIMITROV, G. and DIMITROVA, N. (1974b) Extracellular potential field of an excitable fibre immersed in an anisotropic volume conductor. Electromyogr. Clin. Neurophysiol, 14, 437—450.

DIMITROV, G. and DIMITROVA, N. (1974c) Extracellular potential field of a single striated muscle fibre in an anisotropic volume conductor. Electromyogr. Clin. Neurophysiol., 14, 423—436.

DIMITROV, G., TANKOV, N. and SHAPKOV, J. (1975) Volume conduction of action potentials and velocity of spreading of the excitation along the motor unit muscle fibres in human skeletal muscle. Fisiol. J., (In press) (In russian).

DIMITROVA, N. (1973) Influence of the length of the depolarized zone on the extracellular potential field of a single unmyelinated nerve fibre. Electromyogr. Clin. Neurophysiol., 13, 547—558.

DIMITROVA, N. (1974) Model of the extracellular potential field of a single striated muscle fibre. Electromyogr. Clin. Neurophysiol., 14, 53—66.

DIMITROVA, N. and DIMITROV, G. (1974) Extracellular potential field of a single striated muscle fibre. Electromyogr. Clin. Neurophysiol., 14, 279—292.

GALEOTTI, G. (1902) Über die electrische Leitfähigkeit der tierischen Gewebe. Z. Biol., 43, 289—340.

GEDDES, L.A. and BAKER, L.E. (1967) The specific resistance of biological material-compendium of data for the biomedical engineer and physiologist. Med. Biol. Eng., 5, 271—293.

GYDIKOV, A. and KOSAROV, D. (1972a) Volume conduction of the potentials from separate motor units in human muscle. Electromyography, 12, 127—147.

GYDIKOV, A. and KOSAROV, D. (1972b) Extra-territorial potential field of impulses from separate motor units in human muscles. Electromyography, 12, 283—305.

GYDIKOV, A. and KOSAROV, D. (1973a) The influence of various factors on the shape of the myopotentials in using monopolar electrodes. Electromyogr. Clin. Neurophysiol., 13, 319—343.

GYDIKOV, A. and KOSAROV, D. (1974) Influence of various factors on the length of the summated depolarised area of the muscle fibers in voluntary activating of motor units and in electrical stimulation. Electromyography Clin. Neurophysiol., 14, 79—93.

GYDIKOV, A., KOSAROV, D. and TANKOV, N. (1972) Studying the alpha motoneuron activity by investigating motor units of various sizes. Electromyography, 12, 10—28.

GYDIKOV, A., DIMITROV, G. and KOSAROV, D. (1975a) Influence of the dielectric walls on the volume conduction of potentials from separate motor units upon monopolar recording. (In preparation).

GYDIKOV, A., DIMITROVA, N., KOSAROV, D. and DIMITROV, G. (1975b) Influence of frequency and duration of firing on the shape of the potentials from different types of motor units in human muscle. (In preparation).

GYDIKOV, A., KOSAROV, D. and DIMITROV, G. (1975c) Length of the summated depolarized zone and duration of the depolarization and repolarization proceses in the motor unit upon different conditions. (In preparation).

HÅKANSSON, C.H. (1957) Action potentials recorded intra- and extra-cellularly from the isolated frog muscle fibre in Ringer's solution and in air. Acta Physiol. Scand., 39, 291—312.

JASPER, H. and BALLEM, G. (1949) Unipolar electromyograms of normal and denervated human muscle. J. Neurophysiol., 12, 231—244.

KATZ, B. and MILEDI, R. (1965) Propagation of electric activity in motor nerve terminals. Proc. R. Soc. B., 161, 453—482.

KOSAROV, D. and GYDIKOV, A. (1972) Stimulation vectorelectromyography and vectorelectromyography of impulses from separate motor units under changed functional state of the muscles. Electromyography, 12, 307—324.

KOSAROV, D. and GYDIKOV, A. (1974) Extra-territorial and intra-territorial records of motor unit potentials by means of monopolar concentic and bipolar needle electrodes. Electromyogr. Clin. Neurophysiol. (In press).

KOSAROV, D., GYDIKOV, A. and TANKOV, N. (1974) Improvement of the method of motor units location. Electromyogr. Clin. Neurophysiol., 14, 97—107.

KOSAROV, D., GYDIKOV, A., TANKOV, N. and RADITCHEVA, N. (1971) Examining the work of motor units of various sizes in the muscles of dogs. Agressology, 12, C. 29—39.

LIDDELL, E.E.T. and SHERRINGTON, C.S. (1925) Recruitment and some other features of the reflex inhibition. Proc. R. Soc. B, 97, 488—518.

LORENTE DE NO, R. (1947) A study of nerve physiology. Studies from the Rockefeller Institute for Medical Research 132, New York.

LINDERVOLD, A. and LI, C.L. (1953) Motor units and fibrilation potentials as recorded with different kinds of electrodes. Acta Psychiat. Neurol. Scand. Kopenhagen, 18, 201—212.

PATTLE, R.E. (1971) The external action potential of a nerve or muscle fibre in an extended medium. Phys. Med. Biol., 10, 673—685.

PETERSON, I. and KUGELBERG, E. (1949) Duration and form of action potentials in the normal human muscle. J. Neurol. Neurosurg. Psychiat., 12, 124—128.

PLONSEY, R. (1965) An extension of the solid angle potentials formulation for an active cell. Biophys. J., 5, 663—667.

PLONSEY, R. (1969) Bioelectic phenomena. McGraw Hill Book Co., New York.

ROSENFALCK, P. (1969) Intra- and extra-cellular potential fields of active nerve and muscle fibres. Acta Physiol. Scand. suppl. 321, 1—168.

RUCH, S., ABILDSKOV, S.A. and MCFEE, R. (1963) Resistivity of body tissues at low frequencies. Circulat. Res., 12, 40—50.

SAPENGO, E. (1930) Über die Impedanz und Kapazität des quergestrieften Muskels in Längs- und Querrichtung. Pflügers Arch. Ges. Physiol., 222, 186—211.

STÅLBERG, E. (1966) Propagation velocity in human muscle fibers in situ. Acta Physiol. Scand., 70, suppl. 287, 1—112.

WOODBURY, I.W. (1965) Potentials in a volume conductor. In: (Ruch, I.C., Patton, H.D., Woodbury, I.W. and Towe, A.I. Eds.) Neurophysiology, W.B. Saunders Co., Philadelphia, pp. 83—91.

3

Voluntary control of human motor units

E. HENNEMAN, B.T. SHAHANI and R.R. YOUNG

In 1962, Harrison and Mortensen reported that human subjects could selectively activate ('isolate') any one of several different motor units in a single muscle within the recording range of their EMG electrodes and then maintain activity in that unit. Since then, Basmajian and co-workers (1963, 1967, 1972) have reported on numerous occasions that, when human volunteers are provided with visual and auditory feedback from their active units, they easily learn within 10 or 15 minutes to control the activity of any single motor unit within the recording distance of an EMG electrode. The published records illustrating their results, however, provide no clear support for these claims. This notion, though an interesting one, is in contrast to the widely held concept that higher motor centers do not control the activity of each motoneurone individually. Furthermore, experiments carried out by Henneman et al. (1965a,b) on animals with recordings from ventral root filaments instead of muscle fibers indicate that, under a variety of experimental conditions, single motoneurones can be sequentially activated ('recruited') only in one fixed order determined by the sizes of their cell bodies. The smaller the motoneurone (and presumably its motor unit in the muscle), the more easily it can be discharged; the larger the motoneurone, the greater the amount of excitatory input required to discharge it.

The purpose of the present study was to resolve the controversy as to whether or not the human nervous system can select, out of the available motoneurone pool, any motor unit desired for use according to the wishes or needs of the moment. If true, this would suggest that there is not a completely fixed order of recruitment related to the size of the motor unit. To determine if human subjects can learn to discharge motor units in a selective manner (modifying the natural rank-order determined by the 'size-principle' described above), subjects were asked to discharge single motor units in the extensor indicis proprius muscle by dorsiflexing the index finger. After establishing the normal order of recruitment for two motor units that were clearly distinguishable on the oscilloscope, subjects were instructed either to reverse that normal order or to silence the activity of unit no. 1 without silencing unit no. 2. These simple performances were considered to be crucial tests of the claims for selective control.

Studies were performed on 9 healthy volunteer subjects, 8 male and one female, 23 to 57 years of age. The subjects lay supine on a comfortable couch in a warm room (temperature 24—27°C). Intramuscular electromyographic activity was recorded from the right or left extensor indicis proprius muscle by means of TECA monopolar electrodes (MF25) or single Karma wires, insulated except at the tip, which were inserted using a small hypodermic needle. The muscle extensor indicis proprius was selected for the present study because (a) it has one and only one specific action—extension of the index finger, and (b) Phillips and colleagues have demonstrated that its motoneurone pool (at least in nonhuman primates) receives a relatively large number of monosynaptic connections from pyramidal tract neurones, suggesting a high degree of direct cerebral control (Clough et al., 1968). The recording electrodes were connected to a TECA TE 4 EMG system, and activity was photographed on 100-mm wide paper with the fiber optic graphic recorder, both in the continuous and the sweep modes. In order to study voluntary control over recruitment of single motor unit activity, subjects were asked to produce minimal isometric contraction of the muscle so that only one unit was recruited initially. This task was made possible by 'audio-visual feedback' which consisted of the subject's looking at the oscilloscope screen and listening to the sound produced from the loudspeaker by single motor unit activity. Once reasonable control over the first recruited single motor unit was achieved, subjects were asked to recruit an additional unit by contracting more forcibly to increase tension slightly in the muscle. Finally, the subjects were asked to carry out the tests described above, using audio-visual feedback. Two to 4 pairs of single motor units were studied extensively in each of 11 experiments which lasted approximately 2 hours. In addition, several hundred single motor units were examined for shorter periods of time.

RESULTS

All 9 subjects were able, without difficulty, to isolate single motor units and to control the rate at which they were active. With minimal tension in the muscle, a single motor unit was recruited. The initial frequency of discharge of this unit was usually 3—5 per second and increased to 10—15 per second as the tension in the muscle increased. When the subject was asked to relax, the frequency gradually decreased as the tension was reduced; finally, no activity was seen after the muscle was completely relaxed.

At times, voluntary increases in muscle contraction resulted (in addition to an increase in the frequency of discharge of the first single motor unit) in recruitment of a second motor unit (Fig. 1) which followed the same pattern

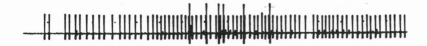

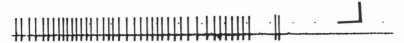

Fig. 1. A continuous recording of activity from single motor units in the human extensor indicis proprius muscle. Note the normal pattern of recruitment in which an increase in discharge frequency in the initial unit is soon joined by the appearance of a second, larger unit. The latter discharges at a lower frequency and ceases activity as the discharge frequency of the first slows. There is no change in configuration of the first motor unit potential during the recording. Calibrations are 1 sec and 500 μV.

as the first. The amplitude of the second recruited unit was usually greater than the first, and its initial discharge frequency of 1—2 per second increased to 10—15 per second as the tension in the muscle was increased further. When the subject was asked to reduce tension in the muscle, the second recruited unit was the first to disappear or 'drop out' followed by progressive decrease in the frequency of the first motor unit the activity of which finally ceased when the muscle was at complete rest. This pattern of recruitment for the pair of motor units could be easily reproduced in all subjects tested in the present study without any special training.

In 6 of the 9 subjects, no changes in the order of recruitment were observed despite 2 hours training with audio-visual feedback. In each experiment, recordings were made from several sites within the extensor indicis proprius muscle, and the subject was encouraged to explore various maneuvers that might lead to alterations in recruitment. At each new site, a minimum of 20—30 minutes was spent in attempting to alter the normal order. In not a single instance out of hundreds of attempts was one of these 6 subjects able to recruit 2 units in their normal order and then turn off unit no. 1 without silencing unit no. 2. It should be emphasized that even under 'isotonic' conditions the most minimal movements of the index finger, scarcely visible to the observers, were associated with activity in both units. The 'critical firing levels' (Henneman et al., 1974) of these pairs of motoneurones probably differed only slightly, and yet no reversals in recruitment order were noted.

The results at most recording sites in the remaining 3 subjects were similar to those just described. In each of these subjects, however, there was one site at which some variability in recruitment order was observed. Although one unit was recruited first and dropped out last in the great majority of tests, the unit which usually was recruited second occasionally was the first to respond and could then be activated repetitively for long periods without any activity in the 'first' unit. These infrequent changes in the recruitment order were accomplished only with great difficulty. Even these 3 subjects could not, on demand, immediately activate either motor unit at will or alternate their activity in a quick, facile fashion. Once the subjects did manage to change the recruitment order, the new pattern appeared to be fixed for some time so that it was difficult for them to change it back to the original pattern on command. When asked how they had succeeded in changing the order of recruitment, none of the subjects could explain how they had achieved it. Attempts to change the recruitment order required a high degree of concentration using audio-visual feedback and all subjects, whether or not they succeeded in changing the recruitment pattern, felt exhausted at the end of the 2-hour period.

DISCUSSION

These results differ radically from Basmajian's report that subjects can easily be trained to 'recall into activity different single motor units by an effort of will while inhibiting the activity of neighbors' (Basmajian, 1963). In the great majority of our trials, there appeared to be a fixed order of recruitment that could not be altered by the subject, at least within the 20—60 minute training period utilized in these studies. None of our subjects were ever able easily to suppress their first trained motor unit and recruit another one. However, our studies obviously agree with numerous previous reports that human subjects can easily be trained to isolate single motor units and control their frequency of activity by following the instructions to 'change the force of contraction' within the muscle. The difference between our findings and Basmajian's reports are not to be explained by differences in recording techniques since we used the same intramuscular fine wire electrodes. For the reasons outlined above, we studied the extensor indicis proprius muscle in detail, but in a series of preliminary experiments, we employed several different recording techniques and recorded from other muscles (in the hand, forearm, and leg). The results were the same as in the more formal study.

In all these situations, it was not difficult to control the frequency of firing of single motor units using audio-visual feedback, but it was very difficult in 3 subjects, and impossible in 6, to change the pattern of recruitment order even of the pairs of motor units whose tension thresholds for activation were close. The very infrequent change of recruitment order appeared at times to be an almost random phenomenon. Once the order did change, the subject was able to maintain the new order for some time. However, there was never evidence of what is ordinarily termed voluntary or conscious control over the change of recruitment order because none of the subjects could, on demand, immediately activate either one of the 2 units in the pair at will. Moreover, when the same subject was asked to repeat the change of recruitment order later in the same experiment performed on a different day, he was unable to do so. Although there is evidence of very infrequent switching in the order of recruitment between motor units whose tension thresholds for firing are close, our studies clearly demonstrate that, on the whole, the pattern of recruitment order in human subjects is relatively fixed, at least for slowly progressive ('ramp' or 'tonic') contractions at low levels of tension. We are, therefore, completely unable to demonstrate the degree of voluntary control of threshold and rate of single motor unit activity reported by Basmajian.

Studies performed by Henneman and colleagues (1965a,b, 1974) have shown that, in the cat spinal cord, it is the size of a motoneurone that determines its threshold and relative excitability. Smaller units are discharged by lower intensity stimulation, regardless of whether (1) the excitatory stimuli arise ipsi-laterally or contra-laterally, (2) physiologic stimuli or electric 'driving' is employed, (3) responses are elicited monosynaptically or polysynaptically, or (4) flexor or extensor motoneurones are studied. It must be conceded that voluntary contraction has not been studied in the cat. In our studies, smaller amplitude units were recruited at a lower voluntary tension threshold than larger amplitude units in most of the pairs of single motor units, but there were a few exceptions. Since we were studying only a restricted area of the muscle, the methods used in the present study are not ideally suited for the demonstration of the 'size-principle'. However, careful studies in human subjects by Stein and his colleagues (Milner-Brown et al., 1973) have confirmed that during voluntary isometric contraction of the first dorsal interosseus muscle, the order of recruitment was constant and single motor units generating lower tension (presumably smaller units) are recruited at a lower threshold than those which generate a higher tension (i.e., larger ones). Although further studies are needed to test these findings (including ours) more extensively, it may be concluded tentatively that, in the situations outlined above, the order of recruitment for motor units is fixed and invariant except rarely when the motoneurones supplying them differ only minimally in size and tension threshold for activation. The variability observed in such cases is not under voluntary control and would appear to have little functional significance in the control of total muscle tension.

In view of these observations, it is difficult to explain Basmajian's findings. It is possible that the muscles selected for his studies are such that they have more than one action so that by producing slight movements in different directions, his subjects are able to recruit different units. This might explain our inability to reproduce his results since we confined our experiments to a muscle in which the action is restricted to movement in one plane at one joint. Further experiments are needed to show to what extent human beings can be trained to isolate and control single motor unit activity by repeated or prolonged effort. By the same token, further reports in which voluntary activation of different motor units is described should be accompanied by appropriate illustrations. These would enable one to ascertain, by the configuration of the single motor unit, that activity had indeed been 'rotated' from the first unit to a second and then back to the first. Otherwise, changes in appearance of single motor units could merely reflect movements of recording electrodes in reference to the muscle fibers.

REFERENCES

BASMAJIAN, J.V. (1963) Control and training of individual motor units. Science, 141, 440—441.
BASMAJIAN, J.V. (1967) Control of individual motor units. Am. J. Phys. Med., 46, 480—485.
BASMAJIAN, J.V. (1972) Electromyography comes of age. Science, 176, 603—610.
CLOUGH, J.F.M., KERNELL, D. and PHILLIPS, C.G. (1968) The distribution of monosynaptic excitation from the pyramidal tract and from primary spindle afferents to motoneurones of the baboon's hand and forearm. J. Physiol., 198, 145—166.
HARRISON, V.F. and MORTENSEN, O.A. (1962) Identification and voluntary control of single motor unit activity in the tibialis anterior muscle. Anat. Rec., 144, 109—116.
HENNEMAN, E., CLAMANN, H.P., GILLIES, J.D. and SKINNER, R.D. (1974) Rank order of motoneurons within a pool: law of combination. J. Neurophysiol., 37, 1338—1349.
HENNEMAN, E., SOMJEN, G. and CARPENTER, D. (1965a) Functional significance of cell size in spinal motoneurons. J. Neurophysiol., 28, 560—580.
HENNEMAN, E., SOMJEN, G. and CARPENTER, D. (1965b) Excitability and inhibitability of motoneurons of different sizes. J. Neurophysiol., 28, 599—620.
MILNER-BROWN, H.S., STEIN, R.B. and YEMMA, R. (1973) The orderly recruitment of human motor units during voluntary isometric contractions. J. Physiol., 230, 359—370.

4

Single fibre electromyography for motor unit study in man

Erik STÅLBERG

The applications of single fibre electromyography for motor unit studies are described. With this method certain motor unit parameters are measured, such as muscle fibre propagation velocity, neuromuscular transmission in single motor end plates, transmission in terminal nerve tree and the muscle fibre arrangement in the motor unit. Results obtained from normal and diseased motor units are presented.

The knowledge concerning the normal and diseased motor unit has increased considerably during recent years with the improvement of experimental techniques. The scattered anatomical arrangement of muscle fibres in the motor unit has been shown in man using electrophysiological techniques (Ekstedt, 1964; Stålberg and Ekstedt, 1973) and in animals with histochemical methods (Kugelberg and Edström, 1968; Brandstater and Lambert, 1969; Doyle and Mayer, 1969). Some principal differences between low- and high-threshold motor units have been shown in animals and man with respect to their histochemical (Warmholts and Engel, 1973) and mechanical characteristics (Edström and Kugelberg, 1968; Milner-Brown et al., 1973a; Burke et al., 1973). The correlation between activation threshold and neurone size and axon diameter has been demonstrated experimentally by Henneman et al. (1965). In man, a correlation between activation threshold and axon diameter (Freund et al., 1973) has been noted. The firing pattern and recruitment order of motor units during voluntary contraction has been studied by many authors (Tokizane and Shimazu, 1964; Grimby and Hannertz, 1968; Petajan and Philip, 1969; Stålberg and Thiele, 1973; Milner-Brown et al., 1973b,c).

Most of these methods are not easily applicable for the study of motor units in man. The most commonly used method is concentric needle electromyography after the introduction of the recording technique by Adrian and Bronk (1929). The action potential recorded with concentric needle electrodes is generated by a number of muscle fibres situated within a few mm of the electrode. Only a portion of all the muscle fibres from a single motor unit contribute to the so-called motor unit potential. The shape of this potential is determined by the particular arrangement of the muscle fibres within the motor unit and the temporal relationship of the single muscle fibre potentials. The position of the recording electrode is thus of great importance, for the characteristics of the recorded action potential can change considerably with slight changes of the electrode position.

In order to obtain more detailed information about the microphysiology of the motor unit, a single fibre electromyography (SFEMG) technique has been developed. (Ekstedt, 1964; Stålberg, 1966; Ekstedt and Stålberg, 1973).

THE SFEMG METHOD

A special electrode is constructed for recordings (Fig. 1). Inside a steel cannula 0.6 mm in diameter, 1—14 platinum wires, (25 μ in diameter) are placed and led out on the side 3 mm behind the tip. Each wire is connected to one of the pins in the plug. The amplifier has an input impedance of the order of 100 Mohm and a frequency response from 500 Hz to 10—20 kHz. The small size of the electrode considerably reduces the pick-up area so that single fibre action potentials can be recorded relatively undistorted without much interference from other muscle fibres of the same motor unit. The single muscle fibre action potential is principally biphasic with a fast posi- tive—negative deflection (100 μsec), a total duration of about 1 msec and an amplitude of 2—20 mV. The amplitude decreases from a maximal value at a short fibre—electrode distance to 10% of this at approximately 5 μ. The recording is usually performed during slight voluntary contraction. In order to maintain as constant a contraction as possible the subject is guided by the oscilloscope recording, the action potential sound and by a ratemeter.

Some SFEMG parameters will be described both in the normal muscle and in some examples of pathological conditions.

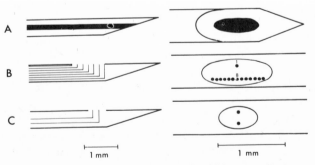

Fig. 1. Concentric needle electrode (A), recording area 580 × 150 μ and single fibre electrodes (B) and (C), recording surface 25 μ in diameter.

PROPAGATION VELOCITY IN SINGLE MUSCLE FIBRES

By means of a multi-electrode with the recording surfaces arranged in two parallel rows 200 μ apart the muscle fibre action potential can be recorded from two sites along the single fibre (e.g. 1—8 in Fig. 1B). The transmission time between the electrodes is measured and the propagation velocity in the fibre is calculated for each discharge. Normally the following is found (Stålberg, 1966):

The propagation velocity decreases during continuous activity, particularly with strong activation. After a pause, the propagation velocity is more or less normalized. This decrease in velocity might explain continuous changes in the EMG frequency spectrum (Kadefors et al., 1968). A decrease in velocity has also been reported by Lindström et al. (1970), with surface electrode measurements. Muscle fibres have different propagation velocity values ranging from 1.5 to 6 m/sec with different mean values for different muscles: m. frontalis 2.0 ± 0.4 m/sec (S.D.), m. extensor digitorum communis 3.15 ± 0.8 m/sec, m. biceps brachi 3.39 ± 0.7 m/sec. Håkansson (1956) has shown with isolated muscle fibres that the velocity is positively correlated to the muscle fibre diameter. The SFEMG method of measuring propagation velocity can therefore be used to give information about the muscle fibre diameter.

In addition to the continuous decrease in velocity there is also a variability in the propagation velocity at consecutive discharges (Stålberg, 1966). For voluntary activation it is generally found that when the preceding interval is short the propagation velocity for the next pulse is increased and when the interval is long the propagation velocity is slowed. In order to obtain the interval—velocity curve, double-pulse stimulation was performed with variable intervals between the stimuli. It was found that for intervals of between 3 and 5 msec the velocity for the second impulse is about 80% of the first impulse. At 10 msec the velocity is similar both for the conditioning and test pulse. At 20—50 msec the test pulse had a velocity of up to 120%. For longer intervals this supernormality gradually decreased and is not seen when intervals exceed one second.

This so-called velocity-recovery function (VRF) reflects an energy-requiring process during the membrane repolarisation and thus gives additional information about the muscle fibre besides that obtained from the propagation velocity.

NEUROMUSCULAR TRANSMISSION

When recording is made from 2 muscle fibres belonging to the same motor unit, the time interval between the 2 action potentials varies slightly at consecutive discharges, typically of the order of 5—50 μsec (expressed as mean of consecutive inter-potential time differences; Fig. 2). This phenome-

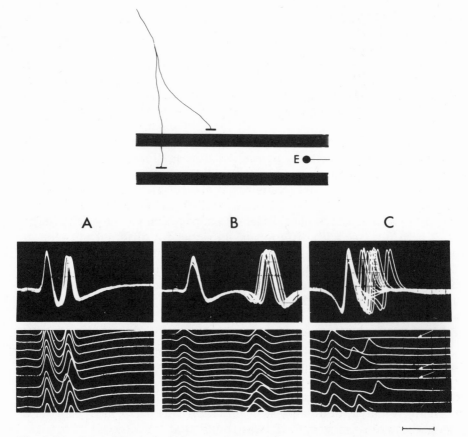

Fig. 2. The jitter. Electrode E is recording activity from 2 muscle fibres belonging to the same motor unit. (A) represents a recording from a normal muscle, (B) and (C) from a myasthenic muscle. The oscilloscope sweep is triggered by the first action potential and interval variability between the potentials is seen as a variable position of the second potential. In the upper row 10—15 action potentials are superimposed. In the lower row the oscilloscope sweep is moved downwards. In (A) normal jitter, in (B) increased jitter but no impulse blockings, in (C) increased jitter and occasional blockings (arrows). Calibration 500 μsec.

non is called the 'jitter' and is, in the normal muscle, mainly due to a variability in the transmission time in the motor end plates as a result of spontaneous fluctuation of the depolarization threshold (Stålberg et al., 1971). Also a variability of the transmission time in the muscle fibres and the nerve twigs contributes to the jitter. Increased jitter is a sign of uncertain impulse transmission in some of these structures. In this situation all impulses are still transmitted and no weakness is present. It is thus possible to detect neuromuscular disturbances before the appearance of any clinical symptoms. When there is clinical weakness partial or nearly total impulse blocking is seen and the jitter is highly increased.

The jitter increases with muscle cooling (Stålberg et al. 1971) and during ischemia (Dahlbäck et al., 1970) probably due to inhibition of acetylcholine synthesis, after non-paralytic doses of curare (Ekstedt and Stålberg, 1969) and during recovery after a succinylcholine block (Stålberg et al., 1973) due to partial receptor block and after intravenous regional injection of local anaesthetics (Ekstedt et al., 1971) due to transmission impairment in the terminal nerve branches as well as in the motor end plate.

The jitter is increased in many neuromuscular disorders, and myasthenia gravis will be described as a typical example.

MYASTHENIA GRAVIS

The diagnosis of myasthenia gravis is based on the presence of neuromuscular blocking which is detected with more or less sensitive clinical and neurophysiological methods, often combined with provocation tests. With the single fibre EMG, it is possible to reveal a disturbed neuromuscular function before any transmission block appears (Stålberg et al., 1974) i.e. before clinical symptoms are present and when conventional neurophysiological investigations are normal. It has been found that when a patient has myasthenic fatigue in any skeletal muscle it is sufficient to make recordings from the extensor digitorum communis muscle. This is even the case when the symptoms are restricted to ocular muscles. Thus, if all 20 recorded potential pairs (representing 40 motor end plates) show a normal jitter for example in the extensor digitorum communis muscle the diagnosis of myasthenia gravis is very unlikely (in our practice 'excluded' even when the suspected symptoms are restricted to other muscles). If the jitter is normal in all motor end plates studied in a muscle with weakness, myasthenia gravis can be excluded.

About 75 patients with myasthenia gravis have been studied in the extensor digitorum communis and other muscles. Some motor end plates in the same muscle are normal, others show increased jitter with or without partial neuromuscular block (Fig. 2). Even motor end plates belonging to the same motor unit may have quite different jitter. The degree of impulse blocking is well correlated to the clinical symptoms.

The degree of blocking increases during activity and is dramatically reduced after intravenous injection of Tensilon in untreated or under-treated patients. In over-treated patients a small dose of Tensilon increases the degree of blocking, and double discharges, initiated in the nerve branches, are also seen. It should be noted that increased jitter and blocking is not pathognomonic of myasthenia but is an indication of disturbed neuromuscular transmission. This can also be found in electrolyte disturbances and in conditions with reinnervation, e.g. post-traumatically, in anterior horn cell disorders and in certain polyneuropathies. Here, other SFEMG parameters will add information and the overall picture may point to a specific disorder.

ARRANGEMENT OF THE MUSCLE FIBRES WITHIN THE MOTOR UNIT

Fibre density

By counting the number of single muscle fibres from one motor unit within the recording area of the electrode (radius about 5 μ) in each of many electrode positions, a measure of the mean fibre density can be calculated (Fig. 3). The electrode is inserted at random positions in the muscle and the action potential from the first recorded muscle fibre is made maximal by small corrections of the electrode position. The number of synchronous spike components with amplitude exceeding 200 μV (when using a low frequency limit of 500 Hz) and having a spiky and constant shape are counted.

In the normal extensor digitorum communis muscle for example, one fibre from an individual motor unit is recorded in 60% of 20 random inser-

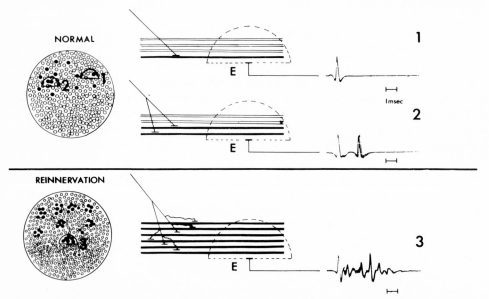

Fig. 3. Single fibre EMG recordings in normal and reinnervated muscle. The diagram illustrates the number of muscle fibres of one motor unit (blackened). The uptake area of the recording electrode is represented as the half circle and E. In the normal (1) and (2) only action potentials from one or two fibres are recorded. In reinnervation (3) many fibre action potentials are recorded due to increased fibre density in the motor unit (right part of figure). (Hakelius and Stålberg, 1974.)

tions, two fibres in about 35% and three or four fibres very seldom. This value corresponds to an average of 1.45 fibres per uptake area of the electrode. The histochemical motor unit mapping in animals has shown a similar anatomical arrangement of the muscle fibres belonging to a single motor unit. The fibre density value in man is increased with age, especially after 60 in this muscle and is about 2.3 in the ninth decade (Stålberg and Thiele, 1975).

IMPULSE TRANSMISSION IN THE TERMINAL NERVE TREE

Axon reflex

Experiments have been performed where the terminal nerves have been stimulated intramuscularly. It was shown that the stimulus gives both orthodromic and antidromic impulses, the latter activating other fibres, perhaps all of them, in that particular motor unit by an axon reflex (Stålberg and Trontelj, 1970). This could also be elicited when stimulating outside the muscle, indicating some nerve branching before the nerve enters to the muscle.

Neurogenic blocking of impulses

When a recording is made from three or more muscle fibres at the same time, sometimes, especially in cases of reinnervation, two or more of the components block together, never independently (Fig. 4). These potentials also show a common and large jitter in relation to the other part of the action potential complex. The phenomenon is due to a transmission impairment (increased neurogenic jitter) and block in the distal nerve branches supplying the muscle fibres from which action potentials are now and then missing (Stålberg and Thiele, 1972). Similar to myasthenia gravis the degree of neurogenic block also increases during continuous activity and can show some improvement after Tensilon. Neurogenic block is usually not seen in myasthenia gravis. Even if multiple potential recordings are obtained in myasthenia the individual spike components show an individual jitter and the components usually block independently of each other.

Reinnervation

When reinnervation after a partial nerve lesion has begun the fibre density is increased due to collateral sprouting and often 3—10 fibres from the same motor unit are recorded with one electrode surface (Fig. 3). Increased fibre density thus indicates an increased number of muscle fibres belonging to the same motor unit within the uptake area. This is seen in ordinary EMG as polyphasic action potentials of increased amplitude. The fibre-density values

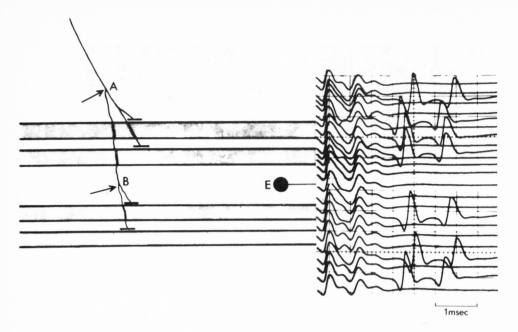

1msec

Fig. 4. Schematic drawing of a recording from 4 muscle fibres belonging to the same motor unit. In the original recording, to the right, it can be seen that potential 3 and 4 generated by the two bottom fibres in this schematic drawing, block simultaneously. The block is situated between A and B. (Stålberg and Thiele, 1972.)

usually increase before any definite signs of abnormality are found in the concentric needle EMG recording. In SFEMG the recorded action potentials are progressively more complex during reinnervation. The spike components initially show a large jitter and blocking which sometimes can be shown to take place in the terminal nerve twig. In many cases it cannot be settled whether the transmission disturbance is localized to the newly formed sprouts or to the anatomically and physiologically immature motor end plates. After 3—6 months the recorded action potential complexes are more stable, show less jitter and little or no impulse blocking (Hakelius and Stålberg, 1974). This is a sign of functional improvement and can serve as a guide when estimating the age of reinnervation potentials in different neuropathies. The increased fibre density however remains.

AMYOTROPHIC LATERAL SCLEROSIS

In amyotrophic lateral sclerosis the degeneration of the anterior horn cell with denervation of all muscle fibres in this motor unit is counteracted by a

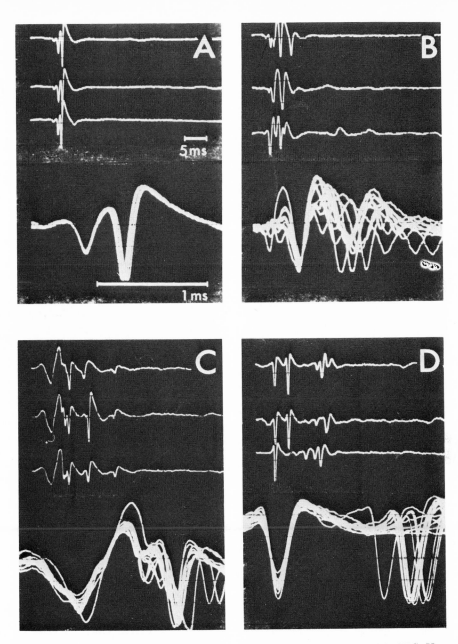

Fig. 5. Four action potentials from the EDC muscle in a patient with ALS. Upper part of each picture shows three consecutive discharges, lower half 8—10 superimpositions of the initial part of the complex with a higher sweep-speed. (A) normal jitter; (B) - (C) great instability, somewhat more complex; (D) complex action potential with single unstable spike-components. (Stålberg et al., 1975.)

regenerative process with peripheral sprouting. With SFEMG fibre-density studies, an average of about 5 spike components from muscle fibres belonging to one motor unit can be seen in a single electrode position. The jitter is considerably increased in most of the spike components and impulse blocking is often seen. It can be assumed that the spike components showing the largest jitter and degree of blocking represent muscle fibres innervated most recently, probably within a few months prior to the investigation. (Fig. 5; Stålberg et al., 1975.)

OTHER PROGRESSIVE SPINAL MUSCULAR ATROPHIES

Similar findings have been made in other progressive spinal muscular atrophies (Fig. 6). Muscles with large jitter and a high degree of blocking might be involved in a disease with faster progress than muscles where the action potential complexes are relatively stable. In the slower forms of progressive spinal muscle atrophies (Kugelberg—Welander), the fibre density is higher, perhaps due to longer survival of the reinnervated motor unit and the potential complexes often have a nearly normal jitter and much less impulse blockings. The described complex potentials can be detected early in the disease when ordinary EMG-signs of disease may be lacking. The SFEMG may give complementary information about progression and prognosis of the disease. The results are summarized in Fig. 7.

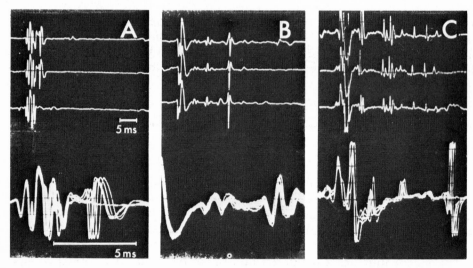

Fig. 6. Complex action potentials from (A) amyotrophic lateral sclerosis, (B) progressive muscular atrophy and (C) syringomyelia. Consecutive discharges are shown at the upper half of the picture. Lower half shows 5 superimpositions with a faster sweep speed demonstrating the initial parts of the complex. There is an increase in complexity but decreasing jitter in (B) and (C). Single components are blocking (Stålberg et al., 1975.)

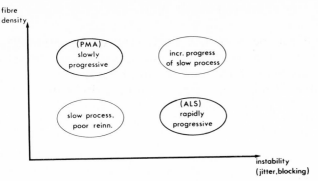

Fig. 7. Schematic illustration of the SFEMG findings in processes with collateral sprouting. Fibre density (morphology) indicates the degree of reinnervation and fibre grouping, typically increased in slow processes allowing time for maturation of the reinnervated motor unit. Instability (functional status) indicates the approximate time since reinnervation has begun of the individual spike components of the recorded action potential. There is a large instability during the first 3 months after reinnervation, a finding thus typical for a rapidly progressive disorder. Intermediate forms are also possible.

POLYNEUROPATHIES

In polyneuropathies with mainly sensory symptoms e.g. diabetes and uremia, the jitter and fibre density is only slightly increased whereas signs of more pronounced reinnervation is seen in alcoholic polyneuropathy with both sensory and motor symptoms. One possible explanation, supported by histological findings, is that in the former types the degenerative process is mainly restricted to the myelin sheath but in the alcoholic polyneuropathies both the myelin and the axons are destroyed (Wallerian degeneration). This axonal degeneration causes denervation followed by collateral reinnervation of the muscle fibres. (Thiele et al., 1973; Thiele and Stålberg, 1975).

GENERAL COMMENTS

With SFEMG it is possible to investigate not only the peripheral part of the motor unit, but also the activity in a single muscle fibre, which can be used to indicate the characteristics of a single ventral horn cell with respect to firing pattern, recruitment order during voluntary contraction and impulse transmission along reflex arcs involving that particular neurone.

The motor unit has a restricted number of reactions in pathological situations. Variations in muscle fibre diameter are observed both in myopathies and neuropathies, neuromuscular defects are found both in myasthenia gravis and after reinnervation and collateral sprouting is seen both in some myopathies and in neuropathies. The SFEMG can be used to characterize the functional status of certain parts of the motor unit and the total information may indicate the type and dynamic changes of pathological processes.

REFERENCES

ADRIAN, E.D. and BRONK, D.W. (1929) The discharge in motor nerve fibres. II. The frequency of discharge in reflex and voluntary contraction. J. Physiol. (Lond.), 67, 119—151.

BRANDSTATER, M.E. and LAMBERT, E.H. (1969) A histochemical study of the spatial arrangement of muscle fibres in single motor units within rat tibialis anterior muscle. Bull. Am. Assoc. Electromyogr. Electrodiagn., 82, 15—16.

BURKE, R.E., TSARIS, P., LEVINE, D.N., ZAJAC III, F.E. and ENGEL, W.K. (1973) Direct correlation of physiological and histochemical characteristics in motor units of cat triceps surae muscle. In: (J.E. Desmedt, Ed.) New Developments in Electromyography and Clinical Neurophysiology, Vol. 1, Karger, Basel, pp. 23—30.

DAHLBÄCK, L-O., EKSTEDT, J. and STÅLBERG, E. (1970) Ischemic effects on impulse transmission to muscle fibres in man. Electroencephalogr. Clin. Neurophysiol., 29, 579—591.

DOYLE, A.M. and MAYER, R.F. (1969) Studies of the motor units in the cat. Cat Bull. Sch. Med. Univ. Maryland, 54, 11—17.

EDSTRÖM, L. and KUGELBERG, E. (1968) Histochemical composition, distribution of fibres and fatiguability of single motor units. J. Neurol. Neurosurg. Psychiat., 31, 424—433.

EKSTEDT, J. (1964) Human single muscle fibre action potentials. Acta Physiol. Scand., 61, suppl. 226, 1—96.

EKSTEDT, J. and STÅLBERG, E. (1969) The effect of non-paralytic doses of D-tubocurarine of individual motor endplates in man, studied with a new electrophysiological method. Electroencephalogr. Clin. Neurophysiol., 27, 557—562.

EKSTEDT, J. and STÅLBERG, E. (1973) Single fibre electromyography for the study of the microphysiology of the human muscle. In: (J.E. Desmedt, Ed.) New Developments in Electromyography and Clinical Neurophysiology, Vol. 1, Karger, Basel, pp. 84—112.

EKSTEDT, J., STÅLBERG, E. and THORN-ALQUIST, A-M. (1971) Impulse transmission to muscle fibres during intravenous regional anaesthesia in man. Acta Anaesth. Scand., 15, 1—21.

FREUND, H.J., DIETZ, V., WITA, C.W. and KAPP, H. (1973) Discharge characteristics of single motor units in normal subjects and patients with supraspinal motor disturbances. In: (J.E. Desmedt, Ed.) New Developments in Electromyography and Clinical Neurophysiology, Vol. 3, Karger, Basel, pp. 242—250.

GRIMBY, L. and HANNERZ, J (1968) Recruitment order of motor units on voluntary contraction: changes induced by proprioceptive afferent activity. J. Neurol. Neurosurg. Psychiat., 31, 565—573.

HAKELIUS, L. and STÅLBERG, E. (1974) Electromyographical studies of free autogenous muscle transplants in man. Scand. J. Plast. Reconstr. Surg., 1—9.

HENNEMAN, E., SOMJEN, G. and CARPENTER, D.O. (1965) Functional significance of cell size in spinal motorneurones. J. Neurophysiol., 28, 560—580.

HÅKANSSON, C.H. (1956) Conduction velocity and amplitude of the action potential as related to circumference in the isolated fibre of frog muscle. Acta Physiol. Scand., 37, 14—34.

KADEFORS, R., KAISER, E. and PETERSÉN, I. (1968) Dynamic spectrum analysis of myo-potentials with special reference to muscle fatigue. Electromyography, 8, 39—74.

KUGELBERG, E. and EDSTRÖM, L. (1968) Differential histochemical effects of muscle contractions on phosphorylase and glycogen in various types of fibres: relation to fatigue. J. Neurol. Neurosurg. Psychiat., 31, 415—423.

LINDSTRÖM, L., MAGNUSSON, R. and PETERSÉN, I. (1970) Muscular fatigue and action potential conduction velocity changes studied with frequency analysis of EMG signals. Electromyography, 10, 341—356.

MILNER-BROWN, H.S., STEIN, R.B. and YEMM, R. (1973a) The contractile properties of human motor units during voluntary isometric contractions. J. Physiol., 228, 285—306.

MILNER-BROWN, H.S., STEIN, R.B. and YEMM, R. (1973b) Changes in firing rate of human motor units during linearly changing voluntary contractions. J. Physiol., 230, 371—390.

MILNER-BROWN, H.S., STEIN, R.B. and YEMM, R. (1973c) The orderly recruitment of human motor units during voluntary isometric contractions. J. Physiol., 230, 359—370.

PETAJAN, J.H. and PHILIP, B.A. (1969) Frequency control of motor unit action potentials. Electroencephalogr. Clin. Neurophysiol., 27, 66—72.

STÅLBERG, E. (1966) Propagation velocity in human muscle fibers in situ. Acta Physiol. Scand. 70, suppl. 287, 1—112.

STÅLBERG, E. and EKSTEDT, J. (1973) Single fibre EMG and microphysiology of the motor unit in normal and diseased muscle. In: (J.E. Desmedt, Ed.) New Developments in Electromyography and Clinical Neurophysiology, Vol. 1, Karger, Basel, pp. 113—129.

STÅLBERG, E. and THIELE, B (1972) Transmission block in terminal nerve twigs. A single fibre electromyographic finding in man. J. Neurol. Neurosurg. Psychiat., 35, 52—59.

STÅLBERG, E. and THIELE, B. (1973) Discharge pattern of motoneurones in humans. In: (J.E. Desmedt, Ed.) New Developments in Electromyography and Clinical Neurophysiology, Vol. 3, Karger, Basel, pp. 234—241.

STÅLBERG, E. and THIELE, B. (1975) Motor unit fibre density in the extensor digitorum communis muscle. A single fibre electromyographic study in normals at different ages. J. Neurol. Neurosurg. Psychiat., 38, in press.

STÅLBERG, E. and TRONTELJ, J. (1970) Demonstration of axon reflexes in human motor nerve fibers. J. Neurol. Neurosurg. Psychiat. 33, 571—579.

STÅLBERG, E., EKSTEDT, J. and BROMAN, A. (1971) The electromyographic jitter in normal human muscles. Electroenceph. Clin. Neurophysiol. 31, 429—438.

STÅLBERG, E., EKSTEDT, J. and BROMAN, A. (1974) Neuromuscular transmission in myasthenia gravis studied with single fibre electromyography. J. Neurol. Neurosurg. Psychiat., 37, 540—547.

STÅLBERG, E., SCHWARTZ, M.S. and TRONTELJ, J.V. (1975) Single fibre electromyography in various processes affecting the anterior horn cell. J. Neurol. Sci., 24, 403—415.

STÅLBERG, E., THIELE, B. and HILTON-BROWN, P. (1973) Effect of succinylcholine on single motor end plates in man. Acta Anaesth. Scand. 17, 108—118.

THIELE, B., STÅLBERG, E. and KARBE, S. (1973) Single fibre EMG findings in polyneuropathy. 8th Internat. Congr. Electroencephalogr. Clin. Neurophysiol., Marseille.

THIELE, B. and STÅLBERG, E. (1975) Single fibre EMG findings in polyneuropathy of different etiology. J. Neurol. Neurosurg. Psychiatr., 38, in press.

TOKIZANE, T. and SHIMAZU, H. (1964) Functional Differentiation of Human Skeletal Muscle. Univ. Tokyo Press, pp. 1—62.

WARMOLTS, J.R. and ENGEL, W.K. (1973) Correlation of motor unit behaviour with histochemical myofiber type in humans by open-biopsy electromyography. In: (J.E. Desmedt, Ed.) New Developments in Electromyography and Clinical Neurophysiology, Vol. 1, Karger, Basel, pp. 35—40.

Afferents, muscle spindles and central excitation

1. Influence of a voluntary innervation on human muscle spindle sensitivity
   by D. Burg, A.J. Szumski, A. Struppler and F. Velho   95

2. Pharmacological blocking of the human fusimotor system
   by J. Mai and E. Pedersen   111

3. Monosynaptic excitation of thoracic motoneurones from both primary and secondary spindle afferents in the anaesthetised cat
   by P.A. Kirkwood and T.A. Sears   117

4. Recurrent inhibition of gamma motoneurones
   by P.H. Ellaway   119

5. Afferent inflow from the human bladder in relation to filling and voiding
   by E. Pedersen and J. Mai   127

Influence of a voluntary innervation on human muscle spindle sensitivity

Doris BURG, Alfred J. SZUMSKI*, Albrecht STRUPPLER
and Francisco VELHO

The influence of a voluntary motor act on muscle spindle sensitivity in the contracting muscle and in remote and relaxed muscles was investigated. Vallbo's finding (1970, 1971), that the majority of muscle spindles are co-activated during an isometric voluntary muscle contraction was confirmed. It was found that the spindle receptor discharge pattern during an isometric voluntary muscle contraction depends on the specific receptor sensitivity, as determined by the receptor response during the relaxation phase of an electrically induced twitch contraction. Muscle spindle receptors with a low dynamic sensitivity were minimally or not affected by the initial muscle shortening during the onset of the contraction and during the muscle lengthening at the end of the contraction, whereas receptors with a high dynamic sensitivity slowed down firing immediately at the beginning of the contraction and responded in a burst-like manner during muscle relaxation at the end of the contraction. When small-amplitude sinusoidal muscle stretches were used as an indicator of receptor sensitivity, static gamma efferents seemed to play a major role in muscle spindle co-activation during the contraction. Present results show that a voluntary motor act also affects muscle spindles in remote and relaxed muscles. For some receptors located in muscles which were not involved in a movement, an increase of the discharge frequency, and a decrease of the receptor threshold to mechanical stimuli could be shown. By specific tests it could be established that a dynamic fusimotor drive contributes to the spindle receptor facilitation in remote muscles.

INTRODUCTION

A voluntary motor act not only affects muscle spindles in the contracting muscle during muscle shortening, but it also affects spindles in remote, non-involved muscles when the movement causes an imbalance of the body or when an unexpected disturbance occurs during the course of the movement.

---

* Alexander von Humboldt Fellow (Germany), on educational leave from the Medical College of Virginia, Virginia Commonwealth University, Richmond, Virginia, U.S.A.

Thus, the performance of a movement is expected to activate not only an increase of the fusimotor drive to muscles involved in order to compensate for the unloading of spindles, it also is expected to activate an appropriate mechanism to enhance the responsiveness of that portion of the musculature which is not voluntarily involved in the movement.

In recent studies in human subjects, Vallbo (1970b, 1971, 1974) could ascertain the suggestion that a voluntary muscle contraction involves both the skeleto- and the fusimotor system, with extrafusal muscle activity apparently preceding the spindle facilitation, and the afferent spindle discharge frequency during the extrafusal muscle contraction being increased above the original firing level. The assistance of skeletomotor activity by the muscle spindle feedback loop during a voluntary muscle contraction is therefore obvious, and the importance of this mechanism is evident in that at least 80% of all muscle spindles recorded to date co-activated during an isometric muscle contraction (Vallbo, 1970b; Burg et al., 1975).

Animal experiments suggest that it is impossible for the dynamic fusimotor drive to overcome an extrafusal muscle shortening and activate muscle spindles above their original discharge level, in spite of a muscle contraction (Lennerstrand and Thoden, 1968). On the basis of these results, it is expected that the muscle spindle discharge pattern during a voluntary muscle contraction, especially during the initial shortening phase, is dependent on the specific muscle spindle sensitivity with spindle co-activation during the muscle contraction resulting from a static gamma drive (Granit, 1970).

The present study was undertaken to test the above suggestion using the muscle spindle response during the twitch contraction (Appelberg and Molander, 1967) and during small-amplitude sinusoidal stretches (Crowe and Matthews, 1964) as an indicator of muscle spindle sensitivity.

The second part of this study investigated the facilitatory influence of a voluntary motor act, not only on muscle spindles in muscles involved in the actual movement but also on muscle spindles in remote, relaxed muscles. Various tests were applied during the widespread fusimotor drive to further identify the specific efferent drive to these remote muscles.

METHODS

Forty-five successful experiments on awake and alert volunteer human subjects are included in the present study. In each experiment only single-unit muscle spindle afferent activity was identified and tested. The single-unit recording technique applied was essentially the same as originally described by Hagbarth and Vallbo (1968) and by Vallbo (1970a, 1972). The impedance of the tungsten electrodes used for the percutaneous recording of single-unit potentials was about 150 kOhms as measured at 1 kHz. A silver plate was used as a reference electrode.

During the experiment subjects rested in a supine position with the arm abducted to about 70°. A firm support of forearm, hand and fingers avoided passive stretch of the corresponding muscles during the experimental procedure. Muscle spindle afferent activity was recorded exclusively from fibers in the median nerve coming from receptors located in the forearm flexor muscles. Further details on subject positioning and precautions are described elsewhere (Burg et al., 1973).

Muscle activity was recorded from forearm muscles and from the remote quadriceps muscle with surface or needle electrodes. The needle electrodes were insulated except for 3 mm of their tip.

Twitch contractions of the muscle of receptor origin were induced electrically through a needle electrode, and were approximately maximal in all experiments. Following the electrical stimulation to produce the twitch, the electrode was used for EMG recording during a voluntary contraction of the corresponding muscle.

In order to localize the muscle receptor site and to identify its threshold for mechanical stimuli, local pressure was applied through an electromagnetic pressure generator having a probe tip diameter of 1.5 mm. The pressure exerted by the tip and the deformation of the tissue was constantly monitored and stored on the tape as analogue signals synchronously with the nerve and muscle activity. The muscle of receptor origin in all experiments was identified by two main tests: (1) by the receptor response to muscle and tendon tapping and (2) by the receptor response to ramp stretches of different slopes and heights as compared to the receptor response following ramp stretches of neighbouring muscles or muscle portions when a finger flexor muscle was concerned. For receptor identification, the same tests and additionally an electrically or reflexly induced twitch contraction was used. Receptor dynamic sensitivity was determined from the receptor afferent response to the discrete muscle lengthening during the relaxation phase of the twitch contraction.

RESULTS

Muscle spindle activity during muscle contraction of receptor origin

In the present study muscle spindle sensitivity was estimated by the response of the receptor to an approximately maximal twitch contraction. Spindles were suggested to have a low dynamic sensitivity when they revealed a poor phasic response with only one or two spikes firing late in the relaxation phase or when they — as in some cases — paused during the twitch and started firing again after muscle relaxation without any dynamic response during the muscle lengthening in the relaxation phase. Receptors were neglected when the estimation concerning their dynamic sensitivity as derived from the twitch relaxation response was obviously not in agreement with the dynamic receptor response during a ramp stretch. In these cases it was suggested that possibly an unfavorable position of the receptor, eccentric to the contracting part of the muscle, did not allow for a reliable determination of receptor sensitivity.

When the EMG activity of the muscle of receptor origin was displayed with high gain, in all experiments included in this study the facilitation of muscle spindle discharge was found to lag behind the extrafusal muscle activity. In particular, the behavior of muscle spindle activity during the onset and at the end of an isometric voluntary muscle contraction, when a muscle shortening and lengthening occured, was taken into consideration. It was observed that, as expected, muscle spindles with a low dynamic sensitivity were not or only minimally affected by the initial muscle shortening at the beginning of an isometric contraction and that they were also unaffected by the muscle lengthening during relaxation. During the maintained contraction usually a marked increase of the receptor discharge frequency was observed. A receptor with a low dynamic sensitivity and an irregular spontaneous activity is illustrated in Fig. 1. As can be seen in Fig. 1(B) during the

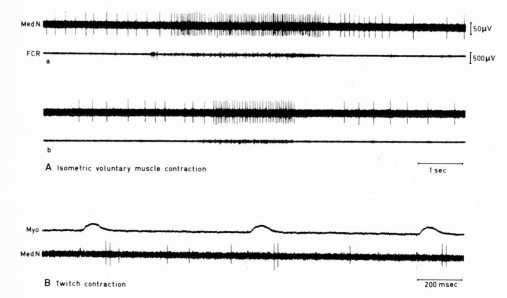

Muscle spindle afferent response

Fig. 1. Muscle spindle afferent response (A) during isometric voluntary muscle contractions (a and b are continous records) and (B) during electrically induced twitch contractions of the flexor carpi radialis muscle (FCR). Upper trace of (A)a and b and lower trace of (B): single unit action potentials recorded from median nerve (Med. N). Lower trace of (A)a and b: FCR EMG. Upper trace of (B): FCR myogram with upward deflection indicating contraction, downward relaxation.

electrically induced twitch contraction this receptor reveals a poor phasic response with two spikes late in the relaxation phase. In Fig. 1(A) the receptor response during two isometric muscle contractions of the muscle of receptor origin is shown in a continuous record. No obvious decrease of receptor activity can be seen at the onset of the contraction and no relaxation burst activity can be seen during relaxation. Following the onset of the extrafusal muscle activity the receptor discharge level was markedly increased above the original firing frequency. This discharge level lasted as long as the contraction was maintained. This type of receptor response was most frequently observed in all experiments.

Following the voluntary muscle contraction the receptor activity was usually decreased below the original firing frequency, as shown in Fig. 1(A)b. The receptor shown in Fig. 1 was classified as a muscle spindle primary since the dynamic response following a twitch contraction, as shown with the subject at rest in Fig. 1(A), was obviously increased when a reinforcement maneuver such as a remote muscle contraction was performed. This test will be shown for the receptor of Fig. 1 in the second part of this study (Fig. 8). The observation that for this receptor a dynamic gamma drive was effective during this test, implies the identity of the receptor as a muscle spindle primary.

Fig. 2 shows another receptor which is co-activated during an isometric voluntary muscle contraction without any slowing during the initial shortening of the muscle at the onset of the contraction and without any bursting activity following muscle relaxation. (A) and (B) are from a continuous record showing the receptor and muscle activity during and between two subsequent contractions. In this record the spindle activity during a test phasic reflex contraction shows an activation of the receptor due to the reflex hammer tap initiating the reflex and a slowing of the receptor during the contraction. No dynamic response occurs during muscle relaxation. For this receptor only a minimal dynamic response was seen during ramp stretches. The receptor was regularly firing at rest and only slowly decreased firing during passive muscle shortening. No increase of firing activity was observed when a reinforcement maneuver was performed during a phasic reflex or during a voluntary muscle contraction. Thus, this receptor was classified as a muscle spindle with a markedly low dynamic sensitivity, possibly a muscle spindle secondary. This receptor which is very strongly facilitated during an isometric voluntary muscle contraction and is not at all influenced by the extrafusal muscle shortening and lengthening at the beginning and at the end of the contraction, seems to be predominantly under a static gamma drive which is further enhanced during voluntary muscle contraction.

During an isometric voluntary muscle contraction the discharge pattern of muscle spindles with a high dynamic sensitivity was found to be different from the pattern shown in Figs 1 and 2. Dynamically sensitive receptors

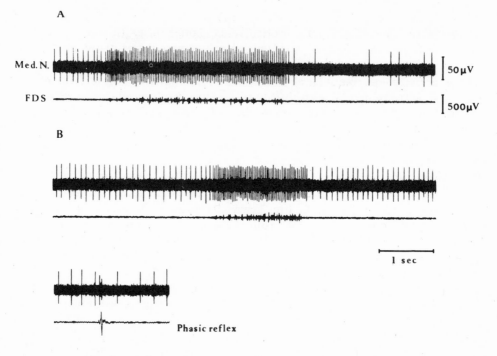

Muscle spindle response during isometric voluntary contraction

Fig. 2. Muscle spindle afferent response during isometric voluntary muscle contraction (A) and (B) and during phasic reflex (lower portion of the figure, upper traces: single-unit action potentials recorded from median nerve. Lower traces: flexor digitorum superficialis (FDS) EMG.

fired spontaneously at rest and decreased firing at the onset of a contraction. During the maintained muscle contraction an increase of the discharge frequency above the original firing level is usually observed in these receptors also. However, the receptor co-activation has usually been found to be more marked in receptors with a lower dynamic sensitivity. During muscle relaxation following the contraction a burst-like response of the receptor was recorded. Fig. 3 demonstrates a typical record of a spindle primary with a high dynamic sensitivity. This receptor responds in a burst-like manner during the relaxation phase of an electrically induced twitch contraction (lower portion of the figure) and during an isometric voluntary muscle contraction (upper portion of the figure). The receptor pauses during the contraction phase of the voluntary isometric contraction and during the electrically induced twitch. During the maintained muscle contraction the discharge frequency of the receptor was slightly increased in comparison to the spontaneous firing frequency.

In order to test the specific spindle drive compensating for the reduced

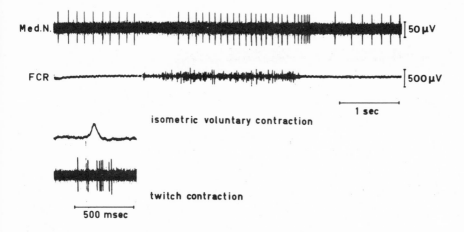

Muscle spindle response

Fig. 3. Muscle spindle afferent response during isometric voluntary muscle contraction (upper portion) and during an electrically induced twitch contraction (lower portion). First trace of the upper and second trace of the lower record: single-unit action potentials recorded from median nerve. Second trace of the upper record: FCR EMG. First trace of the lower record: FCR myogram with upward deflection indicating contraction, downward relaxation.

muscle length and facilitating the spindle frequency during the maintained muscle contraction, sinusoidal stretches of about 3Hz and a displacement of the wrist joint of about 3 degrees when the flexor carpi radialis muscle was concerned, was applied with the subject at rest and superimposed on a slight maintained voluntary contraction of the corresponding muscle. Fig. 4 shows the afferent response of a muscle spindle primary during passive sinusoidal stretches at different amplitudes. The receptor which was firing spontaneously with a frequency of about 5 imp/sec when the subject was at rest, ceased firing completely during a minimal passive muscle shortening and was activated during muscle lengthening. For this receptor a high dynamic sensitivity was established by electrically induced twitch contractions.

Fig. 5 is a record of the same receptor as shown in Fig. 3. Small-amplitude, passive, sinusoidal muscle stretches are applied with the subject at rest in (A) and are superimposed on a slight isometric voluntary contraction of the muscle of receptor origin (flexor carpi radialis muscle) in (B). With the subject at rest the response to sinusoidal muscle stretches reveals a high sensitivity for the change in muscle length with a burst activity reaching an average maximal frequency of 33 imp/sec during the stretching phase and a complete silence during the shortening phases. When the sinusoidal stretch was superimposed on a maintained voluntary contraction of the muscle of

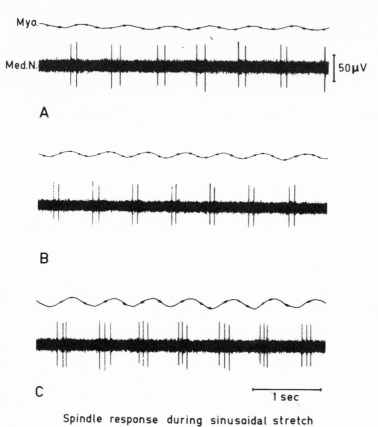

Spindle response during sinusoidal stretch

Fig. 4. Muscle spindle afferent response during passive sinusoidal muscle stretch. Upper traces: myogram of the muscle of receptor origin (FCR) with upward deflection indicating muscle stretch, downward muscle shortening. Lower traces: single-unit action potentials recorded from median nerve.

receptor origin the overall activity of the receptor was increased, although the sensitivity for the change of muscle length was not increased. The passive shortening of the muscle affects the receptor less than at rest and the average maximal frequency reached during the stretching phases was 30 imp/sec and thus slightly lower than at rest. The test illustrated in Fig. 5 was performed in 3 experiments and corresponding results were obtained in all tests.

Muscle spindle activity in relaxed muscles during remote voluntary muscle contraction

Since the description of the Jendrassik handgrip in 1883, it has been suggested that the organisation of a voluntary motor act involves a mechanism increasing the responsiveness of that part of the motor system which

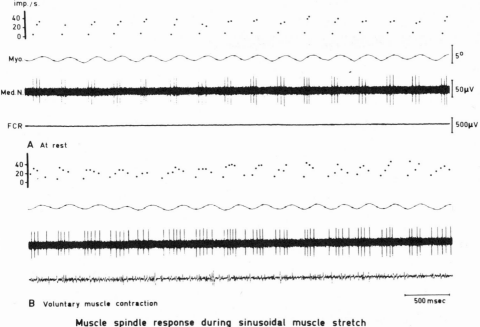

Muscle spindle response during sinusoidal muscle stretch

Fig. 5. Muscle spindle afferent response during passive sinusoidal muscle stretch. Upper traces: instantaneous impulse frequency. Second traces: myogram of the muscle of receptor origin (FCR). Third traces: single-unit action potentials recorded from median nerve. Fourth traces: FCR EMG.

does not participate in the willed movement. The involvement of the muscle spindle system in such a protective mechanism is still under discussion, since the conclusions drawn from indirect approaches, mainly using the comparison between H- and T-reflex excitability, are conflicting (Sommer, 1940; Landau and Clare, 1964). Thus, it seemed to be of interest to record single muscle spindle afferent activity directly during such reinforcement tests.

In the present study it was repeatedly found that muscle spindle afferents — especially those which were spontaneously active — increased their discharge frequency during a remote and restricted voluntary muscle contraction. Fig. 6 shows the afferent activity of a muscle spindle primary in the median nerve and the increase of its discharge frequency during a slight contraction of the remote quadriceps muscle. For this type of facilitation a short latency with a nearly synchronous onset of the remote extrafusal muscle activity and a pronounced after-effect is noteworthy. As can be seen on the lowest trace of Fig. 6, the muscle of receptor origin was silent during the remote quadriceps contraction (second trace). Monitoring the EMG activity of the muscle of receptor origin, the possibility of a concomitant

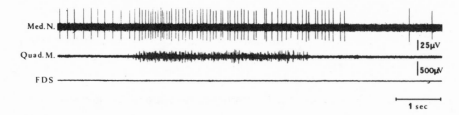

Muscle spindle response during remote voluntary contraction

Fig. 6. Muscle spindle response during remote voluntary muscle contraction. Upper trace: single-unit action potentials recorded from median nerve. Second trace: quadriceps muscle EMG. Third trace: FDS EMG.

extrafusal muscle activity of the forearm muscle was minimized. The degree of spindle facilitation was dependent on the strength of the remote muscular effort and on the number of muscles involved. A decrease of muscle spindle activity in a relaxed muscle during a remote muscle contraction was never observed, no matter whether an ipsi- or contra-lateral muscle, an agonist or an antagonist was contracted, or whether the receptor had a high dynamic or a high static sensitivity. It must, however, be stressed that not all muscle spindles identified have been found to increase their discharge frequency during the remote muscle contraction and that muscle spindles which were silent with the subject at rest only rarely discharged during the remote contraction. In these receptors the observation of the receptor discharge alone is not sufficient to determine whether the receptor is facilitated by a central drive or not, since the fusimotor drive might be insufficient for activation of the receptor. Thus, in a series of experiments, the threshold of spindle receptors to mechanical stimuli causing a well-defined deformation of the tissue overlying the receptor was determined and stimuli were applied which were just below threshold to fire the receptor.

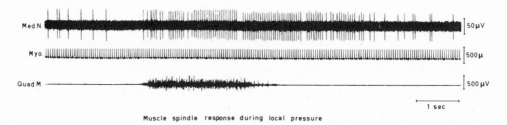

Muscle spindle response during local pressure

Fig. 7. Muscle spindle afferent response during local pressure. Upper trace: single-unit action potentials recorded from median nerve. Second trace: analogue signals of muscle deformation. Third trace: quadriceps muscle EMG.

Fig. 7 shows such an experiment. The upper trace is a record of the activity of a muscle spindle afferent nerve fiber. The middle trace gives the analogue signal of a mechanical stimulus causing a deformation of the tissue overlying the muscle at a frequency of 20 Hz. The third trace shows the EMG of the quadriceps muscle. The mechanical stimulus was applied to the tissue overlying the receptor at a distance of about 10 mm and did not, or rarely, activate the receptor. During the remote quadriceps muscle contraction, however, the receptor threshold was obviously lowered and the receptor followed the mechanical stimulus of 20 Hz. A pronounced after-effect was observed showing that the receptor threshold only slowly and with fluctuations returned to the original level. (It should be noted that the part of the experiment illustrated in Fig. 7 was preceded by a previous remote contraction and the activity which can be seen at the beginning of the trace is part of the after-effect of the preceding reinforcement).

In order to test the specific muscle spindle drive to muscles which are not involved in the performance of a voluntary motor act, the relaxation activity of the receptor during an electrically induced twitch contraction of the muscle of receptor origin was used as a highly reproducible indicator of the receptor dynamic sensitivity. Fig. 8 shows such a record of the receptor which was illustrated in Fig. 1 during a voluntary contraction of the flexor carpi radialis muscle. A slight contraction of the quadriceps muscle, as shown in the lowest trace of B was used as a reinforcement maneuver. The record shows a slight increase of the spontaneous activity and an increased

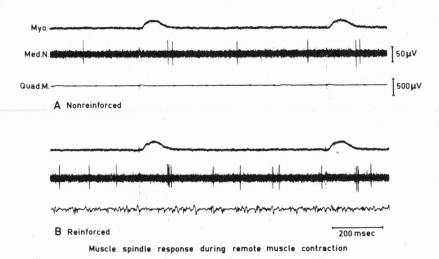

Muscle spindle response during remote muscle contraction

Fig. 8. Muscle spindle afferent response during electrically induced twitch contraction of the muscle of receptor origin. Upper traces: myogram of the muscle of receptor origin (FCR). Second traces: single-unit action potentials recorded from median nerve. Third traces: quadriceps muscle EMG.

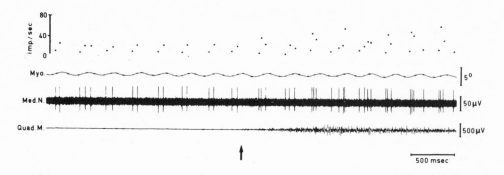

Muscle spindle response during passive sinusoidal muscle stretch

Fig. 9. Muscle spindle afferent response during passive sinusoidal muscle stretch. Upper line: instantaneous impulse frequency. Second line: myogram of the muscle of receptor origin. Third line: single-unit action potentials recorded from median nerve. Fourth line: quadriceps muscle EMG.

dynamic receptor response during twitch relaxation as a result of the reinforcement test. This finding suggests a dynamic fusimotor drive involved in this mechanism.

Identical results were obtained when small-amplitude sinusoidal stretches were used to test the receptor sensitivity during a reinforcement maneuver such as a remote quadriceps muscle contraction. Such an experiment is illustrated in Fig. 9. A muscle spindle with a low and irregular spontaneous activity responded to a small-amplitude sinusoidal muscle stretch with an average maximal discharge frequency of 17 imp/sec during the stretch. During the shortening phases the receptor was silenced. When the passive sinusoidal stretches of the muscle of receptor origin were performed during a slight remote contraction of the quadriceps muscle the receptor response to the sinusoidal stretches was enhanced with an average maximal discharge frequency of 45 imp/sec during the stretching phases, indicating an increased dynamic receptor sensitivity during the remote contraction. However, it also has to be noted that, under these condition, a few spikes were also observed during the shortening phases. Thus, an additional static gamma drive could be involved.

DISCUSSION

The purpose of the present study was to investigate the influence of a voluntary motor act on the fusimotor drive to contracting and to relaxed muscles. The results confirm the earlier results of Hagbarth and Vallbo (1968) and of Vallbo (1970b, 1971, 1974) who showed that the overwhelming muscle spindle afferents recorded in a voluntarily contracted muscle increase their discharge frequency in spite of muscle shortening. An analysis of receptor sensitivity with the subject at rest shows in this study that muscle spindles which reveal a low dynamic sensitivity are usually effectively and with a short latency, co-activated during a voluntary muscle contraction. As expected from animal experiments (Matthews, 1964) receptors with a high dynamic sensitivity decreased firing immediately at the onset of a muscle contraction and were activated in a burst-like manner during muscle relaxation. This response of muscle spindle primaries with a high dynamic sensitivity was predicted by Granit (1970) who considered this behavior 'to be a decisive factor in the assessment and regulation of muscle length when a muscular effort needs to be carried out at constant length'. Muscle receptors with a low dynamic sensitivity were only minimally or not affected by the muscle shortening at the onset, and by the muscle lengthening at the end of the contraction. Usually, however, an increase of receptor firing frequency was observed early in the initial shortening phase of the contraction. Since it was shown by Lennerstrand and Thoden (1968) that an increase of a dynamic fusimotor drive was unable to overcome the silencing effect of muscle shortening on muscle spindle receptors, it can be assumed that the increase of the discharge frequency at the onset of the muscle contraction is due to a specific static gamma drive. It is suggested that receptors with a dominant static gamma drive are co-activated specifically by a further increase of the static fusimotor drive during an isometric voluntary muscle contraction. This interpretation is also compatible with Vallbo's finding (1974) that muscle spindle secondaries are also effectively co-activated during an isometric muscle contraction. Also in our studies a few receptors, which had been tentatively identified as spindle secondaries, were found to be markedly co-activated.

For a few muscle spindles which could be characterized as muscle spindle primaries by their dynamic sensitivity, an attempt was made to identify the specific fusimotor drive responsible for spindle co-activation during a maintained muscle contraction. For this identification small-amplitude muscle stretches were applied and the receptor response with the subject at rest was compared to the response when the same test was superimposed on a maintained slight isometric contraction of the muscle of receptor origin. However, one must be aware that this test is difficult to interpret under these circumstances, since the stiffness of the muscle is altered during the muscle contraction and all that can be said from this experimental approach is that the result obtained does not contradict the suggestion that the main spindle drive accounting for the spindle co-activation during a maintained muscle contraction occurs through the static gamma system. No indication for an increase of the dynamic gamma drive during the muscle contraction was evident using this method. More reliable results may be possible as different frequencies of sinusoidal stretches are used. Current experiments are testing this possibility.

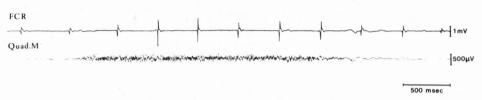

Fig. 10. Phasic reflex response during remote muscle contraction. Upper trace: FCR stretch reflex; lower trace: quadriceps muscle EMG. (From J. Neurol. Neurosurg. Psychiat. 1974, 37, 1015.)

From studies on reflex excitability (Jendrassik, 1883; Hoffman, 1934; Paillard, 1955) it is well known that a restricted voluntary motor act is usually linked to a mechanism which facilitates the reflex responsiveness of parts of the motor system which are not involved in the muscular effort (Sommer, 1940) as shown in Fig. 10. The origin of this facilitatory influence is still under discussion. Comparing H- and T-reflex excitability (Sommer, 1940; Paillard, 1953, 1955; Buller and Dornhorst, 1957) and testing the influence of muscle length on reflex excitability (Struppler and Preuss, 1959), the conclusion was drawn that muscle spindle facilitation via the fusimotor system is the most crucial factor underlying this phenomenon. However, other authors (Landau and Clare, 1964; Clare and Landau, 1964) were unable to find any evidence for an increased gamma drive during a remote muscle contraction.

Present experiments using a direct recording approach of muscle spindle afferent activity in the awake and cooperative subject, show that a voluntary motor act gives rise to a fusimotor drive to muscles which are not involved in the movement and which are electromyographically silent. The time course of this spindle facilitation is identical with the time course observed for reflex reinforcement (Burg et al., 1974) and suggests that both phenomena might be causally related to each other. In this series of experiments not all muscle spindles were facilitated during a remote muscle contraction and receptors which were not spontaneously active at rest were rarely facilitated above their firing threshold. In muscle spindle afferents with poor or no spontaneous activity the receptor threshold to mechanical stimuli was utilized as a more sensitive test to determine the facilitatory influence of a remote voluntary muscle contraction on the fusimotor drive. In these receptors it was found that the receptor threshold was decreased during the remote muscle contraction. This result further supports the suggestion that a fusimotor drive plays a role in reflex reinforcement.

Whereas the co-activation of muscle spindles in a contracting muscle is expected to be predominantly due to a static gamma drive, it is suggested that the fusimotor drive to muscles which are not involved in the movement may have a strong dynamic component, which can be recorded as an increased reflex excitability of these muscles during the remote muscular effort. In the present study, the specific dynamic gamma drive of muscle spindles in relaxed muscles was tested with the subject at rest and during a remote voluntary motor act. The receptor response during the relaxation phase of an electrically induced twitch contraction and during small-amplitude sinusoidal stretches was used for this evaluation. Both tests gave a clear indication of an increased dynamic gamma drive to muscle spindles in relaxed muscles during a remote muscle contraction. These results further support the suggestion of a relationship between the phenomenon of reflex reinforcement, as first described by Jendrassik (1883), and the recorded spindle facilitation during a voluntary motor act. This leads to the conclusion that a restricted muscular effort of a sufficient intensity is accompanied by a widespread fusimotor drive which decreases the reflex threshold of muscles which are not involved in the movement.

Finally, it must be stressed that the present results do not imply that any one of the central effects on muscle spindles is exclusively due to the influence of only one of the fusimotor systems.

ACKNOWLEDGEMENTS

The authors acknowledge the capable technical assistance of Miss Machthild Haberkamp. This work was supported by the Deutsche Forschungsgemeinschaft.

REFERENCES

APPELBERG, B. and MOLANDER, A. (1967) A rubro-olivary pathway. I. Identification of a descending system for control of dynamic sensitivity of muscle spindles. Exp. Brain Res., 3, 372—381.

BULLER, A.J. and DORNHORST, A.C. (1957) The reinforcement of tendon-reflexes. Lancet, 2, 1260—1262.

BURG, D., SZUMSKI, A.J., STRUPPLER, A. and VELHO, F. (1973) Afferent and efferent activation of human muscle receptors involved in reflex and voluntary contraction. Exp. Neurol., 41, 754—768.

BURG, D., SZUMSKI, A.J., STRUPPLER, A. and VELHO, F. (1974) Assessment of fusimotor contribution to reflex reinforcement in humans. J. Neurol. Neurosurg. Psychiat., 37, 1012—1021.

BURG, D., SZUMSKI, A.J., STRUPPLER, A. and VELHO, F. (1975) Observations on muscle receptor sensitivity in the human. Electromyogr. Clin. Neurophysiol., 15, 15—28.

CLARE, M.H. and LANDAU, W.M. (1964) Fusimotor function. V. Reflex reinforcement under fusimotor block in normal subjects. Arch. Neurol., 10, 123—127.

CROWE, A. and MATTHEWS, P.B.C. (1964) Further studies of static and dynamic fusimotor fibres. J. Physiol., 175, 132—151.

GRANIT, R. (1970) The Basis of Motor Control. Academic Press, London, p. 346.

HAGBARTH, K.-E. and VALLBO, A.B. (1968) Discharge characteristics of human muscle afferents during muscle stretch and contraction. Exp. Neurol., 22, 674—694.

HOFFMANN, P. (1934) Die physiologischen Eigenschaften der Eigenreflexe. Ergebn. Physiol. Biol. Chem. Exp. Pharm., 36, 15—108.

LANDAU, W.M. and CLARE, M.H. (1964) Fusimotor function. IV. Reinforcement of the H reflex in normal subjects. Arch. Neurol., 10, 117—122.

LENNERSTRAND, G. and THODEN, U. (1968) Muscle spindle responses to concomitant variations in length and in fusimotor activation. Acta Physiol. Scand., 74, 153—165.

MATTHEWS, P.B.C. (1964) Muscle spindles and their motor control. Physiol. Rev., 44, 219—288.

JENDRASSIK, E. (1883) Beiträge zur Lehre von den Sehnenreflexen. Dtsch. Arch. Klin. Med., 33, 117—199.

PAILLARD, J. (1953) Nouveaux aspects d'une exploration des réflexes tendineux chez l'homme. C.R. Hebd. Séances Acad. Sci., Paris, 236, 1505—1508.

PAILLARD, J. (1955) Analyse électrophysiologique et comparison, chez l'homme, du réflexe de Hoffmann et du réflexe myotatique. Pflügers Arch., 260, 448—479.

SOMMER, J. (1940) Periphere Bahnung von Muskeleigenreflexen als Wesen des Jendrassikschen Phänomens. Dtsch. Ztschr. Nervenheilk., 150, 249—262.

STRUPPLER, A. and PREUSS, R. (1959) Untersuchungen über periphere und zentrale Faktoren der Eigenreflexerregbarkeit am Menschen mit Hilfe des Jendrassikschen Handgriffes. Pflügers Arch., 268, 425—434.

VALLBO, A.B. (1970a) Slowly adapting muscle receptors in man. Acta Physiol. Scand., 78, 315—333.

VALLBO, A.B. (1970b) Discharge patterns in human muscle spindle afferents during isometric voluntary contractions. Acta Physiol. Scand., 80, 552—566.

VALLBO, A.B. (1971) Muscle spindle response at the onset of isometric voluntary contractions in man. Time difference between fusimotor and skeletomotor effects. J. Physiol., 318, 405—431.

VALLBO, A.B. (1972) Single unit recording from human peripheral nerves: muscle receptor discharge in resting muscles and during voluntary contractions. In (G.G. Somjen, Ed.) Neurophysiology Studied in Man, Excerpta Medica, Amsterdam, pp. 281—295.

VALLBO, A.B. (1974) Human muscle spindle discharge during isometric voluntary contractions. Amplitude relations between spindle frequency and torque. Acta Physiol. Scand., 90, 319—336.

Pharmacological blocking of the human fusimotor system

Jesper MAI and Ejner PEDERSEN

Quantitative measurements of the H, T and tonic stretch reflexes, vibration-induced inhibition of the H reflexes, tonic vibration reflex, clonus and voluntary power have been carried out in spastic patients during blocking of alpha- or beta-receptors by thymoxamine and propranolol, respectively. Alpha blockade did not change the H reflexes, but gave rise to a strong reduction in the T reflexes, an increase in the vibration-induced inhibition of the H reflexes, a reduction in the duration of the tonic stretch reflexes, reduction in the T reflexes, a reduction in the duration of the tonic stretch reflexes, reduction in clonus and tonic vibration reflex, while voluntary power remained unchanged. Beta blockade showed unchanged H and T reflexes, prolongation of the tonic stretch reflex, a strong reduction of clonus, no change in voluntary power. Both intra-arterial and intravenous injections were used and revealed evidence of a central action of both drugs. The results might be explained by assuming that alpha blockade inhibits the central connections of the dynamic gamma fibres, while beta blockade centrally inhibits the inflow in the II or Ib afferent fibres.

The aim of the present investigation was to see if the muscle spindles and/or their central connections are influenced by adrenergic drugs. After having had an intravenous injection of propranolol, a paraplegic patient who was severely disabled by clonus reported that his clonus had decreased so much that he was able to get his heels to the floor, which had been impossible before. As a similar effect was also found in other clonus patients, we started a research on the mode of action of anti-adrenergic drugs in the nervous system. We found it reasonable to investigate not only the beta-blocking action, but also an alpha-blocking agent, thymoxamine, which is reported to be able to depress tendon jerks in normal subjects (Phillips et al., 1973).

MATERIAL AND METHODS

So far 22 spastic patients with multiple sclerosis or traumatic paraplegia have been investigated. All were selected and co-operative, with clinically pronounced spasticity, a reasonable voluntary power and ideally a pronounced clonus. They were tested by quantitative measurements of the T reflexes (Achilles tendon), H reflexes, tonic stretch reflexes, clonus tendency, voluntary power and tonic vibration reflex. For details as to the stimulation and recording equipment, see Pedersen et al. (1974a,b).

Of these measurements, as many as possible were made before and after intravenous or intra-arterial injections of the beta-blocking drug propranolol and/or the alpha-blocking drug thymoxamine. All measurements were carried out by the same investigator under basal conditions (Desmedt et al., 1973), and the results were stored on video-tape for later analysis (Pedersen and Klemar, 1974). A total of 15 patients have been tested before and after propranolol injections and 10 patients had intravenous thymoxamine injections. Six patients had injections of both drugs on different days, and three were tested by intra-arterial injections.

RESULTS

The results are summarized in Table I. The alpha-blocking drug thymoxamine did not significantly change the H reflex, while a striking decrease in the T reflex was induced. It was often abolished altogether and always depressed to less than 50% of the control values. The effect started very rapidly after the injection, reached a maximum at 5 minutes, and usually subsided in about 10 minutes, but even so it is a central effect. This was shown by giving a patient with a clear-cut reduction in the T reflex (as shown in a previous investigation) an injection of thymoxamine into the femoral artery. A cuff placed just above the knee was then immediately inflated to a point between the systolic and diastolic pressure. No reduction in the T reflex occurred until after a lapse of 25 minutes, at which time the stasis itself will depress the reflexes as shown in control experiments. To be quite sure, next day we inflated the cuff to above the systolic pressure before an intravenous injection into the arm was given, and this time the previously observed depression of the T reflexes occurred within the normal 5 minutes. We found that the amplitude of the tonic stretch reflex was largely unchanged, while its duration decreased. The clonus was depressed in four of the five patients studied. Voluntary power was unaltered and the tonic vibration reflex, which was found to be very strong and stable in two cases, was abolished in both.

The beta-blocking drug propranolol did not significantly change the H or T reflexes or the amplitude of the tonic stretch reflex. On the other hand, the duration of the tonic stretch reflex increased and, as already mentioned, we found a striking reduction in the clonus. The effect on the clonus seems to be of central origin, as the depression did not recur after intra-arterial injections immediately followed by stasis above the knee. Voluntary power was also unchanged here.

TABLE 1

Changes induced by intravenous thymoxamine and propranolol injections.

	Thymoxamine (0.1 mg/kg, i.v.)				Propranolol (0.1–0.2 mg/kg, i.v.)			
	No. of patients	Increase	Decrease	Unchanged	No. of patients	Increase	Decrease	Unchanged
H reflex	10	1	(3)	6	10	0	0	10
T reflex	10	0	10	0	12	(4)	(2)	6
Tonic stretch reflex (amplitude)	6	1+(1)	1	3	7	1+(1)	2+(1)	2
Tonic stretch reflex (duration)	5	0	4	1	7	6	1	0
Clonus	5	0	4	1	9	0	8	1
Voluntary power	5	(1)	(1)	3	3	0	0	3
Tonic vibration reflex	2	0	2	0	0	0	0	0

DISCUSSION

Where can the actions described then take place? As far as thymoxamine is concerned, there seems to be no doubt that the action is central, as shown by our experiments with stasis and intra-arterial injections, and this is in agreement with the conclusions drawn on a pharmacological basis by Phillips et al. (1973). This drug depresses the reflexes dependent on the dynamic gamma motoneurones or their central connections.

The beta-blocking drug propranolol also showed evidence of a central action, but with regard to the site in the central nervous system at which its action takes place, there are two possibilities. The first is an action exerted on the central connections of the II afferent fibres. This theory fits very well with the action observed on the H, T and tonic stretch reflexes, especially on the duration of the tonic stretch reflex, as it has been shown that the II afferent fibres in the lower extremities inhibit the reflex responses from their agonists (Burke and Lance, 1973). This implies a static component in clonus, which we do not find contradictory.

The second possibility is that the drug exerts its action on the central projections of the Ib afferent inflow; it is not unreasonable to assume that this inflow may be interrupted in some cases of spasticity. If this is the case, it implies that the clasp-knife phenomenon and the cessation of the tonic stretch reflex are caused by Ib afferent discharge, and that a deficient inhibition of this discharge plays a role in the pathophysiology of clonus.

We have obviously also been on the look-out for a beneficial effect of oral treatment with these two drugs, but so far we have found only a limited effect. Propranolol seems capable of reducing the tendency to clonus in some patients, but not in all, and further investigations are needed to show specific indications. Thymoxamine seems to be absorbed in unsuitable form or amounts, or to be much too short-lived in the organism to be of benefit. But with the striking effect on dynamic activity in mind, we think and hope that further research will soon give us an alpha-blocking agent that fulfills the requirements for therapeutic use. Anyhow, the clear-cut physiological actions of the two drugs may make them valuable tools in the determination of the spasticity type of the individual patient and hence lead to a better therapy.

ACKNOWLEDGEMENTS

This study was supported by a grant from the Danish League against Multiple Sclerosis. Thymoxamine was supplied through the courtesy of William R. Warner and Co. Ltd., Eastleigh, England.

REFERENCES

BURKE, D. and LANCE, J.W. (1973) Studies of the reflex effects of primary and secondary spindle endings in spasticity. In (J.E. Desmedt, Ed.) New Developments in Electromyography and Clinical Neurophysiology, Vol. 3, Karger, Basel, pp. 523—537.

DESMEDT, J.E. et al. (1973) A discussion of the methodology of the triceps surae T and H-reflexes. In (J.E. Desmedt, Ed.) New Developments in Electromyography and Clinical Neurophysiology, Vol. 3, Karger, Basel, pp. 773—780.

PEDERSEN, E. and KLEMAR, B. (1974) Recording of physiological measurements based on video technique. Scand. J. Rehab. Med., suppl. 3, 45—50.

PEDERSEN, E., ARLIEN-SØBORG, P. and MAI, J. (1974a) The mode of action of the GABA derivative Baclofen in human spasticity. Acta Neurol. Scand., 50, 665—680.

PEDERSEN, E., DIETRICHSON, P., GORMSEN, J. and ARLIEN-SØBORG, P. (1974b) Measurement of phasic and tonic stretch reflexes in antispastic and antiparkinsonian therapy. Scand. J. Rehab. Med., suppl. 3, 51—60.

PHILLIPS, S.J., RICHENS, A. and SHAND, D.G. (1973) Adrenergic control of tendon jerk reflexes in man. Br. J. Pharmacol., 47, 595—605.

3

Monosynaptic excitation of thoracic motoneurones from both primary and secondary spindle afferents in the anaesthetised cat

P.A. KIRKWOOD and T.A. SEARS

We have recorded afferent impulses from intact intramuscular nerve filaments of the internal intercostal muscle of anaesthetised, paralysed cats. Using these impulses to trigger an averager, we have extracted unitary EPSPs from the intracellularly recorded synaptic noise of antidromically identified expiratory motoneurones of the same spinal segment. Using the same trigger pulses, simultaneous averaging of a surface recording from the dorsal root ganglion gave unitary spikes whose latencies allowed the conduction velocity of each of the afferents to be measured. Two independant criteria identified the connections thus revealed as being monosynaptic: (1) the fast rise time of the EPSPs and (2) the short latencies between the ganglion spikes and the onsets of the EPSPs. The conduction velocities of the afferents giving monosynaptic excitation ranged between 90 and 24 m sec^{-1}. They included fast-conducting units which showed a large dynamic response and slowly conducting units with a relatively small dynamic response to stretch of the intercostal space. We conclude that monosynaptic excitation of these motoneurones derives from both primary and secondary muscle spindle endings.

At the time of going to press these results are still preliminary, although the experiments have now been extended to the triceps surae muscles with the same result, namely monosynaptic excitation of homonymous motoneurones from clearly identified secondary endings of muscle spindles. The references below are further short reports of this work.

REFERENCES

KIRKWOOD, P.A. and SEARS, T.A. (1974) Monosynaptic excitation of motoneurones from secondary endings of muscle spindles. Nature, 252, 243—244.
KIRKWOOD, P.A. and SEARS, T.A. (1975) Monosynaptic excitation of motoneurones

from muscle spindle secondary endings of intercostal and triceps surae muscles in the cat. J. Physiol, 245, 64—66P.

KIRKWOOD, P.A. and SEARS, T.A. (1975) Spike-triggered averaging for the measurement of single-unit conduction velocities. J. Physiol., 245, 58—59P.

4

Recurrent inhibition of gamma motoneurones

P.H. ELLAWAY

In 1945 Leksell firmly established what had been anticipated from Matthews' (1933) experiments that mammalian muscle spindles receive a motor innervation, the gamma motoneurones, which is separate from that to skeletal muscle. This discovery was soon followed by detailed studies of the reflex behaviour of gamma motoneurones and, inevitably, comparison of the reflexes with those of alpha motoneurones which innervate skeletal muscle. One such area of interest concerned the recurrent inhibitory pathway from alpha motoneurone axon collaterals via Renshaw cells back onto the alpha motoneurones themselves. Many groups of workers (Granit et al., 1957; Hunt and Paintal, 1958; Eccles et al., 1960; Voorhoeve and van Kanten, 1962) looked for a similar pathway onto the gamma motoneurones but it was not until 1968 that experiments showed that some gamma motoneurones could be inhibited via the recurrent inhibitory pathway (Ellaway, 1968).

This article attempts to review our present knowledge of recurrent inhibitory control of gamma motoneurones with the readers' attention being drawn to persisting areas of controversy. Finally, recurrent inhibition will be related to another, more controversial, aspect of the reflex control of gamma motoneurones, that of autogenetic inhibition elicited by muscle stretch. The only new contribution to be mentioned here is the work of Judy R. Trott, in this laboratory, which concerns autogenetic control of gammas from stretch and vibration-sensitive receptors in muscle.

NATURE AND INCIDENCE OF RECURRENT INHIBITION OF GAMMA MOTONEURONES

The inhibition was first detected during a study of the rhythmic background discharge of gamma motoneurones in the decerebrate cat. Antidromically conducted impulses were elicited in gamma axons, which had been identified in their parent muscle nerve, in order to see how they disturbed the very regular train of naturally occurring impulses. Often the period of depression following the arrival of an impulse at the cell was longer than could be accounted for by the resetting processes of the spike generator. It then became clear that this extra depression was due to impulses travelling antidromically in other motor axons (Ellaway, 1968, 1972). At about the same time Brown et al. (1968a,b) saw inhibition of spontaneously active units recorded in ventral root filaments in response to antidromic volleys. From their firing characteristics and reflex behaviour these units were almost certainly gamma motoneurones. Other reports of inhibition of gamma moto-neurone discharges in response to antidromic volleys have since appeared (Grillner, 1969; Noth, 1971).

The following is a brief resumé of the salient features of this inhibition. In most respects, save perhaps for its intensity, it resembles that onto alpha motoneurones and can thus be considered as true recurrent inhibition medi-ated via alpha axon collaterals and Renshaw cells. Unless stated otherwise the data presented is drawn from Ellaway (1971).

(1) Approximately three quarters of gamma motoneurones having back-ground discharges in the decerebrate cat (93 studied) received recurrent inhibition. However, in many instances gammas which could be inhibited showed rather brief periods of depression (down to 5—10 msec) following maximal alpha motoneurone volleys in the parent ventral root. Inhibition of the duration seen for tonic alpha motoneurones (Granit et al., 1957) was rarely encountered. It should be borne in mind however that sustained mean frequencies of discharge of gamma motoneurones in the range 50—100 imp/sec are not unusual whereas tonic alphas rarely exceed frequencies of 10—20 imp/sec. The short periods of recurrent inhibition for gammas and longer periods (100 msec plus) for alphas tend to reflect their respective mean intervals of discharge. Thus, in its ability to modify the prevailing discharge, recurrent inhibition may be as effective onto gamma as it is onto alpha motoneurones.

(2) A clear division exists for alpha motoneurones, in which those with fast-conducting axons lack recurrent inhibition while those with slowly con-ducting axons are powerfully affected. No such division exists for gamma motoneurones. The spectrum of axonal conduction velocities of neurones with or without recurrent inhibition overlap completely. This of course does not answer the intriguing question as to whether static and dynamic gamma motoneurones are separately affected; their conduction velocities are known to overlap completely (Brown et al., 1965). In short, both types of gamma efferent appear to receive the inhibition but there are real difficulties in identification of the two types of neurone. This will be considered in more detail below.

(3) The source of recurrent inhibition of gamma motoneurones is un-doubtedly impulses travelling in alpha motoneurone axons. On gradually

increasing the strength of electrical stimulation of a ventral root the onset of inhibition nearly always coincided with excitation of the lowest threshold alpha axons. Estimations of the conduction velocity of the fastest axons eliciting inhibition were always in the alpha range and were never below 50 m/sec. The inhibition was not always maximal, however, at a time when the stimulus began to recruit gamma axons, although one could not exclude the possibility that alpha axons were also still being recruited at this time. Certainly no pronounced increment in inhibition occurred on stimulating the gamma population. This does not, of course, exclude the possibility that impulses in gamma axons might evoke recurrent inhibition which is occluded by that from alpha axons. Indeed, it has been stated recently (Kato and Fukushima, 1973) that, when transmission in alpha axons has been blocked by a certain form of electrical stimulation, then impulses in gamma axons can excite Renshaw cells to discharge.

The origin of the inhibition is not restricted to the parent muscle nerve but, when testing with shocks to the ventral root, is almost invariably confined to the parent ventral root for any one gamma motoneurone. A more powerful inhibition could usually be elicited from the whole tibial division (medial popliteal) of the sciatic nerve than from the parent muscle nerve alone (dorsal roots sectioned). However, in a study of gastrocnemius and soleus gamma motoneurones the degree of inhibition to an antidromic volley in the gastrocnemius medialis branch of the triceps surae nerve supply was found to range from zero up to the maximum that could be evoked on stimulating the whole parent ventral root.

(4) The transmitter between axon collaterals and Renshaw cells is acetylcholine. If antidromic inhibition of gamma motoneurones is, in fact, recurrent inhibition then it should be affected by drugs known to interfere selectively with cholinergic transmission. Eserine, an anticholinesterase which has been found to exert a rather variable potentiation of recurrent inhibition to alphas (Eccles et al., 1954), was found to increase the duration of inhibition in four out of eight gammas.

Mecamylamine, an autonomic ganglionic blocker, is an effective blocking agent of the recurrent inhibitory pathway (Henatsch, personal communication). Recent experiments in this laboratory (Ellaway and Trott, unpublished observations) have shown that mecamylamine reduces antidromic inhibition of gamma motoneurones. Strychnine, a blocker of post-synaptic inhibition also blocks the inhibition of both alpha and gamma motoneurones following antidromic volleys. These similarities of pharmacology strongly suggest that antidromic inhibition of gammas is mediated via the recurrent inhibitory pathway.

(5) The efficacy of recurrent inhibition of gamma motoneurones depends upon the integrity of descending spinal cord pathways. The inhibition is depressed in much the same way as is recurrent inhibition of alphas (Holmqvist and Lundberg, 1959) following spinal cord section. In certain instances

quite marked recurrent inhibition of a gamma motoneurone in the decerebrate cat can disappear completely following spinal cord section.

DISTRIBUTION OF RECURRENT INHIBITION TO STATIC AND DYNAMIC GAMMA
MOTONEURONES

Gamma motoneurones are classified as static or dynamic according to the
effect they have on the response of muscle spindle primary afferents to
stretch of the muscle (Matthews, 1962). When recording from the cut central
end of a gamma motoneurone there is no direct way of telling to which
category it belongs. In the decerebrate cat with an intact spinal cord both
static and dynamic neurones may exhibit background discharges to both
extensor (Jansen and Matthews, 1962) and flexor muscles (Jansen and
Rudjord, 1965; Ellaway, 1971) although there is usually only a very low
level of fusimotor activity to flexor muscles. The position is clearer in the
spinal cat, however, particularly for flexor muscles where only dynamic
neurones are likely to have background discharges. Static gammas are quiet
but may be induced to fire by intravenous injection of L-Dopa which simultaneously depresses the discharge of dynamic gammas (Bergmans and Grillner, 1969). If we try to use these criteria in the spinal cat to identify as static
or dynamic those gamma motoneurones receiving recurrent inhibition we
meet two problems: (a) a background discharge is necessary to test for the
inhibition but the static neurones are not firing, and (b) in the spinal state
the inhibition may be depressed or even absent. However, by noting the
presence or absence of a discharge in the decerebrate animal both before and
after spinal section and then again following treatment with L-Dopa it did
prove possible to distinguish between dynamic and static gamma motoneurones of flexor muscles and to show that both are subject to recurrent
inhibition.

With extensor muscles identification of the two types of neurone is more
uncertain. The distinction has been made in the spinal cat that dynamic
neurones have background discharges whereas static gammas do not (Alnaes
et al., 1965). Here L-Dopa cannot be used to distinguish between the two
categories since both are excited by the drug (Grillner, 1969). Any classification on the basis of the presence or absence of a background discharge is
tentative (e.g. see Fromm and Noth, 1974). It must be borne in mind that
few extensor gamma motoneurones discharge in the spinal cat and classification of those just below threshold for tonic firing as static and those firing at
a few impulses a second as dynamic is rather arbitrary. Such a classification
could be erroneous since it is quite possible for neurones close to the firing
threshold to discharge intermittently. This difficulty may account for the
discrepancy in the reports concerning extensor gammas. Grillner (1969) saw
recurrent inhibition of both types of neurone (sample of 4) and yet, dealing

with a larger number (sample of 8), Fromm and Noth (1974) maintain that the inhibition is restricted to static gamma motoneurones.

AUTOGENETIC INHIBITION OF GAMMA MOTONEURONES AND THE RECURRENT PATHWAY

Confirmation of the existence of autogenetic inhibition of gamma motoneurones by stretch-sensitive afferents in muscle has been sought after for many years ever since the first description by Hunt (1951) that it was present in the decerebrate cat. The subject has received new interest following the discovery of recurrent inhibition of gamma motoneurones. Clearly one might expect to see recurrent inhibition of gammas following muscle stretch which excited alpha motoneurones to discharge. Gamma motoneurone discharges recorded in ventral root filaments were seen to be inhibited by selective activation of spindle primary endings during low-amplitude vibration of the triceps surae which also excited alpha motoneurones (Brown et al., 1968a). The destination of the gamma motoneurones was not known and thus these particular results cannot support the idea of autogenetic inhibition. However, in the same study, these authors did see recurrent inhibition of some of the gammas inhibited by vibration. If stretch-dependent inhibition of gammas is mediated via the recurrent inhibitory pathway it might explain why Hunt and Paintal (1958) could not find evidence of autogenetic inhibition in the spinal animal. Here the recurrent inhibitory pathway both to alpha and gamma motoneurones is depressed (Holmqvist and Lundberg, 1959; Ellaway, 1971).

On recording from gamma motoneurones identified in their muscle nerve evidence has recently been offered that a length-dependent autogenetic inhibition to muscle stretch can be seen in the decerebrate cat (Fromm et al., 1974). Furthermore, these authors found that only those gammas (9 out of 25) inhibited by muscle stretch were subject to recurrent inhibition. Since stretch of the muscle in their experiments also excited alpha motoneurones to discharge they concluded that inhibition due to stretch is, at least in part, mediated by recurrent collaterals. A further study, this time in the spinal cat (Fromm and Noth, 1974), showed that when the quiet majority of gammas was excited to discharge by intravenous injection of L-Dopa, once again it was those and only those neurones receiving recurrent inhibition that could be inhibited by muscle stretch. (In this preparation L-Dopa potentiates both recurrent inhibition (Anden et al., 1966) and the stretch reflex (Grillner, 1969)). In this case however, the inhibitory effects of muscle stretch were more pronounced than those obtained by antidromic activation of alpha axons and it was concluded that recurrent inhibition could be only partly responsible for the autogenetic effect.

THE AFFERENT PATHWAY INVOLVED IN AUTOGENETIC INHIBITION

Stretch-dependent inhibition of gammas could involve either the muscle spindle afferents or Golgi tendon organs. The experiments of Brown et al., (1968a) suggested that selective excitation of primary spindle afferents can inhibit gamma discharges recorded in ventral roots (see also Proske and Lewis, 1972). Recent work in this laboratory (Trott, unpublished), however, discounts the possibility that it is impulses in primary spindle afferents that are responsible for autogenetic inhibition of gamma motoneurones as seen by Hunt (1951) and Fromm et al. (1974). A preliminary study largely confirmed the results of Brown et al., (1968a) in that of 30 units recorded in ventral root filaments, and tentatively identified as gamma axons, seven were inhibited (2 only slightly) by vibration and by stretch of the triceps surae muscles while eighteen remained unaffected. (The remaining five neurones were, in fact, excited by the vibration but only one markedly so. Their other reflex properties did not suggest that these five could have been alpha motoneurones). A second study went on to examine the effect of vibration of the muscle on the discharge of gamma motoneurones isolated from the parent muscle nerve and identified by their conduction velocities. Twenty-eight gamma motoneurones of the gastrocnemius medialis muscle were studied. Vibration of the muscle at 100—200 Hz at an amplitude of 50—200 μm was found to powerfully excite most primary spindle endings whilst leaving secondary endings unaffected. The stimulus always excited considerable alpha discharge (only a small part of the gastrocnemius medialis nerve had been cut for recording purposes) but never inhibited gamma motoneurone discharges. Weak excitation of gammas was seen, however, in many instances. It would thus appear that primary endings of muscle spindles are not a source of autogenetic inhibition and neither is it evident that alpha motoneurone discharge automatically leads to recurrent inhibition of gamma motoneurones.

CONCLUSIONS

The controversy as to whether recurrent inhibition is responsible for the stretch-evoked inhibition of gamma motoneurones highlights a need for further investigations into the physiological conditions that can reflexly inhibit gamma axons via the recurrent pathway. The danger of assuming that recurrent inhibition as revealed by electric shocks to motor axons, is of physiological importance, should be obvious to all. But equally well it should not be assumed that, because in gamma motoneurones there is an apparently weak or rather short-lasting action, the inhibition is unimportant. As argued above, such an effect on a neurone with a high frequency of discharge gives quite a substantial modulation of the discharge.

REFERENCES

ALNAES, E., JANSEN, J.K.S. and RUDJORD, T. (1965) Fusimotor activity in the spinal cat. Acta Physiol. Scand., 63, 197—212.
ANDÉN, N.E., JUKES, M.G., LUNDBERG, A. and VYKLICKY, L. (1966) The effect of Dopa on the spinal cord. 1. Influence on transmission from primary afferents. Acta Physiol. Scand., 67, 373—386.
BERGMANS, J. and GRILLNER, S. (1969) Reciprocal control of spontaneous activity and reflex effects in static and dynamic gamma motoneurones revealed by injection of Dopa. Acta Physiol. Scand., 77, 106—124.
BROWN, M.C., CROWE, A. and MATTHEWS, P.B.C. (1965) Observations on the fusimotor fibres of the tibialis posterior muscle of the cat. J. Physiol., 177, 140—159.
BROWN, M.C., LAWRENCE, D.G. and MATTHEWS, P.B.C. (1968a) Reflex inhibition by Ia afferent input of spontaneously discharging motoneurones in the decerebrate cat. J. Physiol., 198, 5—7P.
BROWN, M.C., LAWRENCE, D.G. and MATTHEWS, P.B.C. (1968b). Antidromic inhibition of presumed fusimotor neurones by repetitive stimulation of the ventral root in the decerebrate cat. Experientia, 24, 1210—1211.
ECCLES, J.C., ECCLES, R.M., IGGO, A. and LUNDBERG, A. (1960) Electrophysiological studies on gamma motoneurones. Acta Physiol. Scand., 50, 32—40.
ECCLES, J.C., FATT, P. and KOKETSU, K. (1954) Cholinergic and inhibitory synapses in a pathway from motor-axon collaterals to motoneurones. J. Physiol., 126, 524—562.
ELLAWAY, P.H. (1968) Antidromic inhibition of fusimotor neurones. J. Physiol., 198, 39—40P.
ELLAWAY, P.H. (1971) Recurrent inhibition of fusimotor neurones exhibiting background discharges in the decerebrate and the spinal cat. J. Physiol., 216, 419—439.
ELLAWAY, P.H. (1972) The variability in discharge of fusimotor neurones in the decerebrate cat. Exp. Brain. Res., 14, 105—117.
FROMM, Chr., HAASE, J. and NOTH, J. (1974) Length-dependent autogenetic inhibition of extensor gamma motoneurones in the decerebrate cat. Pflügers Arch., 346, 251—262.
FROMM, Chr. and NOTH, J. (1974) Autogenetic inhibition of gamma motoneurones in the spinal cat uncovered by Dopa injection. Pflügers Arch., 349, 247—256.
GRANIT, R., PASCOE, J.E. and STEG, G. (1957) The behaviour of tonic alpha and gamma motoneurones during stimulation of recurrent collaterals. J. Physiol., 138, 381—400.
GRILLNER, S. (1969) The influence of Dopa on the static and dynamic fusimotor activity to the triceps surae of the cat. Acta Physiol. Scand., 77, 490—509.
HOLMQVIST, B. and LUNDBERG, A. (1959) On the organisation of the supraspinal inhibitory control of interneurones of various spinal reflex arcs. Arch. Ital. Biol., 97, 340—356.
HUNT, C.C. (1951) The reflex activity of mammalian small nerve fibres. J. Physiol., 115, 456—469.
HUNT, C.C. and PAINTAL, A.S. (1958) Spinal reflex regulation of fusimotor neurones. J. Physiol., 143, 195—212.
JANSEN, J.K.S. and MATTHEWS, P.B.C. (1962) The effects of fusimotor activity on the static responsiveness of primary and secondary endings of muscle spindles in the decerebrate cat. Acta Physiol. Scand., 55, 376—386.
JANSEN, J.K.S. and RUDJORD, T. (1965) Fusimotor activity in a flexor muscle of the decerebrate cat. Acta Physiol. Scand., 65, 236—246.

KATO, M. and FUKUSHIMA, K. (1974) Effect of differential blocking of motor axons on antidromic activation of Renshaw cells in the cat. Exp. Brain Res., 20, 135—144.

LEKSELL, L. (1945) The action potential and excitatory effects of the small ventral root fibres to skeletal muscle. Acta Physiol. Scand., 10, Suppl. 30, 1—84.

MATTHEWS, B.H.C. (1933) Nerve endings in mammalian muscle. J. Physiol., 78, 1—53.

MATTHEWS, P.B.C. (1962) The differentiation of two types of fusimotor fibre by their effects on the dynamic response of muscle spindle primary endings. Q. J. Exp. Physiol., 47, 324—333.

NOTH, J. (1971) Recurrente Hemmung der Extensor-Fusimotoneurone? Pflügers Arch., 329, 23—33.

PROSKE, U. and LEWIS, D.M. (1972) The effects of muscle stretch and vibration on fusimotor activity in the lightly anaesthetised cat. Brain Res., 46, 55—69.

Afferent inflow from the human bladder in relation to filling and voiding

Ejner PEDERSEN and Jesper MAI

Afferent inflow from the human bladder during filling and voiding was recorded by quantitative measurements of the H, T and flexor reflexes. At least two different types of bladder receptors may influence the spinal cord, viz. detrusor stretch receptors, active during bladder filling, increasingly active during voiding and inactive after the voiding phase. The extensor alpha moto-neurones were stimulated by this receptor type as evidenced by increasing H and T reflexes during filling and voiding, while it had the opposite effect on the flexor alpha motoneurones as seen by decreasing flexor reflexes. The other receptor type was active only in some cases, and only after a certain degree of bladder filling; it stimulated the flexor alpha motoneurones and thus the flexor reflexes, and this activity was correlated with difficulties in initiating voiding.

The afferent inflow from the human bladder as well as that from receptors in muscles, tendons, skin, etc. is of general interest.

Special interest attaches to the bladder, as it is a common clinical experience that in spastic conditions bladder filling may promote flexor spasms in the lower extremities. Thus, it is possible that the well-known 'spontaneous' fluctuations in the H and T reflexes during investigations of longer duration may, at least in part, be explained by changes in the inflow from the bladder receptors. We have encountered these problems in our studies of the patho-physiology of spasticity. As few investigations on the influence of the human bladder on spinal reflexes are available, we have studied this influence on the three reflexes most commonly used in our laboratory, viz. the T reflex (Achilles tendon), H reflex and flexor reflex.

MATERIAL AND METHODS

The series studied consisted of 53 adults comprising both normal subjects and patients with spasticity as well as urological complaints. During the recording of a pressure — volume curve of the bladder ('cystometry') indicated by other causes, 30 of them were investigated in the supine position at every 100 ml of filling of the bladder. The remaining 23 were investigated during natural bladder filling and voiding, sitting in a specially designed chair permitting reflex measurements and voiding at the same time. The micturition pattern was measured by a Disa mictiometer placed under the chair. The T reflexes were elicited by means of a hammer, which could give well-defined and reproducible taps at the Achilles tendon (Pedersen et al., 1974b). The H reflexes were elicited by square-wave pulses of a duration of 1 msec (Veale et al., 1973) from a Disa ministim fed through a Grass constant-current unit to a modified Simon electrode (Simon, 1962) placed in the popliteal fossa over the posterior tibial nerve. An unchanged M response was required for inclusion in the study.

The flexor reflexes were elicited by the same Disa ministim by means of trains of five stimuli, each of a duration of 1 msec and delivered at 10-msec intervals. Now the stimulating electrode, Disa 13K62, was placed over the posterior tibial nerve behind the medial malleolus (Pedersen, 1954). In all investigations, an attempt was made to maintain basal conditions, and the recommendations given by Desmedt et al. (1973) were followed. Furthermore, the person under test was asked to empty his bladder before the investigation (Pedersen and Mai, 1974, 1975).

RESULTS

Bladder filling

The monosynaptic reflexes were studied in 37 persons. The T and H reflexes always changed in the same direction and usually in parallel. The monosynaptic reflexes increased in 21 and decreased in 12, often preceded by an initial increase. Four cases were unclassifiable. Flexor reflexes were studied in 19 persons. Nine showed a decrease in the duration of the flexor reflex; six revealed an increase, and again four were unclassifiable. In three cases, both the flexor reflexes and monosynaptic reflexes were measured in the same investigation. Two of these three patients showed increasing monosynaptic reflexes and a decreasing flexor reflex, whereas the third revealed decreasing monosynaptic reflexes and an increasing flexor reflex.

Voiding phase

During voiding, monosynaptic reflexes were measured in 16 cases. Here, too, the H and T reflexes changed in the same direction and largely in parallel. In 11 cases, a steep increase was observed, and all showed a satisfactory flow curve. Eight of them had increasing reflexes during bladder filling, and in 10 voiding was easily initiated. Five showed unchanged monosynaptic reflexes or a slight decrease during micturition. They all revealed decreasing reflexes during bladder filling and all had difficulties in initiating voiding; towards the end of the bladder filling they expressed an intense 'desire to void' localized at the outlet of the bladder. Flexor reflexes were measured only in four cases during voiding, and they all showed a decrease in this reflex during voiding. Three of them had decreasing flexor reflexes during filling of the bladder and easily initiated voiding. The fourth had difficulties in initiating voiding and increasing flexor reflexes during bladder filling, but when the voiding was properly started, the flexor reflex decreased.

Post-voiding phase

After micturition, the monosynaptic reflexes remained at the voiding level for some time and then fell below the initial value, which was again reached after a varying period of time. The flexor reflexes were difficult to assess because of the intervals required between the individual measurements in order to avoid habituation (Pedersen et al., 1974a) and because of the light euphoria often seen after voiding, giving rise to movements, etc.

DISCUSSION AND CONCLUSION

In all our experiments, both during bladder filling, voiding and in the post-voiding phase, the T and H reflexes changed in the same direction in the individual case. Thus, we found no evidence of an action of the bladder receptors on the gamma loop as claimed by McPherson and Skorpil (1966) on the basis of H reflex studies in 16 normal volunteers. The fact that the flexor reflex always changed in the opposite direction of the monosynaptic reflexes, as seen both in the three subjects in whom both reflex types were measured in the same investigation and in a subsequent study in which it was seen that the sphincter muscles and the flexors of the lower extremities are influenced in parallel and opposite to monosynaptic extensor reflexes (Mai and Pedersen, 1975), also points to a direct action of the inflow from the bladder receptors on the alpha motoneurones.

In some of the individuals studied, we found increasing monosynaptic and/or decreasing flexor reflexes during bladder filling, while others showed the reverse picture. When applied to a group such opposite changes tend to cancel out each other. This may explain why McPherson and Skorpil (1966) found unchanged H reflex in a group, but they did extend their studies of the filling phase only over 10 minutes, while our study was for 30 minutes. The question is then why the reflex changes during bladder filling fell in two opposed groups. In the investigations in which the subjects were requested to void it was a striking feature that those who showed decreasing monosynaptic and/or increasing flexor reflexes towards the end of the bladder filling expressed a very intense 'desire to void' localized at the outlet of the bladder. The same subjects had great difficulty in initiating voiding. Once voiding was started, the flow was poor, and there was no or only a slight increase in the monosynaptic reflexes and/or a decrease in the flexor reflex until the flow improved towards the end of the voiding, accompanied by a simultaneous increase in the monosynaptic reflexes. The decrease in the monosynaptic reflexes during bladder filling was often preceded by an initial increase. On the other hand, the second group with increasing monosynaptic reflexes and/or decreasing flexor reflexes during bladder filling experienced a sensation of normal bladder tension at the end of the filling; voiding was easily initiated, usually resulting in a satisfactory flow accompanied by a steep increase in the monosynaptic reflexes and/or a decrease in the flexor reflexes during voiding. It then appeared that the start of micturition could be correlated with the type of reflex changes during voiding: an increase in the monosynaptic and/or a decrease in the flexor reflexes most frequently occurred in patients with easy initiation of voiding, whereas decreasing monosynaptic and/or increasing flexor reflexes were usually seen in patients with difficulty in initiating voiding ($P < 0.01$).

Therefore, our conclusion is that two different types of bladder receptor exert their influences on the central nervous system. One type which is active during the entire filling and during voiding facilitates the extensor motoneurones and thus increases the monosynaptic extensor reflexes during bladder filling, reaching a maximum during voiding, whereas the stimulation by these receptors is abolished when the bladder is empty.

The steep increase in the monosynaptic reflexes during voiding is in agreement with the observations reported by McPherson and Skorpil (1966), who found increasing H reflexes during this phase.

The stretch receptors placed in series with the detrusor muscle demonstrated in cats by Iggo (1955) will, if such receptors are also present in man, be capable of responding in this way, both to passive stretching during bladder filling and to active detrusor contraction during the act of voiding.

The second type of receptor, which comes into action at a later stage of the filling, may be localized at the outlet of the bladder. In individuals without lesions of the centripetal pathways of these receptors, this inflow is perceived as a sensation that 'voiding is imminent' and result in hyperactivity of the alpha motoneurones to the flexors of the lower extremities and to the muscles of the pelvic floor. It is still an unclarified question whether it is these receptors which in spastic states, where the impulses are not always perceived because of central lesions, may be one of the underlying causes of the flexor spasms and the hyperactivity of the muscles of the pelvic floor. But the activation of the motoneurones of the flexors and sphincters is not abolished — even in spastic patients with hyperactivity of the muscles of the pelvic flor — until the uroflow is properly started. This suggests that, also in such patients, the active receptors are situated at or close to the outlet of the bladder.

In conclusion it may be said that in protracted reflex studies in which bladder filling occurs, the subject must be requested to empty his bladder before the experiment is started. In addition, slight changes in the H, T and flexor reflexes should be interpreted with due regard to the experimental data presented here, especially if the subject under test reports a sensation of a full bladder or an intense 'desire to void'.

ACKNOWLEDGEMENTS

This study was supported by a grant from the Danish League against Multiple Sclerosis.

REFERENCES

DESMEDT, J.E. et al. (1973) A discussion of the methodology of the triceps surae T and H-reflexes. In (J.E. Desmedt, Ed.) New Developments in Electromyography and Clinical Neurophysiology, Vol. 3, Karger, Basel, pp. 773—780.

IGGO, A. (1955) Tension receptors in the stomach and the urinary bladder. J. Physiol., 128, 593—607.

MAI, J. and PEDERSEN, E. (1975) Central effect of bladder filling and voiding. (In press).

McPHERSON, A. and SKORPIL, V. (1966) Effects of micturition on leg reflexes. Lancet, 2, 309—312.

PEDERSEN, E. (1954) Studies on the central pathway of the flexion reflex in man and animal. Thesis. Acta Psychiat. Neurol. Scand., suppl. 188, 81p.

PEDERSEN, E. and MAI, J. (1974) L'influence de la vessie et de la miction sur le réflexe monosynaptique. Réunion de la Soc. Belge d'Electromyogr. Neurophysiol. Clin., Liège.

PEDERSEN, E. and MAI, J. (1975) Influence of bladder filling and micturition on monosynaptic reflexes. Electromyogr. Clin. Neurophysiol., 15, 57—66.

PEDERSEN, E., ARLIEN-SØBORG, P. and MAI, J. (1974a) The mode of action of the GABA derivative Baclofen in human spasticity. Acta Neurol. Scand., 50, 665—680.

PEDERSEN, E., DIETRICHSON, P., GORMSEN, J. and ARLIEN-SØBORG, P. (1974b) Measurement of phasic and tonic stretch reflexes in antispastic and antiparkinsonian therapy. Scand. J. Rehab. Med., suppl. 3, 51—60.

SIMON, J.N. (1962) Dispositif de contention des electrodes de stimulation pour l'étude du réflexe de Hoffmann chez l'homme. In (P. Pinelli, F. Buchthal and F. Thiebaut, Eds.) Progr. Electromyogr. Electroenceph. Clin. Neurophysiol., 22, 174—176.

VEALE, J.L., REES, S. and MARK, R.F. (1973) Renshaw cell activity in normal and spastic man. In (J.E. Desmedt, Ed.) New Developments in Electromyography and Clinical Neurophysiology, Vol. 3, Karger, Basel, pp. 523—537.

Reflex physiology

1. Human brainstem reflexes
   by M. Bratzlavsky   135

2. Behaviour of human brainstem reflexes in muscles with antagonistic function
   by M. Bratzlavsky   155

3. The effects of caloric vestibular stimulation on the tonic vibration reflex in man
   by P.J. Delwaide, M. Dessalle and M. Juprelle   163

4. Reflex physiology in man
   by P.J. Delwaide   169

5. Effects of vibration on human spinal reflexes
   by G.C. Agarwal and G.L. Gottlieb   181

6. Effect of vibration on the F response
   by B.T. Shahani and R.R. Young   189

7. Single muscle spindle afferent recordings in human flexor reflex
   by A. Struppler and F. Velho   197

1

Human brainstem reflexes

M. BRATZLAVSKY

The cranial somatic motor functions reach a degree of complexity which is rarely encountered in other parts of the body. This is especially true in man with the development of speech and mimicry. In no other part of the body is the spatial arrangement of different muscle groups so compact while the diversity of the performed motor functions is so vast. As a consequence, cranial muscles are often involved in several completely different motor functions. If, for example, both the superior and the inferior facial musculature in man contribute to the realisation of mimicry, each muscle group has well-defined and distinct functions related to its involvement in oculo-facial and oro-facial motor activities, respectively. The presence of a series of specialized sense organs at the cranial level and the occurrence of continuous mucosal and cutaneous contacts during some cranial motor activities, result in an enormous amount of sensory information reaching the central nervous system through the cranial nerves. For all these reasons it is not surprising that the characteristics of brainstem reflexes differ in many aspects from those of spinal reflexes. Moreover, several features of cranial motor organisation such as the frequent bilateral synergic action of identical muscles, the poor or absent gravitational relations of several muscle groups, the atypical, rather primitive, types of sensory endings often encountered in cranial muscles (Hosokawa, 1961) and the presumed lack of axon collaterals at a bulbar level (Cajal, 1909; Lorente de No, 1933), account for the peculiarities of brainstem reflexes.

OCULO-FACIAL MUSCULATURE

Extrinsic eye muscles

The extra-ocular muscles of man and of the artiodactyl branches of the ungulates (i.e. goat, sheep and pig) have been shown to contain muscle spindles (Cilimbaris, 1910; Cooper and Daniel, 1949). Types of tendon organs have been described in the eye muscles of mammals including man (Huber, 1900; Cooper and Daniel, 1949). In sheep the extra-ocular muscle spindles have nuclear bag and chain fibers and receive both primary and secondary innervation (Harker, 1972). Primary and secondary spindle afferent discharges were obtained upon stretching goat and pig extra-ocular muscles (Cooper et al., 1951; Lennerstrand and Bach-y-Rita, 1974). In artiodactyls both electrophysiological (Whitteridge, 1958; Lennerstrand and Bach-y-Rita, 1974) and anatomical (Harker, 1972) evidence has been provided of the presence of a static and a dynamic fusimotor control of eye muscle spindles. Even those animals, such as the cat, whose extra-ocular muscles lack spindles have ocular muscles richly supplied with a variety of afferent nerve endings whose sensitivity to stretch has been clearly demonstrated (Cooper and Fillenz, 1955; Bach-y-Rita and Murata, 1964).

Since the time of Sherrington controversy has continued over several aspects of the functional organisation of the proprioceptive message arising in extra-ocular muscles. A first point concerns the mode of entry of the ocular proprioceptive fibers into the brainstem, as well as the location of their cell bodies. The existence of species differences is likely to have contributed to some confusion in the past. In the cat it has been demonstrated that extra-ocular muscle afferents run to the brainstem via oculomotor nerves (Bach-y-Rita and Murata, 1964). Nevertheless, some data show that a part of these afferents joins the ophthalmic nerve and reaches the brainstem through the V (Cooper and Fillenz, 1955; Batini and Buisseret, 1974). The location of the cat's extra-ocular proprioceptive soma remains unclear. In artiodactyls some evidence has been presented that the cell bodies of the eye muscle spindles are located in the medial dorso-lateral part of the trigeminal ganglion (Manni et al., 1971a). Their peripheral processes reach the ophthalmic nerve through anastomotic branches with the eye muscles (Winckler, 1937). Their central processes have been suggested to project to the brainstem through the sensory trigeminal root, to run in the descending trigeminal tract and to end in the homonymous nucleus (Manni et al., 1971b). In man no unequivocal data are available concerning the afferent pathway of extra-ocular proprioceptive fibers. The anatomical similarities between man and artiodactyls in regard both to the presence of extra-ocular muscle spindles (Cooper and Daniel, 1949) and of ophthalmic anastomotic branches to eye muscles (Winckler, 1956) could suggest that the trigeminal nerve is the main afferent limb of human extra-ocular muscle proprioception. However such considerations still remain speculative.

A second point of controversy concerning extra-ocular proprioception, relates to the existence of a stretch reflex in extrinsic eye muscles. Most of the recent experimental results obtained from animals, show that little or no reflex organisation exists in these muscles (McCouch and Adler, 1932; Keller and Robinson, 1971; Baker and Precht, 1972). However, several electromyographical studies on the extra-ocular muscles in man present contradictory arguments on the existence of proprioceptive influences in these muscles (Breinin, 1957; Sears et al., 1959; Maruo, 1964). Irrespective of the many reports on the absence of stretch reflexes in extrinsic eye muscles, Granit (1970) considers the linearity of length—tension curves, reported in human extra-ocular muscles over a wide range of following movements (Robinson et al., 1969), as strongly indicative of a feedback mechanism controlling these muscles. Besides, certain results obtained from experimental animals still suggest that a form of reflex organisation exists in the extra-ocular muscles. For instance, some authors presented evidence of inhibitory responses elicited in oculomotor neurons upon stimulation of ocular muscle nerves (Sasaki, 1963) or upon stretching of extra-ocular muscles (Bach-y-Rita, 1972). Furthermore, a number of investigations in experimental animals (see reviews of Granit, 1970 and Bach-y-Rita, 1971) emphasize the possible contribution of extra-ocular proprioceptive information to motor control via the cerebellum as well as through interactions with vestibular, visual and neck muscle afferent impulses.

Tonic neck reflexes have been recognized in human extra-ocular muscles (de Kleyn and Stenvers, 1941). However, these positional reflexes from the neck seem to a large extent to be obscured by highly developed visual and labyrinthine postural mechanisms (Ford and Walsh, 1940).

Eyelid muscles

The principal muscles concerned with eyelid function are the m. orbicularis oculi and the m. levator palpebrae. The blink reflex is by far the most intensively studied reflex at the palpebral level. Much data pertaining to this reflex have been derived from human experimentation. Its first description stems from Overend (1896), who evoked a blink response in man upon tapping the supra-orbital region and considered it as a skin reflex. Kugelberg (1952) reviewed the extensive literature which was subsequently published on this subject. The tap-induced blink reflex was successively suggested to have a periostal origin, a bone origin, a perichondral origin and a myotatic origin. This profusion of contradictory hypotheses undoubtedly pertains to the close anatomical interrelation of different peri-orbital tissues, making particularly difficult any selective stimulation at this level. By electromyographic registration it was later proved in man (Kugelberg, 1952) and in cats (Tokunaga et al., 1958) that the blink reflex is composed of two successive discharges in the m. orbicularis oculi: a homolateral response of short latency and fairly synchronized aspect, and a bilateral response of longer latency and longer duration. Mechanical as well as electrical peri-orbital stimulation were proved efficient in evoking both blink reflex components, the late one being elicitable upon stimulation of the entire face (Kugelberg, 1952; Rushworth, 1962). The early component was considered as a monosynaptic myotatic reflex, while the late component was identified as a polysynaptic cutaneous reflex (Kugelberg, 1952). However, this mixed interpretation of the blink reflex still remained unsatisfactory in view of the lack of histological correlation. In fact, only simplified muscle spindles have occasionally been reported in facial muscles of man (Kadanoff, 1956) and of experimental animals (Bowden and Mahran, 1956). In the last few years both the early and the late blink reflex components were suggested to result from activation of cutaneous mechanoreceptors in man (Shahani and Young, 1968) and in cats (Lindquist and Mårtensson, 1970). Indeed, several arguments were presented against the myotatic origin of the early blink reflex component. In man, this component is elicitable by percutaneous electrical stimulation within a wide region corresponding to the first trigeminal division, even in areas without underlying musculature (Shahani and Young, 1968); furthermore, single motor unit potentials activated in the first blink reflex component show latency fluctuations which are incompatible with a monosynaptic response (Shahani, 1970; Trontelj and Trontelj, 1973). In cat the first blink reflex component can be evoked by tapping a skin flap dissected free from the underlying muscle, but not by tapping the muscle itself (Lindquist and Mårtensson, 1970); moreover, its central relay time indicates that it is mediated through a polysynaptic reflex arc (Lindquist and Mårtensson, 1970; Tanaka et al., 1971).

Early and late blink reflex discharges have much the same threshold and were suggested to have afferent fibers of equal diameter, travelling centrally through the trigeminal nerve (Kugelberg, 1952; Tokunaga et al., 1958). Few investigations were devoted to the problem of the central pathway of the blink reflex components. In cats the early reflex seems to be relayed to the main sensory trigeminal nucleus, possibly through a bi-synaptic arc (Tanaka et al., 1971). The late component could be transmitted through the spinal tract and nucleus of the trigeminal nerve (Tokunaga et al., 1958). In man, Kugelberg (1952) reported that trigeminal tractotomy does not affect the first component but raises the threshold of the second component. Kimura and Lyon (1972) showed in cases of Wallenberg syndrome that the early reflex is generally within normal limits, while the late reflex is affected in the majority of the cases. These findings suggest that the first order neurones responsible for the bilateral late component terminate in the homolateral spinal nucleus of the trigeminal nerve without significant crossing over to the same structure on the other side.

Concerning the functional significance of the blink reflex components, several points remain unsettled. While an early orbicularis oculi discharge is seen only following mechanical or electrical stimulation of the peri-orbital skin, a late discharge is also produced by a puff of air or other corneal stimuli (Magladery and Teasdall, 1961) or a loud noise or flash of light (Rushworth, 1962). It has not yet been excluded that some of these late responses have a cortical or a subcortical pathway. Habituation and sensitisation of the late blink-reflex discharges have been recognized (Rushworth, 1962). Their nociceptive function is not disputed. On the contrary, the significance of the first component of the tap-induced blink reflex remains obscure. A possible function of this early discharge could be to reinforce and shorten the latency of the blink reflex when a noxious mechanical stimulus approaches the orbital area. However, this does not coincide with the observation that the early blink reflex is practically not contributing to the downward movement of the eyelid (Shahani and Young, 1972). It has been suggested that blink-reflex afferents, being activated upon contraction of the underlying musculature, may be involved in some form of continuous facial motor control (Lindquist and Mårtensson, 1970). Still, this hypothesis remains to be confirmed by direct proof.

Uncertainty persists concerning the existence of a proprioceptive control at a facial level. The demonstration of the cutaneous origin of the early blink reflex left this question unanswered. Attempts to record afferent impulses of a proprioceptive character, either in the trigeminal or in the facial nerve of cats, have given negative results (Lindquist and Mårtensson, 1970). Still, this does not exclude the possibility that proprioceptive afferents contribute to facial motor control. Anatomical evidence has been presented in man and in the experimental animal of the presence of several types of sensory nerve endings in facial muscles (Bowden and Mahran, 1956; Kadanoff, 1956). Besides, some studies indicate that periostal receptors could fulfill a powerful proprioceptive function at the facial level (Sakada, 1971). Another question relates to the pathway for an eventual facial proprioception. Whether in man the facial nerve carries some proprioceptive fibers, or whether they are carried exclusively in the trigeminal nerve has not yet been clearly established. In cats, stimulation of high-threshold afferents in the facial nerve has been reported to evoke reflex responses in facial motoneurons (Lindquist and Mårtensson, 1970; Kitai et al., 1971). The origin and method of action of the involved afferent fibers is still unknown. An important problem which remains unsolved is whether or not facial motor function really requires a steady peripheral control. In respect to this, postural reflex activities have been reported in human facialis superior musculature (Bratzlavsky, 1973a). Neck propioceptors were postulated to exert a tonic reciprocal reflex influence on the orbicularis oculi and frontalis muscles, favoring widening of the palpebral fissure at the side toward which the head is rotated, and narrowing of the opposite palpebral fissure.

Most of the electrophysiological work on reflex control of eyelid movements has been focused on the orbicularis oculi muscle. In the present volume it is reported that the m. levator palpebrae in man is the site of an early and a late bilateral pause in its activity, upon exteroceptive peri-orbital stimulation (see next Chapter). The experimental method does not allow us to differentiate between motoneuronal disfacilitation and true post-synaptic inhibition. The late levator pause mostly appears simultaneously with the late orbicularis oculi discharge and can therefore be postulated to represent the latter's reciprocal equivalent. On the contrary, the early levator pause is quite distinctive from the early orbicularis oculi reflex in having a lower threshold and a bilateral character.

ORO-FACIAL MUSCULATURE

(a) Jaw muscles

Reflexes arising in the oro-facial mucosa and skin   Miller and Sherrington (1915) described in decerebrated cats a trigeminal reflex in response to lingual nerve stimulation which consisted of a brisk opening of the jaws. Afterwards it was pointed out that mechanical or electrical stimulation of the gums, teeth, hard palate, tongue and lips could produce this jaw-opening reflex (Sherrington, 1917; Schoen and Koeppen, 1931; Lubinska, 1932). The jaw-opening movement was attributed mainly to the contraction of the digastric muscle. The bilateral character of this reflex, even when elicited by light stimuli, has been emphasized (Lubinska, 1932). Sherrington (1917) demonstrated in cats presenting decerebrated rigidity, that even after section of the digastric muscles, intra-oral stimulation resulted in a jaw depression. He attributed this effect to a reflex inhibition of the hypertonic jaw elevators, and concluded that the jaw-opening reflex exhibits reciprocal innervation. Interest has been focused in recent times on this inhibitory component of the jaw-opening reflex. In man, Hoffmann and Tönnies (1948) reported a suppression of the jaw-closing muscle activity upon painful stimulation of the lingual surface. Later investigators (Goldberg and Nakamura, 1968; Kidokoro et al., 1968a) showed in cats that electrical stimulation of low-threshold lingual nerve or inferior alveolar nerve afferents evokes a long-lasting hyperpolarisation of masseter motoneurones, presenting a short and a long latency component. Similarly in man it has been shown that peri-oral exteroceptive stimulation, especially at the labial level, induces an early and a late bilateral pause in the masseter activity, the first of which has a lower threshold (Bratzlavsky, 1972; Yu et al., 1973). In the present volume both pauses are suggested to result from a post-synaptic motoneurone inhibition (see next Chapter). In cats the early IPSP in jaw-closing motoneurones is likely to be conveyed by a di-synaptic pathway through the nucleus supratrigeminalis (Goldberg and Nakamura, 1968; Kidokoro et al., 1968b). The long latency inhibition of cat jaw-closing motoneurones has been suggested to travel along a polysynaptic pathway through the bulbar reticular formation mainly via the subnucleus interpolaris (Sumino, 1971). Less information is available concerning the excitatory components of the jaw-opening reflex. In cats, the afferent fibres responsible for the digastricus response upon infra-orbital nerve stimulation were reported to range from high-threshold A-alpha fibers to A-delta fibers (Keller et al., 1972; Thexton, 1974). The earliest digastricus responses to inferior alveolar nerve stimulation were suggested to have a di-synaptic pathway and to travel through the subnucleus oralis and interpolaris of the spinal trigeminal tractus (Sumino, 1971). In healthy man this excitatory digastricus reflex seems quite difficult to demonstrate (Yemm, 1972). Inhibitory digastricus responses on the contrary are more readily elicited upon exteroceptive peri-oral stimulation. Several authors emphasized the possible contribution of the jaw-opening reflex to rhythmic chewing movements (Sherrington, 1917; Jerge, 1964; Kidokoro et al., 1968a). Hoffmann and Tönnies (1948) believed the reflex inhibition of jaw-closing muscles to act as a protective mechanism for the tongue. Reconciling, as it were, both views, it has been suggested that in man the late exteroceptive masseter inhibition performs a nociceptive function, while the early exteroceptive inhibition contributes more continuously to the integration of oral motor functions (Bratzlavsky, 1972; Yu et al., 1973).

In addition to the jaw-opening reflex, Sherrington (1917) described in cats a jaw-closing reflex upon stroking the dorsum of the tongue near its tip. More recently a masked short-latency excitatory response has been observed in cat masseter motoneurones after stimulation of the lingual or inferior alveolar nerve (Goldberg and Nakamura, 1968; Kidokoro et al., 1968a; Sumino, 1971). This early facilitation was suggested to have a di-synaptic pathway involving excitatory interneurones in the trigeminal spinal tract nucleus. Subsequently several authors were able to isolate short- and long-latency excitatory reflex responses in cat jaw-closing muscles upon stimulation of low-threshold oro-facial exteroceptive afferents (Goldberg, 1972; Thexton, 1974). In man too, excitatory reflex responses could be elicited in the masseter muscle by stimuli applied to the oral mucosa (Goldberg, 1971; Achari and Thexton, 1974). Thus it appears that excitatory as well as inhibitory exteroceptive reflex pathways are available both to jaw-opening and to jaw-closing muscles. The way in which these different pathways are activated and interact is not yet well understood. It seems to depend both on central and peripheral factors such as the state of jaw muscle activation, jaw position, site and character of the stimulus. Several data indicate that, at a masticatory level, the laws of reciprocal reflex innervation are far from being strictly applicable. In contrast to Sherrington's (1917) observation, Schoen and Koeppen (1931) noticed in cats that in many instances during reflex jaw-opening the jaw elevators either do not present any obvious influence or contract simultaneously with the jaw depressors. In this regard, some results obtained in last few years suggest that, at a masticatory level, the exteroceptive reflex control is mediated through independent pathways to jaw-opening and to jaw-closing motoneurones (Kidokoro et al., 1968a; Sumino, 1971; Thexton, 1974).

Reflexes arising in the jaw muscles The jaw-closing muscles in man and in experimental animals are richly supplied with muscle spindles (Voss, 1935; Freiman, 1954; Karlsen, 1965) whose primary afferents mediate the myotatic reflex of jaw-closing muscles or jaw jerk. Experiments in the cat have shown that the afferent fibers of this reflex run in the portio minor of the trigeminal nerve, their soma being constituted of large unipolar cells, located in the trigeminal mesencephalic nucleus and relayed monosynaptically to the trigeminal motor nucleus (Cajal, 1909; Corbin, 1940; Corbin and Harrison, 1940; Szentagothai, 1948; McIntyre, 1951). In man it has been proved that both afferent and efferent limbs of the jaw jerk run in the trigeminal motor root (McIntyre and Robinson, 1959), which suggests that the central connections of the reflex are much the same as those described in the experimental animal. The latency of the human jaw jerk averages 7.5 msec (Kugelberg, 1952) and calculation of its central relay time makes a monosynaptic pathway likely (McIntyre and Robinson, 1959). During active jaw closing, the jaw jerk or the twitch contraction of the masseter muscle is followed by a silent period, which was originally suggested to result from a crossed autogenic inhibition arising in Golgi tendon organs (Hufschmidt and Spuler, 1962). More recently it has been shown that this jaw-closing muscle silent period is confined to the homolateral side and can be explained on the sole basis of the pause of jaw-closing muscle-spindle afferent discharges (Bratzlavsky, 1972). Most investigators were unable to demonstrate in cats clear heterolateral effects of low-threshold jaw muscle proprioceptors at trigeminal mesencephalic or at trigeminal motor level (Corbin and Harrison, 1940; McIntyre and Robinson, 1959; Nakamura et al., 1973). The behaviour of primary spindle afferent impulses upon passive manipulation of jaw muscles has been studied at mesencephalic level in cats (Corbin and Harrison, 1940; Cody et al., 1972) and in several other experimental animals. Fewer data have been published concerning the function of secondary spindle afferents of jaw-closing muscles, although they were identified both anatomically (Karlsen, 1965) and physiologically (Cody et al., 1972). Both dynamic and static fusimotor innervation of jaw muscle spindles has been demonstrated (Cody et al., 1972; Matsunami and Kubota, 1972). In order to elucidate their functional significance, several investigators analysed the behaviour of spindle afferent discharges from jaw elevators during natural oral motor functions in experimental animals (Matsunami and Kubota, 1972; Taylor and Cody, 1974). Recent work (Goodwin and Luschei, 1974) performed on monkeys, has shown that selective loss of spindle afferent control of jaw muscles does not result in a significant disturbance of the temporo-spatial activation pattern of these muscles during chewing. These findings indicate either that other oro-facial afferent systems can quite easily compensate for the lack of spindle control, or that the pattern of mastication is exclusively generated at a central level and does not require an additional peripheral control.

A paucity of observations have been published about Golgi tendon organs in jaw-closing muscles (Szentogothai, 1948; Jerge, 1964; Kawamura, 1974) and nothing is known about their possible central connections. Szentagothai (1948) demonstrated in cats that lesions of the trigeminal mesencephalic nucleus cause no degeneration of Golgi tendon organs in jaw-closing muscles and he suggested that their afferents travel centrally through the trigeminal sensory root. Indirect electrophysiological observations (Cody et al., 1972) confirm Szentagothai's view. It remains, however, that until now no tendon organ afferent impulses have been recorded from the trigeminal sensory root or ganglion (Beaudreau and Jerge, 1968). Kidokoro and co-workers (1968a) were unable to elicit any IPSP in jaw-closing motoneurones upon masseter nerve stimulation, which could be indicative of input from Golgi tendon organ afferents. On the basis of the presumed different pathway of group Ia and group Ib afferent fibers of jaw elevators, attempts were made in man to disclose reflex influences of both origins, by studying subjects with selective section of the trigeminal sensory root (McIntyre and Robinson, 1959; Hufschmidtt and Spuler, 1962). A number of works have been published in recent years concerning reflex influences of high-threshold masseter afferents on lingual nerve afferents and on hypoglossal and trigeminal motoneurones in the cat. Until now, no corresponding findings have been reported in man.

In subprimates the digastric muscle seems to be devoid of muscle spindles (Baum, 1900; Szentagothai, 1948) and they have been found only rarely in other muscles which open the jaw. In man only a few muscle spindles have been described in the anterior belly of the digastric muscle (Voss, 1956). No myotatic digastric reflex has been reported. The function of this muscle, which can be regarded as a flexor muscle, possibly accounts for these negative results. However, nothing is known about eventual connections of the digastric muscle with the trigeminal mesencephalic tract and nucleus. Furthermore, no positive proof has been obtained that the digastric motoneurones have any monosynaptic connections (Szentagothai, 1948). Proprioceptive afferents of jaw-closing muscles have not been reported to influence digastric motoneurones and no proprioceptive effects of the digastric muscle were shown to affect masseter motoneurones (Kidokoro et al., 1968a). Nevertheless, some electrophysiological work in cats indicates that the nerve of the anterior m. digastricus contains proprioceptive afferents capable of inducing primary afferent depolarization of lingual and glossopharyngeal nerve terminals (Sauerland and Thiele, 1970). If these findings are confirmed, the question which still remains to be answered relates to the type or types of the proprioceptors involved.

Reflexes arising in and around the teeth   The periodontal tissues in man are supplied with several specialized sensory nerve endings which have been variously described (Anderson et al., 1970). Numerous histological studies in experimental animals have also been published. Large and small diameter nerve fibers arise at a periodontal level. Periodontal mechanoreceptor activity has been recorded in the peripheral dental nerves of experimental animals (Pfaffmann, 1939; Ness, 1954). Both rapidly and slowly adapting units and spontaneously firing units, were identified by pressure being applied to the teeth. Most of the dental mechanosensitive units have a low threshold and show a directional sensitivity. As previously mentioned, Sherrington (1917) was able to elicit reflex jaw opening in cats by mechanical stimulation of the teeth. This reflex involved excitation of the jaw-opening muscles as well as inhibition of the jaw-closing muscles. Since the demonstration of afferent activity arising in periodontal mechanoreceptors, it is widely accepted that these receptors are the site of origin of the reflex described by Sherrington (Corbin, 1940; Jerge, 1964). More recent evidence has been provided that periodontal stimulation can produce reflex contraction of the digastric muscle in cats (Hannam and Matthews, 1969). In man, a transient, bilateral, short-latency suppression of the jaw-closing muscle activity occurs during chewing (Schaerer et al., 1967; Ahlgren, 1969) and during tooth tapping in centric occlusion (Griffin and Munro, 1969; Hannam et al., 1969). These effects also appear upon selective and controlled tooth stimulation and are abolished by local tooth anaesthesia (Beaudreau et al., 1969; Sessle and Schmidt, 1972). This proves that the reflexogenic site is located in the periodontium. Following a conditioning mechanical tooth stimulation in man, the monosynaptic masseter-reflex exhibits a phase of suppression, whose time course closely corresponds to that of the dentally evoked masseter pause (Bratzlavsky, unpublished observation). This suggests that the reflex is set up by post-synaptic inhibition of jaw-closing motoneurones. The central pathway of the periodontal reflexes is not yet definitively established. Histological (Corbin, 1940) as well as electrophysiological studies (Corbin and Harrison, 1940; Cody et al., 1972) in experimental animals, show evidence for the presence of first-order neurones of periodontal afferents in the trigeminal mesencephalic nucleus. The pathway of the central processes of these neurones is not exactly known. On the other hand, response to mechanical stimulation of teeth were recorded in Gasserian ganglion cells (Kerr and Lysac, 1964; Beaudreau and Jerge, 1968). Furthermore, dental pressoreceptors are represented in the homolateral main sensory trigeminal nucleus and in the subnucleus oralis (Eisenman et al., 1963). Thus, the periodontal reflex pathway may involve the trigeminal mesencephalic nucleus as well as the trigeminal ganglion. It appears that the supratrigeminal nucleus could function as a relay in this pathway (Eisenman et al., 1963; Jerge, 1963). In view of its short latency the reflex is likely to be oligosynaptic.

In man, tapping the teeth during isometric contraction of the jaw-closing muscles evokes a short-latency excitatory masseter-reflex, preceding the inhibitory response (Goldberg, 1971; Sessle and Schmitt, 1972). This reflex has been assumed to arise at the periodontal level. Its neuronal pathway is still speculative. Excitatory responses in jaw-closing muscles have also been obtained in the rat upon stimulation of periodontal receptors, and were suggested to travel centrally through the trigeminal mesencephalic nucleus (Funakoshi and Amano, 1974). It should be pointed out that, just as is the case for exteroceptive jaw reflexes, the human jaw depressor muscles do not seem actively involved in periodontal reflexes. Upon mechanical tooth stimulation in man, only a reflex pause in the digastric activity has been reported (Beaudreau et al., 1969).

The functional significance of periodontal reflexes is a matter of contro-versy. Some investigators have proposed that these reflexes contribute to the cyclic movements of normal chewing (Jerge, 1964). In this regard, peri-odontal stimulation in rabbits has been reported to evoke a lateral jaw move-ment reflex, related to the specific chewing pattern of this animal (Lund et al., 1971). Periodontal afferents were also suggested to be involved in the reflex regulation of swallowing by producing presynaptic depolarization of laryngeal afferents (Sessle and Storey, 1972). Observations have been re-ported indicating that periodontal sensory control is not essential for the production of normal masticatory cycles in man. This led some authors to conclude that periodontal reflexes rather contribute to the regulation of chewing force in accordance with the physical characters of food, and to the protection of the teeth by avoiding development of excessively strong jaw-closing forces (Kawamura, 1974).

In the cat, electrical stimulation of tooth pulpal nerves elicits a nocicep-tive jaw-depressing reflex by excitation of the digastric muscles (Mahan and Anderson, 1970; Keller et al., 1972). To our knowledge no reports have been published on this subject in man.

Reflexes arising in the temporo-mandibular joint capsule   Histological studies in man (Thilander, 1961; Ishibashi, 1966) and in several experimental animals, revealed that the temporo-mandibular joint (TMJ) capsule is rich-ly innervated: free, complex and encapsulated nerve endings have been described. Upon mechanical stimulation of the cat's TMJ capsule both inhibitory and excitatory reflex effects (mostly of tonic character) were evoked in jaw muscles and in their motoneurones (Greenfield and Wyke, 1966; Kawamura et al., 1967). Furthermore, reflex inhibition of jaw muscles (Klineberg et al., 1970) and reflex jaw opening (Shwaluk, 1971) were reported upon stimulation of peripheral nerves subserving the TMJ. A recent work (Lowe and Sessie, 1973) attributed reflex influences of passive jaw opening on cat's hypoglossal motoneurones, to TMJ receptors. In man as well, afferent input from the TMJ is likely to participate in the reflex control of masticatory muscles, although objective data are very scarce. Local anaes-thesia of the human TMJ has been reported to produce impairment of mandi-bular positioning (Thilander, 1961). Furthermore, the duration of the pro-prioceptive masseteric silent period was observed to be significantly in-creased in patients with TMJ pain — dysfunction syndrome (Bessette et al., 1971). The central pathway of TMJ reflexes has not yet been studied inten-sively. In man the TMJ is chiefly innervated by the auriculo-temporal nerve, which projects to the main trigeminal sensory nucleus (Thilander, 1961). Afferent impulses have been recorded in this nucleus in cats upon move-ments of an isolated TMJ (Kawamura et al., 1967). Neither anatomical (Cor-bin, 1940) nor physiological studies (Cody et al., 1972) provide arguments for a representation of TMJ receptors at the trigeminal mesencephalic level.

Several suggestions have been made concerning the functional significance of TMJ reflexes. Distinctive reflex effects are elicitable according to the anterior or posterior location of the stimulated TMJ capsule receptors (Kawamura et al., 1967). Some of these influences were suggested to participate closely in the regulation of cyclic chewing movements. Other TMJ reflexes could have a protective character. In this respect, Posselt and Thilander (1965) showed that maximal jaw opening could be increased by anaesthesia of the TMJ. They suggested that TMJ reflexes restrict excessive jaw opening, as in yawning, to prevent subluxation of the condyle.

(b) Tongue muscles

In decerebrated cats a licking movement of the tongue tip accompanied by a tongue retraction has been described following stimulation of the lingual nerve and of the tongue mucosa (Sherrington, 1917; Schoen and Koeppen, 1931). Blom and Skoglund (1959) and Blom (1960) recorded efferent discharges in the cat's hypoglossal nerve upon lingual nerve stimulation, and concluded that a crossed polysynaptic connection exists between the two nerves. This they described as the linguo-- hypoglossal reflex. Subsequently, synaptic responses were recorded intracellularly in the hypoglossal nucleus following single lingual nerve stimuli (Porter, 1965). It was shown that such stimuli act differently on tongue-protruding motoneurones and on tongue-retractive motoneurones, evoking inhibitory post-synaptic potentials in the former and excitatory post-synaptic potentials in the latter (Morimoto et al., 1968). The rapidly adapting mechanoreceptors associated with the filiform papillae of the cat's tongue have been suggested to act as the most efficient triggers of the linguo—hypoglossal reflex (Porter, 1967). In man, Carleton (1937) reported that local anaesthesia of the surface of the tongue and the inside of the mouth removes the ability to detect tongue position. Other authors found that the human tongue is not atactic after bilateral anaesthesia of the lingual nerve (Weddell et al., 1940; Adatia and Gehring, 1971) but noticed that articulation becomes more difficult in such circumstances (Weddell et al., 1940). These clinical data make it seem likely that lingual nerve afferents contribute to the motor control of the tongue. Recently a bilateral pause in the activity of the tongue-protruding genioglossal muscle has been reported in human subjects upon electrical stimulation of the lingual surface (Bratzlavsky and vander Eecken, 1974). This observation suggests that, in man as well, crossed linguo—hypoglossal connections of exteroceptive origin do exist. In view of its latency, the reflex is likely to be polysynaptic. Possibly, reciprocal excitatory pathways connect human lingual nerve afferents and tongue-retracting motoneurones, as has been shown to be the case in the cat (Morimoto et al., 1968). This reflex could be effective in preventing tongue injuries during mastication. In experimental animals the linguo—hypoglossal reflex has been reported to contain two components, the first of which has the lowest threshold (Blom and Skoglund, 1959; Blom, 1960). A di-synaptic arc (Porter, 1967) and a tri-synaptic arc (Morimoto et al., 1968) respectively have been suggested for the short-latency reflex response. The anatomy of its central circuit is not yet clearly established. Cajal (1909) described in cats a di-synaptic pathway of lingual nerve afferents to hypoglossal motoneurones, with the second order neurone located in the main trigeminal sensory nucleus. On the other hand, connections have been traced between the spinal trigeminal nucleus and the hypoglossal nucleus (Stewart and King, 1963) which may be concerned with the linguo—hypoglossal reflex (Porter, 1967).

In experimental animals, several other exteroceptive influences on the tongue musculature have been reported. Repeated hypoglossal discharges and repeated tongue movements occur in cats following intra-oral stimulation (Schoen and Koeppen, 1931; Blom, 1960). This reflex seems related to the food-positioning response described by Miller and Sherrington (1915), whose purpose should be to transfer substances to the back of the mouth for swallowing. The jaw elevator muscle tonus was reported to be in some way antagonistic to the repeating hypoglossal reflex activities (Blom, 1960). Involvement of hypoglossal motoneurones in reflex deglutition has been documented in cats by Sumi (1969). Recently, low-threshold laryngeal stimulation was shown to evoke a tongue-protrusion reflex which is modulated by oro-facial sensory information (Schmitt et al., 1973). No reports are available concerning similar influences on human tongue muscles.

Muscle spindles have been found in the extrinsic and intrinsic tongue muscles of man and Rhesus monkey (Cooper, 1953; Bowman, 1968). The tongue muscles of several subprimates lack spindles (Blom, 1960) but are supplied with a series of less organized afferent nerve endings (Law, 1954). Afferent discharges originating in tongue muscle spindles have been recorded in the distal portion of the Rhesus monkey's hypoglossal nerve (Bowman and Combs, 1968). These impulses were suggested to reach the central nervous system via C2 or C3 dorsal root or both, which they join through hypoglosso—cervical anastomoses (Corbin and Harrison, 1939; Bowman and Combs, 1969). Similarly in man, several indirect arguments suggest that the hypoglossal nerve contains the tongue muscle spindle afferents (Weddell et al., 1940; Adatia and Gehring, 1971). In subprimates, upon stretching the tongue, afferent discharges were recorded in the hypoglossal nerve beyond its connection with the lingual nerve (Hanson and Widen, 1970). These discharges probably arise in the atypical tongue proprioceptors described by Law (1954). All these data clearly indicate that the hypoglossal nerve in mammals carries primary afferent fibers originating in stretch-sensitive tongue proprioceptors. However, the location of their cell bodies is still speculative. Moreover, the existence of connections to hypoglossal motoneurones is equivocal. No reports are available concerning monosynaptic projections into hypoglossal motoneurons. Blom (1960) did not succeed in evoking any stretch reflex in cat tongue muscles. In man neither mechanical nor electrical stimulation of the tongue nor of the hypoglossal nerve have been efficient in eliciting any proprioceptive lingual reflex (Bratzlavsky and van-der Eecken, 1974). Only in the monkey has a bilateral short-latency reflex discharge been reported in the hypoglossal nerve upon stimulation of the C2 dorsal root, which was proposed to result from excitation of group Ia lingual spindle afferents (Bowman and Combs, 1969). No data have been reported in man concerning high-threshold hypoglosso—hypoglossal reflexes similar to those described in the cat (Hanson and Widen, 1970).

Concerning the postural reflex control of the tongue musculature, Sauerland and Mitchell (1970) observed in human subjects a marked increase in tonic genioglossal activity when the head is tilted to the supine position. These effects could arise in neck proprioceptors or in labyrinth receptors and be involved in preservation of free air passage to the lungs.

(c) Lip muscles

The peri-oral facial muscles are actively involved in several motor functions such as articulation, mastication and facial mimicry. Not enough attention has been given to the problems of afferent control of the lip muscles. It has long been known that mechanical stimulation of the peri-oral area could give rise to reflex contraction of the human lip musculature. Although the tap-induced lip reflex was first described in 1898 by Escherich, it was not subjected to an electrophysiological analysis until 1952 (Kugelberg, 1952; Ekbom et al., 1952). These investigators showed that the human lip-tap-reflex consists of two components, an early homolateral and a late bilateral discharge. The afferent limb of both reflexes involves the trigeminal nerve (Ekbom et al., 1952; Prechtl et al., 1967). Reflex responses have also been elicited in the cat's orbicularis oris muscle, upon stimulation of A-alpha fibres of the infra-orbital nerve (Keller et al., 1972). In agreement with their speculations about the origin of the blink reflex components, Kugelberg and co-workers (Kugelberg, 1952; Ekbom et al., 1952) considered the early component of the tap-induced lip reflex as a monosynaptic proprioceptive reflex. At the present time this hypothesis seems questionable, due to the demonstration of the cutaneous origin of both blink reflex components (Shahani and Young, 1968; Lindquist and Mårtensson, 1970). However, it appears no less risky merely to conclude from the latter findings that both tap-induced lip reflexes are of exteroceptive nature. Unlike the blink reflex, no data were reported indicating that electrical stimulation of the peri-oral skin is able to set up the orbicularis oris reflex components. The only orbicularis oris reflex evokable in healthy man by exteroceptive electrical stimulation has a rather long latency (25—40 msec), an inconstant character and only appears upon strong painful peri-or intra-oral stimulation (Bratzlavsky, 1973b). When set up at an intra-oral level, the optimal area of elicitation of this reflex is the anterior tongue mucosa and the labial gums and mucosa, which suggests that it is organised to protect intra-oral structures against external noxious stimuli. Although in cats stimulation of A-delta fibers of the tooth pulp does not evoke any reflex response in the lip musculature (Keller et al., 1972), peri-oral muscles were shown to respond to stimulation of nociceptive fibers in the hypoglossal nerve (Hanson and Widen, 1970). In man, the late electrically induced lip reflex appears to be quite distinctive from the late component of the lip-tap-reflex, the latter having a rather low threshold and a more constant character, especially when evoked against a background of slight voluntary activity. The central connections of the tap-induced lip reflexes are as yet unknown, but their latencies suggest that both are mediated through a polysynaptic arc. As to the origin of the lip-tap-reflexes, at the present time any suggestion could only be speculative. At least, it seems probable that they do not arise in superficially located cutaneous receptors. In this regard, suggestive evidence has been presented in human subjects that afferent information arising in intradermal or intramuscular peri-oral receptors contributes to the integration of normal articulatory EMG patterns of the lip muscles (Leanderson and Persson, 1972).

REFERENCES

ACHARI, N.K. and THEXTON, A.J. (1974) A masseteric reflex elicited from the oral mucosa in man. Arch. Oral Biol., 19, 299—302.
ADATIA, A.K. and GEHRING, E.N. (1971) Proprioceptive innervation of the tongue. J. Anat. (Lond.), 110, 215—220.
AHLGREN, J. (1969) The silent period in the EMG of the jaw muscles during mastication and its relationship to tooth contact. Acta Odontol. Scand., 27, 219—227.
ANDERSON, D.J., HANNAM, A.G. and MATTHEWS, B. (1970) Sensory mechanisms in mammalian teeth and their supporting structures. Physiol. Rev., 50, 171—195.
BACH-Y-RITA, P. (1971) Neurophysiology of eye movements. In (P. Bach-y-Rita, C.C. Collins and J.E. Hyde, Eds.) The Control of Eye Movements, Academic Press, New York, pp. 7—45.
BACH-Y-RITA, P. (1972) Extra-ocular muscle inhibitory stretch reflex during active contraction. Arch. Ital. Biol., 110, 1—15.
BACH-Y-RITA, P. and MURATA, K. (1964) Extra-ocular proprioceptive responses in the VI nerve of the cat. Quart. J. Exp. Physiol., 49, 408—415.
BAKER, R. and PRECHT, W. (1972) Electrophysiological properties of trochlear motoneurons as revealed by IVth nerve stimulation. Exp. Brain Res., 14, 127—157.
BATINI, C. and BUISSERET, P. (1974) Sensory peripheral pathway from extrinsic eye muscles. Arch. Ital. Biol., 112, 18—32.
BAUM, J. (1900) Beiträge zur Kenntnis der Muskelspindeln. Anat. Hefte, 13, 249—305.
BEAUDREAU, D.E. and JERGE, C.R. (1968) Somatotopic representation in the Gasserian ganglion of tactile peripheral fields in the cat. Arch. Oral Biol., 13, 247—256.
BEAUDREAU, D.E., DAUGHERTY Jr, W.F. and MASLAND, W.S. (1969) Two types of motor pause in masticatory muscles. Am. J. Physiol., 216, 16—21.

BESSETTE, R.W., BISHOP, B. and MOHL, N.D. (1971) Duration of masseteric silent period in patients with TMJ syndrome. J. Appl. Physiol., 30, 864—869.

BLOM, S. (1960) Afferent influences on tongue muscle activity. A morphological and physiological study in the cat. Acta Physiol. Scand., 49, suppl. 170, 1—97.

BLOM, S. and SKOGLUND, S. (1959) Some observations on the control of tongue muscles. Experientia, 15, 12—13.

BOWDEN, R.E.M. and MAHRAN, Z.Y. (1956) The functional significance of the pattern of innervation of the muscle quadratus labii superioris of the rabbit, cat and rat. J. Anat., 90, 217—227.

BOWMAN, J.P. (1968) Muscle spindles in the intrinsic and extrinsic muscles of the Rhesus monkey's (macaca mulatta) tongue. Anat. Rec., 161, 483—485.

BOWMAN, J.P. and COMBS, C.M. (1968) The discharge patterns of lingual spindle afferent fibers in the hypoglossal nerve of the Rhesus monkey. Exp. Neurol., 21, 105—119.

BOWMAN, J.P. and COMBS, C.M. (1969) The cerebrocortical projection of hypoglossal afferents. Exp. Neurol., 23, 291—301.

BRATZLAVSKY, M. (1972) Pauses in activity of human jaw closing muscle. Exp. Neurol., 36, 160—165.

BRATZLAVSKY, M. (1973a) Tonic neck reflexes in facial muscles controlling eyelid position in man. Exp. Neurol., 39, 355—358.

BRATZLAVSKY, M. (1973b) Afferent control of human lip musculature. Electroencephalogr. Clin. Neurophysiol., 34, 805.

BRATZLAVSKY, M. and VANDER EECKEN, H. (1974) Afferent influences upon human genioglossal muscle. J. Neurol. — Z. Neurol., 207, 19—25.

BREININ, G.M. (1957) Electromyographic evidence for ocular muscle proprioception in man. A.M.A. Arch. Ophthalmol., 57, 176—180.

CAJAL, S.R. y. (1909) Histologie du Système Nerveux de l'Homme et des Vertébrés. Vol. I, A. Maloine, Paris.

CARLETON, A. (1937) Observations on the problem of the proprioceptive innervation of the tongue. J. Anat. (Lond.), 72, 502—507.

CILIMBARIS, P.A. (1910) Histologische Untersuchungen über die Muskelspindeln der Augenmuskeln. Arch. Mikr. Anat., 75, 692—747.

CODY, F.W.J., LEE, R.W.H. and TAYLOR, A. (1972) A functional analysis of the components of the mesencephalic nucleus of the fifth nerve in the cat. J. Physiol. (Lond.), 226, 249—261.

COOPER, S. (1953) Muscle spindles in the intrinsic muscles of the human tongue. J. Physiol. (Lond.), 122, 193—202.

COOPER, S. and DANIEL, P.D. (1949) Muscle spindles in human extrinsic eye muscles. Brain, 72, 1—24.

COOPER, S. and FILLENZ, M. (1955) Afferent discharges in response to stretch from the extra-ocular muscles of the cat and monkey and the innervation of these muscles. J. Physiol. (Lond.), 127, 400—413.

COOPER, S., DANIEL, P.D. and WHITTERIDGE, D. (1951) Afferent impulses in the oculomotor nerve from the extrinsic eye muscles. J. Physiol. (Lond.), 113, 463—474.

CORBIN, K.B. (1940) Observations on the peripheral distribution of fibers arising in the mesencephalic nucleus of the fifth cranial nerve. J. Comp. Neurol., 73, 153—177.

CORBIN, K.B. and HARRISON, F. (1939) The sensory innervation of the spinal accessory and tongue musculature in the Rhesus monkey. Brain, 62, 191—197.

CORBIN, K.B. and HARRISON, F. (1940) Function of mesencephalic root of the fifth cranial nerve. J. Neurophysiol., 3, 423—435.

DE KLEYN, A. and STENVERS, H.W. (1941) Tonic neck-reflexes on the eye muscles in man. Proc. K. Nederl. Akad. Wet. (Biol. Med.), 44, 385—396.

EISENMAN, J., LANDGREN, S. and NOVIN, D. (1963) Functional organization in the main sensory trigeminal nucleus and in the rostral subdivision of the nucleus of the spinal trigeminal tract in the cat. Acta Physiol. Scand., 59, suppl. 214, 4—44.

EKBOM, K.A., JERNELIUS, B. and KUGELBERG, E. (1952) Peri-oral reflexes. Neurology (Minn.), 2, 103—111.

ESCHERICH, Th. (1898) in (Masson et al., Eds.) Traité des Maladies de l'Enfance, Vol. IV, Paris, pp. 750—789.

FORD, F.R. and WALSH, F.B. (1940) Tonic deviations of the eyes produced by movements of the head. Arch. Ophthalmol., 23, 1274—1284.

FREIMANN, R. (1954) Untersuchungen über Zahl und Anordnung der Muskelspindeln in den Kaumuskeln des Menschen. Anat. Anz., 100, 258—264.

FUNAKOSHI, M. and AMANO, N. (1974) Periodontal jaw muscle reflexes in the albino rat. J. Dent. Res., 53, 598—605.

GOLDBERG, L.J. (1971) Masseter muscle excitation induced by stimulation of periodontal and gingiva receptors in man. Brain Res., 32, 369—381.

GOLDBERG, L.J. (1972) An excitatory component of the jaw-opening reflex in the temporal and masseter muscles of cats and monkeys. Experientia, 28, 44—46.

GOLDBERG, L.J. and NAKAMURA, Y. (1968) Lingually induced inhibition of masseteric motoneurons. Experientia, 24, 371—373.

GOODWIN, G.M. and LUSCHEI, E.S. (1974) Effects of destroying spindle afferents from jaw muscles on mastication in monkeys. J. Neurophysiol., 37, 967—981.

GRANIT, R. (1970) The basis of motor control. Academic Press, London, p. 346.

GREENFIELD, B.E. and WYKE, B. (1966) Reflex innervation of the temporo-mandibular joint. Nature (Lond.), 211, 940—941.

GRIFFIN, C.J. and MUNRO, R.R. (1969) Electromyography of the jaw-closing muscles in the open-close-clench cycle in man. Arch. Oral Biol., 14, 141—149.

HANNAM, A.G. and MATTHEWS, B. (1969) Reflex jaw opening in response to stimulation of periodontal mechanoreceptors in the cat. Arch. Oral Biol., 14, 415—419.

HANNAM, A.G., MATTHEWS, B. and YEMM, R. (1969) Changes in the activity of the masseter muscle following tooth contact in man. Arch. Oral Biol., 14, 1401—1406.

HANSON, J. and WIDEN, L. (1970) Afferent fibers in the hypoglossal nerve of cat. Acta Physiol. Scand., 79, 24—36.

HARKER, D.W. (1972) The structure and innervation of sheep superior rectus and levator palpebrae extraocular musles. II. Muscle spindles. Invest. Ophthalmol., 11, 970—979.

HOFFMANN, P. and TÖNNIES, J.F. (1948) Nachweis des völlig konstanten Vorkommens des Zungen-Kieferreflexes beim Menschen. Pfluegers Arch., 250, 103—108.

HOSOKAWA, H. (1961) Proprioceptive innervation of striated muscles in the territory of the cranial nerves. Tex. Rep. Biol. Med., 19, 405—464.

HUBER, G.C. (1900) Sensory nerve terminations in the tendons of the extrinsic eye-muscles of the cat. J. Comp. Neurol., 10, 152—158.

HUFSCHMIDT, H.J. and SPULER, H. (1962) Mono- and polysynaptic reflexes of the trigeminal muscles in human beings. J. Neurol. Neurosurg. Psychiatry, 25, 332—335.

ISHIBASHI, K. (1966) Studies on innervation of human mandibular joint. Jap. J. Oral Biol., 8, 46—57.

JERGE, C.R. (1963) The function of the nucleus supratrigeminalis. J. Neurophysiol., 26, 393—402.

JERGE, C.R. (1964) The neurological mechanism underlying cyclic jaw movements. J. Prosthet. Dent., 14, 667—681.

KADANOFF, D. (1956) Die sensiblen Nervenendigungen in der mimischen Muskulatur des Menschen. Z. Mikrosk.- Anat. Forsch., 62, 1—15.

KARLSEN, K. (1965) The location of motor end plates and the distribution and histological structure of muscle spindles in jaw muscles of the rat. Acta. Odontol. Scand., 23, 521—547.

KAWAMURA, Y. (1974) Neurogenesis of mastication. In (Y. Kawamura Ed.) Frontiers of Oral Physiology, Vol. 1, S. Karger, Basel, pp. 77—120.

KAWAMURA, Y., MAJIMA, T. and KATO, I. (1967) Physiologic role of deep mechano-receptor in temporomandibular joint capsule. J. Osaka Univ. Dent. Sch., 7, 63—76.

KELLER, E.L. and ROBINSON, D.A. (1971) Absence of a stretch reflex in extraocular muscles of the monkey. J. Neurophysiol., 5, 908—919.

KELLER, O., VYKLICKY, L. and SYKOVA, E. (1972) Reflexes from A-delta and A-alpha trigeminal afferents. Brain Res., 37, 303—332.

KERR, F.W.L. and LYSAK, W.R. (1964) Somatotopic organization of trigeminal-ganglion neurones. Arch. Neurol., 11, 593—602.

KIDOKORO, Y., KUBOTA, K., SHUTO, S. and SUMINO, R. (1968a) Reflex organization of cat masticatory muscles. J. Neurophysiol., 31, 695—708.

KIDOKORO, Y., KUBOTA, K., SHUTO, S. and SUMINO, R. (1968b) Possible interneurons responsible for reflex inhibition of motoneurons of jaw-closing muscles from the inferior dental nerve. J. Neurophysiol., 31, 709—716.

KIMURA, J. and LYON, L.W. (1972) The orbicularis oculi reflex in the Wallenberg syndrome: alteration of the late reflex by lesions of the spinal tract and nucleus of the trigeminal nerve. J. Neurol. Neurosurg. Psychiatry, 35, 228—233.

KITAI, S.T., AKAIKE, T., BANDO, T., TANAKA, T., TSUKAHARA, N. and YU, H. (1971) Antidromic and synaptic activation of the facial nucleus of cat. Brain Res., 33, 227—232.

KLINEBERG, I.J., GREENFIELD, B.E. and WYKE, B.D. (1970) Contribution to the reflex control of mastication from mechanoreceptors in the temporomandibular joint capsule. Arch. Oral Biol., 21, 73—83.

KUGELBERG, E. (1952) Facial reflexes. Brain, 75, 385—396.

LAW, E. (1954) Lingual proprioception in pig, dog and cat. Nature (Lond.), 174, 1107—1108.

LEANDERSON, R. and PERSSON, A. (1972) The effect of trigeminal nerve block on the articulatory EMG activity of facial muscles. Acta Otolaryngol., 74, 271—278.

LENNERSTRAND, G. and BACH-Y-RITA, P. (1974) Spindle responses in pig eye muscles. Acta Physiol. Scand., 90, 795—797.

LINDQUIST, C. and MÅRTENSSON, A. (1970) Mechanisms involved in the cat's blink reflex. Acta Physiol. Scand., 80, 149—159.

LORENTE DE NO, R. (1933) Action potential of the motoneurons of the hypoglossal nucleus. J. Cell. Comp. Physiol., 29, 207—288.

LOWE, A.A. and SESSLE, B.J. (1973) Tongue activity during respiration, jaw opening, and swallowing in cat. Can. J. Physiol. Pharmacol., 51, 1009—1011.

LUBINSKA, L. (1932) Contribution à l'étude des réflexes non-itératifs (Le réflexe linguo-maxillaire). Ann. Physiol. Physicochim. Biol., 8, 668—759.

LUND, J.P., McLACHLAN, R.S. and DELLOW, P.G. (1971) A lateral jaw movement reflex. Exp. Neurol., 31, 189—199.

MAGLADERY, J.W. and TEASDALL, R.D. (1961) Corneal reflexes. Arch. Neurol., 5, 269—274.

MAHAN, P.E. and ANDERSON, K.V. (1970) Jaw depression elicited by tooth pulp stimulation. Exp. Neurol., 29, 439—448.

MANNI, E., PALMIERI, G. and MARINI, R. (1971a) Peripheral pathway of the proprioceptive afferents from the lateral rectus muscle of the eye. Exp. Neurol., 30, 46—53.

MANNI, E., PALMIERI, G. and MARINI, R. (1971b) Extraocular muscle proprioception and the descending trigeminal nucleus. Exp. Neurol., 33, 195—204.

MARUO, T. (1964) Electromyographical studies on stretch reflex in human extraocular muscle. Jap. J. Ophthalmol., 8, 97—111.

MATSUNAMI, K. and KUBOTA, K. (1972) Muscle afferents of trigeminal mesencephalic tract nucleus and mastication in chronic monkeys. Jap. J. Physiol., 22, 545—555.

McCOUCH, G.P. and ADLER, F.H. (1932) Extraocular reflexes. Am. J. Physiol., 100, 78—88.

McINTYRE, A.K. (1951) Afferent limb of the myotatic reflex arc. Nature (Lond.), 168, 168—169.

McINTYRE, A.K. and ROBINSON, R.G. (1959) Pathway for the jaw jerk in man. Brain, 82, 468—474.

MILLER, F.R. and SHERRINGTON, C.S. (1915) Some observations on the bucco-pharyngeal stage of reflex deglutition in the cat. Quart. J. Exp. Physiol., 9, 147—186.

MORIMOTO, T., TAKATA, M. and KAWAMURA, Y. (1968) Effect of lingual nerve stimulation on hypoglossal motoneurones. Exp. Neurol., 22, 174—190.

NAKAMURA, Y., NAGASHIMA, H. and MORI, S. (1973) Bilateral effects of the afferent impulses from the masseteric muscle on the trigeminal motoneuron of the cat. Brain Res., 57, 15—27.

NESS, A.R. (1954) The mechanoreceptors of the rabbit mandibular incisor. J. Physiol. (Lond.), 126, 475—493.

OVEREND, W. (1896) Preliminary note on a new cranial reflex. Lancet, 1, 619.

PFAFFMANN, C. (1939) Afferent impulses from the teeth due to pressure and noxious stimulation. J. Physiol. (Lond.), 97, 207—219.

PORTER, R. (1965) Synaptic potentials in hypoglossal motoneurones. J. Physiol. (Lond.), 180, 209—224.

PORTER, R. (1967) The synaptic basis of a bilateral lingual-hypoglossal reflex in cats. J. Physiol. (Lond.), 190, 611—627.

POSSELT, U. and THILANDER, B. (1965) Influence of the innervation of the temporo-mandibular joint capsule on mandibular border movements. Acta Odontol. Scand., 23, 601—613.

PRECHTL, H.F.R., GRANT, D.K., LENARD, H.G. and HRBEK, A. (1967) The lip-tap-reflex in the awake and sleeping newborn infant. A polygraphic study. Exp. Brain Res., 3, 184—194.

ROBINSON, D.A., O'MEARA, D.M., SCOTT, A.B. and COLLINS, C.C. (1969) Mechanical components of human eye movements. J. Appl. Physiol., 26, 548—553.

RUSHWORTH, G. (1962) Observations on blink reflexes. J. Neurol. Neurosurg. Psychiatry, 25, 93—108.

SAKADA, S. (1971) Response of Golgi-Mazzoni corpuscles in the cat periostea to mechanical stimuli. In (R. Dubner and Y. Kawamura, Eds.) Oral-facial Sensory and Motor Mechanisms, Appleton-Century-Crofts, New York, pp. 105—122.

SASAKI, K. (1963) Electrophysiological studies on oculomotor neurons of the cat. Jap. J. Physiol., 13, 287—302.

SAUERLAND, E.K. and MITCHELL, S.P. (1970) Electromyographic activity of the human genioglossus muscle in response to respiration and to postural changes of the head. Bull. Los Angeles Neurol. Soc., 35, 69—73.

SAUERLAND, E.K. and THIELE, H. (1970) Presynaptic depolarisation of lingual and glossopharyngeal nerve afferents induced by stimulation of trigeminal proprioceptive fibers. Exp. Neurol., 28, 344—355.

SCHAERER, P., STALLARD, R.E. and ZANDER, H.A. (1967) Occlusal interferences and mastication: An electromyographic study. J. Prosthet. Dent., 17, 438—449.

SCHMITT, A., YU, S.-K.J. and SESSLE, B.J. (1973) Excitatory and inhibitory influences from laryngeal and orofacial areas on tongue position in the cat. Arch. Oral Biol., 18, 1121—1130.

SCHOEN, R. and KOEPPEN, S. (1931) Untersuchungen über Zungen- und Kieferreflexe. II. Mitteilung: Exterozeptive Reflexe und ihre wechselnde Schaltung. Arch. Exp. Pathol. Pharm., 160, 343—368.

SEARS, M.L., TEASDALL, R.D. and STONE, H.H. (1959) Stretch effects in human extraocular muscle; an electromyographic study. Bull. Johns Hopkins Hosp., 104, 174—178.

SESSLE, B.J. and SCHMITT, A. (1972) Effect of controlled tooth stimulation on jaw muscle activity in man. Arch. Oral. Biol., 17, 1597—1607.

SESSLE, B.J. and STOREY, A.T. (1972) Periodontal and facial influences on the laryngeal input to the brainstem of the cat. Arch. Oral. Biol., 17, 1583—1595.

SHAHANI, B. (1970) The human blink reflex. J. Neurol. Neurosurg. Psychiatry, 33, 792—800.

SHAHANI, B. and YOUNG, R.R. (1968) A note on blink reflexes. J. Physiol. (Lond.), 198, 103P—104P.

SHAHANI, B.T. and YOUNG, R.R. (1972) Human orbicularis oculi reflexes. Neurology (Minn.), 22, 149—154.

SHERRINGTON, C.S. (1917) Reflexes elicitable in the cat from pinna, vibrissae and jaws. J. Physiol. (Lond.), 51, 404—431.

SHWALUK, S. (1971) Initiation of reflex activity from the temporomandibular joint of the cat. J. Dent. Res., 50, 1642—1646.

STEWART, W.A. and KING, R.B. (1963) Fiber projections from the nucleus caudalis of the spinal trigeminal nucleus. J. Comp. Neurol., 121, 271—286.

SUMI, T. (1969) Synaptic potentials of hypoglossal motoneurons and their relation to reflex deglutition. Jap. J. Physiol., 19, 68—79.

SUMINO, R. (1971) Central neural pathways involved in the jaw-opening reflex in the cat. In (R. Dubner and Y. Kawamura, Eds.) Oral-facial sensory and motor mechanisms, Appleton-Century-Crofts, New York, pp. 315—329.

SZENTAGOTHAI, J. (1948) Anatomical considerations of monosynaptic reflex arcs. J. Neurophysiol., 11, 445—453.

TANAKA, T., YU, H. and KITAI, S.T. (1971) Trigeminal and spinal inputs to the facial nucleus. Brain Res., 33, 504—508.

TAYLOR, A. and CODY, F.W.J. (1974) Jaw muscle spindle activity in the cat during normal movements of eating and drinking. Brain. Res., 71, 523—530.

THEXTON, A.J. (1974) Jaw opening and jaw closing reflexes in the cat. Brain Res. 66, 425—433.

THILANDER, B. (1961) Innervation of the temporo-mandibular joint capsule in man. Trans. R. Sch. Dent., Stockholm, Umea, 2, 1—67.

TOKUNAGA, A., OKA, M., MURAO, T., YOKIO, H., OKUMURA, T., HIRATA, T., MIYASHITA, Y. and YOSHITATSU, S. (1958) An experimental study on facial reflex by evoked electromyography. Med. J. Osaka Univ., 9, 397—411.

TRONTELJ, M. and TRONTELJ, J.V. (1973) First component of human blink reflex studied on single facial motoneurones. Brain. Res., 53, 214—217.

VOSS, H. (1935) Ein besonderes reichliches Vorkommen von Muskelspindeln in der tiefen Portion des M. masseter des Menschen und der Arthropoiden. Anat. Anz., 81, 290—292.

VOSS, H. (1956) Zahl und Anordnung der Muskelspindeln in den oberen Zungenbein-muskeln, im M. trapezius und M. latissimus dorsi. Anat. Anz., 103, 443—446.

WEDDELL, G., HARPMAN, J.A., LAMBLEY, D.G. and YOUNG, L. (1940) The innervation of the musculature of the tongue. J. Anat. (Lond.), 74, 255—267.

WHITTERIDGE, D. (1958) The motor nerve supply to the extra-ocular muscle spindles. Electroencephalogr. Clin. Neurophysiol., 10, 353.

WINCKLER, G. (1937) L'innervation sensitive et motrice des muscles extrinsèques de l'oeil chez quelques ongulés. Arch. Anat. Histol. Embryol., 23, 219—234.

WINCKLER, G. (1956) L'innervation proprioceptive des muscles extrinsèques du globe oculaire chez l'homme. C.R. Ass. Anat., 43, 848—857.

YEMM, R. (1972) Reflex jaw opening following electrical stimulation of oral mucous membrane in man. Arch. Oral Biol., 17, 513—523.

YU, S.-K.J., SCHMITT, A. and SESSLE, B.J. (1973) Inhibitory effects on jaw muscle activity of innocuous and noxious stimulation of facial and intra-oral sites in man. Arch. Oral Biol., 18, 861—870.

2

Behaviour of human brainstem reflexes in muscles with antagonistic function

M. BRATZLAVSKY *

The way in which reflex integration takes place in antagonistic muscles at the cranial level is far from being well understood. From this point of view the most frequently investigated muscles are the jaw muscles. Whereas in the past, classical reciprocal reflex actions have been described in jaw muscles of cats (Sherrington, 1917), more recent experimental data have been reported concerning the afferent control of these muscles, which do not fit in the scheme of reciprocal reflex innervation (Kidokoro et al., 1968; Thexton, 1974). The purpose of the present study was to investigate some of these problems in man.

Brainstem reflexes were analysed in healthy adults by recording simultaneously through co-axial needle electrodes, the EMG activity of a pair of antagonistic muscles at the oro-facial level (the masseter and the anterior digastric muscles) and at oculo-facial level (the levator palpebrae and the orbicularis oculi muscles). Reflex responses were elicited in both muscle groups by graded single-shock electrical stimulation of the labial and the peri-orbital skin, through two flat, silver disc electrodes. Rectangular impulses of 0.5 msec duration and of 5—80 V intensity were delivered by a constant voltage insulated stimulator. The myotatic masseter reflex was evoked by tapping the chin down with an electrodynamic type force generator (mini-shaker, Bruël & Kjaer, type 4810). The evoked muscular responses were displayed after amplification on a cathode-ray oscilloscope and filmed on direct-print paper.

As has been reported previously (Bratzlavsky, 1972; Yu et al., 1973) a light electrical stimulus delivered to the peri-oral skin during active jaw closing induces, after a latency varying between 10 and 15 msec, a suppression of both ipsi-lateral and the contra-lateral masseter muscle activities lasting 10—20 msec (Fig. 1A). This short latency reflex pause of the jaw-closing muscle activity remains very stable when evoked repeatedly at 1 c/sec. If the

* Supported by a grant from the Belgian Nationaal Fonds voor Wetenschappelijk Onderzoek.

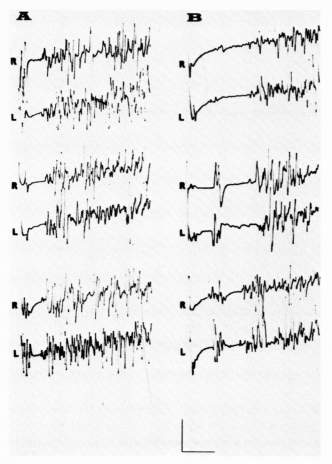

Fig. 1. EMG activity of right (R) and left (L) masseter muscle. (A) Repeated light stimulation (10 V) of left peri-oral skin at frequency of 1 c/sec; (B) Repeated painful stimulation (50 V) of same area at frequency of 1 c/sec. Calibration : 2 mV; 40 msec.

stimulus is made stronger a second bilateral pause appears in the masseter muscle which has a latency of between 30 and 60 msec and a duration of 10—50 msec (Fig. 1B). Contrasting with the early masseter pause the late masseter pause shows fluctuations in latency and duration when evoked repeatedly at 1 c/sec. When elicited by strong stimuli, the early and the late masseter pauses often fuse into a single long-lasting suppression of the masseter activity. Just as has been shown to be the case in cat (Goldberg and Nakamura, 1968; Kidokoro et al., 1968), both the early and the late masseter pauses are likely to result from a post-synaptic reflex inhibition of jaw-closing motoneurones, since the monosynaptic masseter-reflex tested following a conditioning, peri-oral, exteroceptive stimulus exhibits two phases of

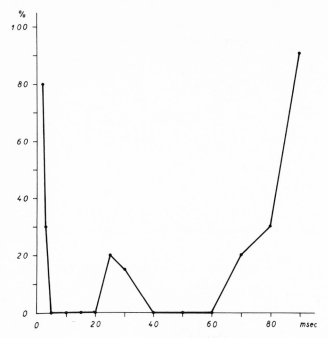

Fig. 2. Time course of variations in amplitude of myotatic masseter reflex following conditioning exteroceptive peri-oral stimulation (30V) during jaw closure- Ordinate: reflex amplitude as percent of control. Abscissa: time interval between conditioning and test stimulus.

suppression whose time course closely corresponds to that of the masseter pauses (Fig. 2).

In cats, exteroceptive peri-oral stimulation has been reported to induce, besides a jaw-closing muscle inhibition, a reciprocal excitation of the jaw-opening digastric muscle (Sherrington, 1917). However, it must be emphasized that these animals were tested in decerebrated conditions. In healthy man, as a general rule, neither tactile nor painful stimulation of the peri-oral area is successful in eliciting a reflex contraction in the anterior digastric muscle (Fig. 3). Besides, a clear jaw-opening movement is practically never observed in such circumstances. The only constant reflex response elicitable in the anterior digastric muscle is a pause in its activity produced by painful peri-oral exteroceptive stimulation during active jaw opening (Fig. 3B). The digastricus pause has a latency of 12—15 msec and a duration of 20—60 msec. In many instances it seems to be composed of an early and a late response.

At the palpebral level, a tactile peri-orbital stimulation evokes an early bilateral pause in the activity of the m. levator palpebrae with a latency of 10—14 msec and a duration of 10—15 msec (Fig. 4A1). If the stimulus is

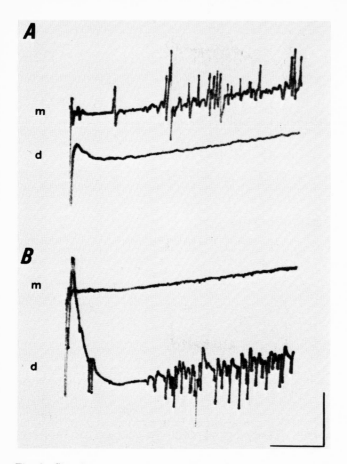

Fig. 3. Simultaneous registration of EMG activity in m. masseter (m) and m. digastricus (anterior belly) (d). (A) Painful peri-oral stimulation (50 V) during active-jaw closing. (B) Painful peri-oral stimulation (60 V) during active jaw opening. Calibration: 2 mV; 40msec.

made stronger, a second bilateral pause is observed in the levator activity (Fig. 4A2). It has a latency of 30—40 msec and a duration of 10—60 msec. The late pause is elicitable upon stimulation of the entire face (Fig. 4A3). Just as is the case in the m. masseter, the early levator pause remains very stable when elicited repeatedly at 1 c/sec, while the late levator pause shows fluctuations both in duration and in latency (Fig. 4B). A tactile peri-orbital stimulus evoking the early levator pause does not elicit any response in the m. orbicularis oculi (Fig. 5). Upon stronger peri-orbital stimulation, the second levator pause is evoked while both the early and the late excitatory blink reflex components appear in the m. orbicularis oculi. Slight variations can be observed in the threshold of these different responses. However, an

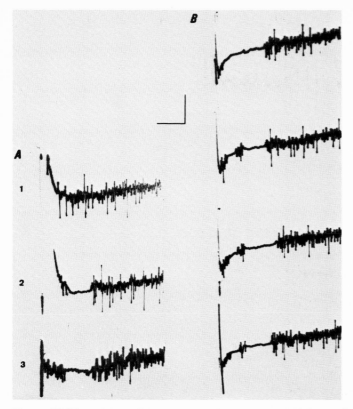

Fig. 4. EMG activity of levator palpebrae muscle. (Al) Tactile supra-orbital stimulation (15 V). (A2) Painful supra-orbital stimulation (30 V). (A3) Painful peri-oral stimulation (50 V). (B) Repeated painful supra-orbital stimulation at frequency of 1 c/sec. Calibration: 0.1 mV; 40 msec.

orbicularis oculi response never occurs at lower threshold than a levator palpebrae response. On the contrary, in most instances the pauses in the levator activity precede the orbicularis oculi reflexes. No clear myotatic reflex was elicitable in the m. levator palpebrae, therefore it was not possible to test the excitability of the levator motoneurones after exteroceptive stimulation or to decide whether the levator pauses are induced by a moto-neuronal disfacilitation or by post-synaptic motoneurone inhibition.

The present results allow us to draw some comparisons between the exteroceptive reflex behaviour of antagonistic muscles at the oro-facial and at oculo-facial levels in healthy man. It appears that in both areas the tested muscles are subjected to a differential exteroceptive reflex control, extensor-type muscles being influenced more readily and at a lower threshold than the flexor-type muscles. The late inhibition in the masseter and levator pal-

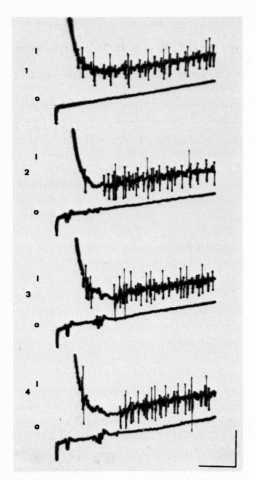

Fig. 5. Simultaneous registration of EMG activity in m. levator palpebrae (I) and m. orbicularis oculi (pars palpebralis) (o). Electrical stimulation of homolateral supra-orbital skin with progressively increasing intensity (1: tactile stimulus, 2,3,4). Calibration: 0.2 mV; 40 msec.

pebrae muscles seems part of a generalised cranial nociceptive reflex, while the early inhibition could be involved in some form of continuous motor control, especially at the oro-facial level.

REFERENCES

BRATZLAVSKY, M. (1972) Pauses in activity of human jaw-closing muscle. Exp. Neurol., 36, 160—165.

GOLDBERG, L.J., and NAKAMURA, Y. (1968) Lingually induced inhibition of masseteric motoneurones. Experientia, 24, 371—373.

KIDOKORO, Y., KUBOTA, K., SHUTO, S., and SUMINO, R. (1968) Reflex organisation of cat masticatory muscles. J. Neurophysiol., 31, 695—708.

SHERRINGTON, C.S. (1917) Reflexes elicitable in the cat from pinna vibrissae and jaws. J. Physiol. (Lond.), 51, 404—431.

THEXTON, A.J. (1974) Jaw opening and jaw closing reflexes in the cat. Brain Res., 66, 425—433.

YU, S.-K.J., SCHMITT, A., and SESSLE, B.J. (1973) Inhibitory effects on jaw muscle activity of innocuous and noxious stimulation of facial and intra-oral sites in man. Arch. Oral Biol., 18, 861—870.

3

The effects of caloric vestibular stimulation on the tonic vibration reflex in man

P.J. DELWAIDE, M. DESSALLE and M. JUPRELLE

The tonic vibration reflex (TVR) is studied in man in four muscles of the lower limb: quadriceps, short biceps, soleus and tibialis anterior. The TVR is not affected in flexor muscles (short biceps and tibialis anterior) by injection of water into the ear canal at 30, 37 or 44°C. The TVR of extensor muscles (quadriceps and soleus) is potentiated during the duration of injection. The facilitation persists during the nystagmic phase. With stimulation at 37°C, a facilitation is observed during the injection but this effect disappears immediately upon cessation. A mixed effect of reticulo- and vestibulo-spinal tracts may be hypothesized. Some discrepancies with the known facts of animal physiology are pointed out.

It is well known that caloric vestibular stimulation in man causes a deviation of the axis of the body. Therefore, it is legitimate to look for a modification of tone in the muscles of the lower extremity. Unfortunately it is rather difficult to directly record muscular tone in human subjects. Inversely, the excitability of the myotatic arcs offers the opportunity to easily study tone (Sherrington, 1906; Lloyd, 1943; Paillard, 1955).

In man, a myotatic reflex arc can be activated by phasic and tonic stimuli. The tendon reflex and the Hoffmann reflex are examples of phasic stimulations (Magladery et al., 1951; Paillard, 1955) while the tonic vibration reflex (TVR), due to the permanent stimulation of the muscle spindles constitutes an example of tonic stimulation (Eklund and Hagbarth, 1965, 1966; Lance, 1965; Delwaide, 1971, 1974). It has been suggested that the TVR represents an adequate technique to study muscle tone in man (de Gail et al., 1966). A supplementary advantage of this technique is that the tonic vibration reflex may be obtained without difficulty in all the limb muscles (Eklund and Hagbarth, 1966). In contrast to this, under normal conditions the tendon reflexes are inexcitable in the tibialis anterior muscle.

In this study, the influence of caloric vestibular stimulation on TVR has been investigated both in flexor and extensor muscles of the lower limb.

TECHNIQUE

Eight subjects were examined while sitting. The knee was positioned in 45 degrees of flexion; the head was inclined 35° towards the rear, so that a semi-circular canal was in the vertical plane. The caloric stimulation was accomplished by injections of water at 44 or 30°C. Controls were made with water at body temperature. The injection was carried out with a constant flow for one minute. In each study, the nystagmus was recorded. The TVR was provoked by application of a vibrator (Keydon) to the tendons of the quadriceps, biceps femoris, tibialis anterior and soleus muscles, respectively. The excursion of the vibrator was 1 mm (Eklund, 1971) with a constant frequency of 100 c/sec.

The TVR was recorded by cutaneous electrodes attached over the muscle at some distance from the vibrator.

RESULTS

Vibratory stimulation was applied continuously throughout the duration of the experiment. It is useful to consider the experimental maneuver in distinct stages. At the beginning of the experiment, it is necessary to wait until the intensity of the evoked TVR is almost constant (see Fig. 1, control). We did not retain subjects in whom the reflex could not be evoked during resting conditions or those in whom the activity was too widely fluctuating. A new phase may be defined from the start of the injection to its end. The nystagmus does not appear immediately but in general a few seconds before the injection is completed. It persists for more than one minute after the injection phase and progressively diminishes in amplitude. Thus, a third phase corresponds to the duration of the nystagmus. Finally, after the disappearance of this third phase one can define a period of post-test control.

The injection of water at 44 or 30°C into the external auditory canal does not cause the appearance of electromyographic activity in the four muscles studied.

Flexor muscles: tibialis anterior and biceps femoris

As shown in the upper part of the figure, neither during the period of injection nor during the period of nystagmus is there a clear modification of the TVR in either of these muscles. There appears to be neither facilitation nor inhibition of the electromyographic activity.

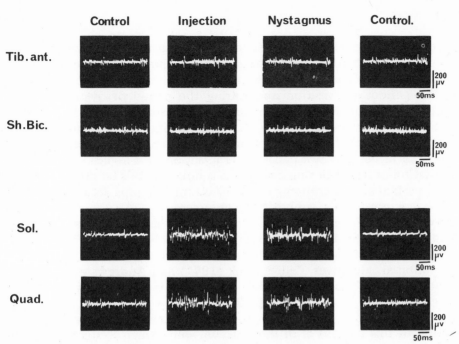

Fig. 1. Examples of TVR recordings in four muscles of the lower limb. It is useful to consider four distinct phases. In flexors, there are no modifications either during the injection phase or during the nystagmic phase. In extensors, during the injection, a clear facilitation appears which persists during the nystagmus. In quadriceps, EMG activity is grouped in bursts during the nystagmus.

Extensor muscles: soleus and quadriceps

The results are similar in these two muscles, as shown in the lower part of the figure. From the start of the injection, there is an important facilitation of the TVR. This facilitation clearly persists after the injection and during the phase of nystagmus. In addition, as can be easily seen in the figure, the electromyographic activity is grouped in bursts with the same frequency as the nystagmus movements. When the nystagmus ceases, electromyographic activity is found with the same amplitude as that which is seen during the pre-test control. The same results are observed with injections of water at 44 and 30°C but it is difficult to estimate any possible quantitative difference.

When the water temperature is at 37°C, there is a clear facilitation of the TVR during the period of injection. However, contrary to the results observed with caloric stimulation, the facilitation disappears immediately at the end of the injection.

COMMENTARY

The results indicate distinctly different effects in the flexor and extensor muscles resulting from the same stimulation. No modification of activity is observed in the flexor muscles although facilitation of the extensors is seen during the period of injection and during the period of nystagmus. The facilitation during the period of injection is equally provoked by injection of water at 37°C. This result suggests that the facilitation is related to cutaneous stimulation of the auditory canal or mechanical stimulation of the eardrum. This effect does not persist after injection. It is logical to think that the facilitation observed during nystagmus is linked to this labyrinthic stimulation. In particular, the grouping of the electromyographic activity in bursts relative to eye movements, supports this argument.

The vestibular influences on the motoneurones and segmental pathways of the lumbo-sacral cord of the cat are now well known (Grillner and Hongo, 1972). Extensor motoneurones are facilitated while those of the flexors are chiefly inhibited. Moreover, Gillies et al. (1971) and Andrews et al. (1973) have studied the mechanism by which electrical stimulations of various sites of the cat brainstem modify the TVR. This reflex is reduced to 20% by ablation of the lateral vestibular nucleus and, inversely, is potentiated by stimulation of this nucleus or of the vestibulo-spinal tract. Systematic exploration of the brainstem disclosed that the TVR of the triceps surae could be consistently inhibited by stimulation of the medullary reticular formation and potentiated by stimulation of the caudal part of the pons. It is of interest to point out that facilitation obtained from the medulla is bilateral and affects both flexors and extensors.

However, the validity of transferring the result of animal studies to humans must be questioned. Our results show some discrepancies with the known facts of animal physiology. We observe a reflex facilitation in the extensors but no clear effect in the flexors. The similarity of results after warm and cold caloric stimulation of the same labyrinth is another striking fact which must be pointed out. A mixed effect of reticulo- and vestibulo-spinal tracts may be hypothesized.

The use of the TVR, besides permitting the study of all muscles, seems to be strongly indicated in the study of modifications of tone because of its tonic rather than phasic character. Unfortunately it does not offer a useful tool for the analysis of implied physiopathological mechanisms. Indeed the TVR is dependent upon facilitation of motoneurones via a direct monosynaptic pathway but there is more and more evidence which suggests a facilitation via a polysynaptic pathway (de Gail et al., 1966; Delwaide, 1971). Therefore, the observed facilitation can arise, in principle, from three mechanisms: direct facilitation of alpha motoneurones, facilitation of gamma neurones modifying the sensitivity of muscle spindles and facilitation of interneurones activated by Ia afferents. Analytical studies on cats have shown that all three mechanisms may be influenced (Grillner and Hongo, 1972).

It is important to note that the facilitation observed in the extensor muscles arises from a different mechanism than the facilitation observed following a Jendrassik maneuver. In fact, the facilitation recorded during this maneuver affects the flexor and extensor muscles in the same way and not selectively the extensors.

REFERENCES

ANDREWS, C., KNOWLES, L. and HANCOCK, J. (1973) Control of the tonic vibration reflex by the brain stem reticular formation in the cat. J. Neurol. Sci., 18, 217—226.

De GAIL, P., LANCE, J.W. and NEILSON, P.D. (1966) Differential effects on tonic and phasic reflex mechanisms produced by vibration of muscles in man. J. Neurol. Neurosurg. Psychiatry, 29, 1—11.

DELWAIDE, P.J. (1971) Etude experimentale de l'hyperréflexie tendineuse en clinique neurologique. Editions Arscia. S.A. Bruxelles, p.324.

DELWAIDE, P.J. (1974) Le stimulus vibratoire en neurophysiologie clinique: aspects physiologiques et physiopathologiques. Rev. d'E.E.G. Neurophysiol., 4, 539—553.

EKLUND, G. (1974) Some physical properties of muscle vibrators used to elicit tonic proprioceptive reflexes in man. Acta Soc. Med. Upsalla, 76, 271—280.

EKLUND, J. and HAGBARTH. K.E. (1965) Motor effect of vibratory muscle stimuli in man. Electroencephogr. Clin. Neurophysiol., 19, 619.

EKLUND, G. and HAGBARTH, K.E. (1966) Normal variability of tonic vibration reflexes (TVR) in man. Exp. Neurol., 16, 80—92.

GILLIES, J.D., BURKE, D. and LANCE, J.W. (1971) The tonic vibration reflex in the cat. J. Neurophysiol., 34, 252—262.

GRILLNER, S. and HONGO, T. (1972) Vestibulospinal effects on motorneurones and interneurones in the lumbo-sacral cord. In (A. Brodal and O. Pompeiano, Eds.) Basic Aspects of Central Vestibular Mechanisms, Elsevier Publishing Company, p. 656; Progr. Brain Res. 37, 243—262.

LANCE, J.W. (1965) The mechanism of reflex irradiation. Proc. Aust. Assoc. Neurol., 3, 77—82.

LLOYD, D.P. (1943) Conduction and synaptic transmission of reflex response to stretch in spinal cats. J. Neurophysiol., 6, 317—326.

MAGLADERY, J.W., PORTER, W.E., PARK, A.M. and TEASDALL, R.D. (1951) Electrophysiological studies of nerve and reflex activity in normal man. IV. The two-neurone reflex and identification of certain action potentials from spinal roots and cord. Bull. Johns Hopkins Hosp., 88, 499—519.

PAILLARD, J. (1955) Réflexes et régulations d'origine proprioceptive chez l'homme. Thèse Fac. Sci. Paris (Sér. A., nr. 2858-3729) Arnette, Paris, p. 293.

SHERRINGTON, C.S. (1906) The integrative action of the nervous system. Yale University Press, New Haven.

4

Reflex physiology in man

P.J. DELWAIDE

The electrophysiological study of human reflexes may offer very specific information about the physiopathology of most neurological syndromes. However, this approach is limited as far as methodology is concerned because of ethical problems. Without being exhaustive, this paper discusses several of the possible and commonly used procedures of clinical reflexology in order to: (1) attain stimulations as selective as possible: by selection of the nervous trunks; anesthesia; microneuronography; experimental search for effective stimuli; pharmacology, and (2) interpret the observed results in the individual in toto: by comparison of the H reflex and the tendon reflex; comparison of monosynaptic and polysynaptic reflexes, and comparison of the results obtained on extensor and flexor muscles.

Over the past thirty years, the neurophysiology of the spinal cord has been uncovered in stages. Neurophysiologists have primarily used cats as their experimental subjects, the preparations most often being decerebrated or spinalized (Renshaw, 1941; Lloyd, 1943; Eccles, 1964; Lundberg, 1967). Moreover, the techniques available have become more and more sophisticated.

Evidently, it is of the greatest interest to know to what extent the results obtained from cats are applicable to man, in the normal state and in pathological conditions. Notable peculiarities exist in man, e.g., bipedal posture, unique development of the pyramidal system and the cerebellum and, inversely, involution of the rubro-spinal system. In the areas of physiology and psychophysiology, there are good reasons to specifically study spinal cord functions in man.

However, it is in the area of physiopathology that the study of spinal reflex in man is the most useful. For more than a century, clinicians have been very much interested in tendinous and exteroceptive reflex changes, especially in cases of pyramidal syndrome. Modifications of these reflexes offer a unique opportunity to study the physiopathology of the clinical syndrome. In fact, it is difficult, if not impossible, to achieve accurate models of spasticity in experimental animals. This is also true for the majority of the habitual neurological syndromes. These reasons explain and justify the development of the electrophysiological study of reflexes in man, so-called 're-flexology'. This approach is necessary if one wants to understand better the human nervous system and its pathological perturbations.

Clinical reflexology does not offer the possibility of equalling the precision and sophistication of animal physiology. These limitations are related to the fact that clinical studies must be carried out without injuring the patient or allowing him to run the slightest risk. Obviously one cannot conduct de-afferentations or de-efferentations. Moreover, the afferent discharge of muscular and joint receptors which follows a reflex contraction (re-afferentation) must be taken into account for interpretation of excitability changes. Another difficulty resides in the fact that electrical shocks, normally used as a stimulus, are most often applied to mixed nerves and not to purely motor or sensory nerves. Therefore, one can legitimately question the value of the findings that clinical reflexology can bring to the study of physiopathology.

Without being exhaustive, we will discuss several of the possible and commonly used procedures of clinical reflexology in order to attain stimulations that are as selective as possible and to interpret the observed results in the individual in toto.

THE CONTROL OF AFFERENTS

It is often possible to control both qualitatively and quantitatively the afferent messages to the spinal cord. There are several techniques which achieve this and one can try to adapt one or more of the following procedures to the problem under study.

Selection of the nervous trunks

In man, it is possible to activate purely motor or purely sensory nerve fibres. In this way, Hugon (1967) employed graduated stimulation of the sural nerve, a nerve which is purely sensory. By modifying the intensity of the stimulation, he was able to evoke two types of polysynaptic reflexes in the short biceps femoris. Moreover, he was able to relate each of these reflexes to stimulation of group II or group III cutaneous fibres of the sural nerve: RA II and RA III.

Another example of the benefit which may be derived from the proper choice of human anatomical structures is offered by analysis of the blink reflex (Shahani and Young, 1972a,b). The afferent pathway of this reflex is made up of the sensory fibres of the fifth cranial nerve while the motoneurones follow the seventh cranial nerve. Because of the segregation between the afferent and the efferent pathways, it is possible to activate the nucleus by two

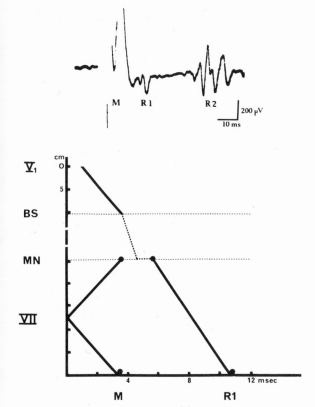

Fig. 1. The upper part of graph shows an example of a blink reflex (R1 and R2) preceded by the maximal motor response (M) in the same muscle. The stimulation of the supra-orbital nerve is applied 1 msec after the stimulation of the facial nerve (VII). The first components of the reflex (R1) are present and not inhibited. The lower part is a diagram showing that the motoneurons are able to transmit the reflexogenic volleys applied on V_1 some msec after receiving antidromic stimulation applied on the seventh cranial nerve. Distance and conduction velocities were estimated according to the data of Kugelberg and of Shahani.

distinct modes: orthodromic stimulation of the fibres of nerve V and anti-dromic stimulation of the fibres of nerve VII. By combining these two types of stimulation, it is possible to test the refractory period of the motor nucleus. This nucleus may be orthodromically activated by stimulation of the supra-orbital nerve. Supramaximal antidromic stimulation of the seventh cranial nerve is then applied utilizing progressively longer delays between the two stimuli. By recording from the orbicularis oculi muscle, one observes that the blink reflex occurs 5—6 msec after the direct motor response (Fig. 1, upper part). This result indicates that the refractory period of the motoneurone is extremely brief if taking into account the antidromic conduction time (Fig. 1, lower part). This result is not compatible with the duration of a recurrent inhibition of the Renshaw type such as has been described at the spinal level (Penders and Delwaide, 1973).

There remain surely possibilities of judicious selection of nervous trunks which have not been fully explored to this date: stimulation of the digital nerves in relation to the motor activity of the upper extremities; of the femoral-cutaneous nerve in relation to the quadriceps muscle, etc.

Anesthesia

Matthews and Rushworth (1957) have shown that progressive anesthesia of a nerve with procaine can, at least with certain concentrations of the anesthetic, selectively suppress the activity of small diameter fibres without affecting large diameter fibres. By this technique, one is able to block the gamma fibres and therefore to appreciate the contribution of the muscle spindle system. Since 1960, this technique has been frequently used (Rushworth, 1960; Knutsson et al., 1973) although it has been the object of some criticism (Gassel and Diamantopoulos, 1964).

The fusimotor system can also be depressed in a selective manner by local cooling of the muscle (Eldred et al., 1960). Knutsson and Mattsson (1969) have employed this technique in the para-clinical examination of spastic patients. However, as in the case of procaine, criticism can be directed at this method (Delwaide et al., to be published). Local ischemia has also been used to anesthetize peripheral receptors (Goodwin et al., 1972). Finally, certain cutaneous territories or sensory nerves can be anesthetized.

In summary, anesthesia may be used in various combinations to try to clarify an experimental situation.

Microneuronography

Hagbarth and his colleagues have developed an ingenious technique which allows the recording in man of the activity of nervous fibres. With this technique, one may also specify the type of receptor in which these fibres originate. This technique is actually utilised by many researchers to study the patterns of afferent discharges (Hagbarth and Vallbo, 1968; Gybels and Van Hees, 1972; Struppler and Ervel, 1972).

In man, this technique allows the analysis of complex experimental situations. Thus, Burg et al. (1975) were able to demonstrate modifications in the discharge of Ia fibres during a Jendrassik maneuver. Gybels and Van Hees (1972) have analysed the discharge of afferent C fibres following painful cutaneous stimulation. Hagbarth et al. (1973) have studied afferent impulses following percussion of the Achilles tendon in spastic patients. Hagbarth et al., (1970) have also shown modifications in the discharge of Ia fibres in Parkinson's disease.

Although the technique is both new and difficult, it is currently of great usefulness.

EXPERIMENTAL SEARCH FOR EFFECTIVE STIMULI

It is sometimes possible to look for the effective stimulus in a complex experimental situation. For example, in clinical neurophysiology, the interpretation of vibratory inhibition of monosynaptic reflexes is very difficult (Lance et al., 1966). When a vibratory stimulus is applied to the tendon of the soleus muscle, one can assume that it activates muscle spindles of this muscle but also that it diffuses to the antagonist muscle and that it provokes a significant cutaneous stimulation. However, in creating a simpler experimental situation producing the same effect but utilizing fewer kinds of afferents, one may look for those afferents which are directly responsible for the inhibition of the tendon reflex. To do this, we have replaced the vibratory stimulus by passive mobilisation at variable speeds of the ankle. With these conditions, the muscles of the anterior and posterior compartments of the leg are alternately stretched. This stretching provokes as with the vibratory stimulus a stimulation of the muscle spindle receptors of both soleus and tibialis anterior, especially of their primary endings. But, contrary to the vibrations, the cutaneous stimulation is reduced or even absent. We have been able to establish that this maneuver provokes an inhibition of the monosynaptic reflex (Fig. 2A) which is related chiefly to the stretching of the posterior compartment of the leg. If vibration is applied during passive stretching of the soleus, there is no reinforcement of the inhibition. This inhibition seems to be caused by the same mechanism as that following vibration and this result suggests that an occlusion would intervene between the two inhibiting mechanisms. One may thus conclude that the cutaneous stimulus is of little importance in producing the vibratory inhibition (Delwaide, 1971). In a later experiment, we designed another maneuver to verify that the effective inhibitory afferents come from posterior rather than the anterior compartment of the leg. With this in mind, we have studied the influence of a progressive and selective stretching of the triceps muscle. This stretching is realized with the ankle immobilised using a progressive and regular pressure on the Achilles tendon (Delwaide, 1971). This stretching causes stimulation of the muscle spindles only in the triceps surae. The skin is anesthetised at the site of pressure. If it is carried out at a slow speed, the stretching of the triceps muscle also provokes inhibition of the monosynaptic reflex. This inhibition is not reinforced by application of the vibratory stimulus. This second step in the analysis of vibratory stimulation allows the affirmation that the majority of inhibitory influx comes from the spindles of the posterior compartment of the leg (Delwaide, 1971). Starting from a complex situation (stimulation of at least three kinds of afferents), we were able to restrict the effective inhibitory afferents to the spindles of the posterior compartment of the leg.

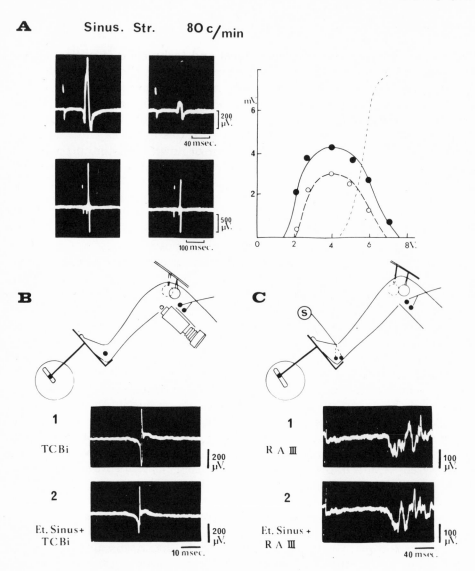

Fig. 2. (A) The monosynaptic reflexes of the soleus are inhibited during the sinusoidal movement of the ankle at 80 cycles/min. Upper row: tendon reflex; lower row: H reflex. On the right, comparison of recruitment curves of the H reflex; plain line: control values; dotted line: during the maneuver. (B) The monosynaptic reflex of the short biceps femoris is also inhibited. Schema of the experimental procedure and examples of control value (1) and test value (2). (C) The polysynaptic reflex evoked in the short biceps by painful stimulation of the sural nerve is not inhibited (compare 1 and 2) during the maneuver shown on the top of graph.

Pharmacology

The use of drugs in man involves ethical and technical difficulties. However, it can be hoped that this method of research will allow progression in the analysis of afferent pathways. Succinylcholine has already been used in man to provoke the discharge of the primary spindle endings (Brune et al., 1960). The results obtained by this pharmacological activation strongly resemble those obtained by vibratory stimulation. Unfortunately, one cannot hope for a selective activation of either a flexor or extensor group, and the possibility of action at the spinal and supraspinal level must be questioned in each instance.

ANALYSIS OF THE RESULTS

The difficulty in selectively activating medullary afferents does not constitute the only problem in clinical reflexology. Moreover, numerous mechanisms both inhibitory and facilitory, capable of modifying the amplitude of the reflex are known to exist in the central nervous system. Even with the proper selection of afferents, numerous questions must be systematically raised in order to interpret the results. In other words, the experimental situation is often comparable to the solution of an equation with several unknowns. This analogy may raise the fear that no solution is possible. However, as in the case of this type of equation, an answer may be found by using a system of equations containing the same unknowns. This is why it is always interesting to study the effects of a conditioning maneuver on the largest possible battery of spinal tests rather than on one predetermined test such as the Hoffman reflex, tendon reflex, etc.

Pragmatically, what are the most interesting tests to be carried out together for interpreting reflex changes?

Comparison of the H reflex and the tendon reflex

The Hoffman reflex is provoked by electrical stimulation of Ia afferent fibres of sciatic nerve, proximal to the muscle spindles of the soleus muscle. Schematically, one can say that variations of amplitude of the Hoffman reflex are independent of fluctuations of spindle tone. The tendon reflex, on the contrary, is dependent upon modifications of spindle tone and thus upon the gamma system. Therefore, comparison of the results of a conditioning maneuver on the H and the tendon reflex may reveal the activity of the spindle system.

Paillard (1955) has demonstrated the interest of this comparison which is now largely used (Gassel, 1973; Pierrot-Deseilligny and Lacert, 1973). However, the differences between tendon and H responses may not be exclusively attributed to the action of the gamma neurones. Other factors, notably the duration of the afferent message which is clearly longer and asynchronous following percussion of the tendon, must be taken into consideration.

Comparison of monosynaptic and polysynaptic reflexes

It is possible to simultaneously activate certain motor nuclei by mono-synaptic and by polysynaptic pathways (Young, 1973). This is the case for the motor nucleus of the biceps femoris (Hugon, 1967) and for the motor nucleus of the soleus (Delwaide, 1971). Comparison of results obtained by these two types of stimulation may be of interest in two situations:

1) If the monosynaptic reflex is inhibited while the polysynaptic reflex is augmented, one may postulate an inhibitory action affecting on the myotatic arc to the motoneurones. Such a result suggests the intervention of pre-synaptic inhibition acting on the Ia fibres (Delwaide, 1971).

2) If the monosynaptic reflex is facilitated, while the polysynaptic reflex is inhibited, one is drawn to the conclusion that an inhibitory action is being exercised on the interneurones.

The comparison of mono- and polysynaptic responses has been advocated for the study of spinal mechanisms in the cat (Pompeiano, 1968). The criticism that may be made of this technique, however, is that it is not certain that the two reflexes excite the same motoneurones (Henneman et al., 1965; Ashworth et al., 1967; Grimby and Hannertz, 1968).

Comparison of the results obtained on extensor and flexor muscles

The motor nuclei of extensor and flexor muscles are influenced different-ly by certain peripheral afferents. The Ia fibres originating in a particular muscle facilitate the homonymous motoneurones but, reciprocally, inhibit the antagonistic motor nucleus. Irrespective of the muscle they originate from, the group II afferents for their part facilitate the flexor nuclei and inhibit the extensor nuclei (Lloyd, 1946; Brock et al., 1951; Laporte and Lloyd, 1952). Their role is often questioned when inhibition of the Achilles reflex is observed following stretching of the triceps surae muscle. In addi-tion, one must consider that the FRA (Lundberg, 1964) is made up of various afferents (muscular and cutaneous) which specifically facilitate the flexor motor nuclei. Comparison of effects produced by the same maneuver on a flexor and an extensor reflex, respectively, may thus be of interest. We used this methodology to interpret the influence of a sinusoidal movement of the ankle on the excitability of the H reflex (Fig. 2).

In this maneuver, inhibition of the monosynaptic reflexes of the soleus is observed in relation to the stretching of the posterior compartment of the leg. To establish if the group II afferents play a role in this inhibition, we have studied the influence of ankle movement on the monosynaptic reflex of the biceps femoris muscle. It must first be ascertained that the movement of the foot does not stretch the muscles of the thigh. When the technical conditions are optimal, an inhibition of 20% is observed in the tendon reflex of the biceps femoris (Fig. 2B). The polysynaptic RA II reflex is also inhibited while the nociceptive RA III reflex is not modified (Fig. 2C). The exploration of biceps femoris muscle seems to negate the existence of an important discharge in the group II fibres of muscular origin coming from the leg. In this case, a facilitation and not an inhibition of the monosynaptic reflex of the biceps femoris would be expected (flexor muscle).

Other possibilities still exist for interpreting the results of reflexologic explorations in man, notably the study of occlusion phenomena. For example, distinct experimental maneuvers which, when performed separately, cause a reflex inhibition, may or may not contribute an inhibitory influence on a given response when performed together. If the resulting inhibition corresponds to the sum of the inhibitions observed after each maneuver, one is drawn to the conclusion that two distinct mechanisms operate. On the contrary, if no additional inhibition is observed, it would seem that both maneuvers induce inhibition by the same circuit.

It seems that pharmacological studies are raising some hope for future research. Several interesting results have already been obtained in this way. For example, de Gail et al. (1966) have shown by the use of barbiturates that the neuronal pathway responsible for the tonic vibration reflex is polysynaptic and distinct from that which causes the vibratory inhibition of phasic monosynaptic reflexes. Diazepam may be used to reinforce presynaptic inhibition (Schmidt et al., 1967; Delwaide, 1971).

At this time, there have been few reflex studies in man utilizing clonidine although this product is employed in animal neurophysiology (Forssberg and Grillner, 1973) and extensively utilised in clinical medicine. It must, however, be recalled that the effects induced by drugs are most often multiple and complex and not easily analyzed.

COMMENTS

Criticisms may be formulated in regard to the clinical neurophysiology of human reflex studies. This approach is not as analytical as in animal experiments and some physiologists are reluctant to accept it (Matthews, 1972; Granit and Burke, 1973). Of course, in human reflexology, the evidence is sometimes indirect and the conclusions in some instances must remain speculative. However, certain tests have been thoroughly analyzed and permit satisfactory exploration of specific spinal circuits. Moreover, one may stress the specific advantage of studies in humans, notably the possibility of collaboration with the subject.

Despite their limitations, the electrophysiological studies of human spinal circuits prove to be indispensable in the physiopathological analysis of most of the motor syndromes. More severe criticisms may be formulated against the validity of experimental models. In order to improve the reliability of exploration in humans, it is necessary that the protocol is as close as possible to the requirements of animal neurophysiology. Moreover, a very strict methodology is indispensable due to the number of possible variables (Hugon, 1973). If such a methodology is followed, it is possible to obtain regularly reproducible quantitative results.

It is striking to note the satisfactory concordance existing between the conclusions deduced from experimentation in man, despite the technical limitations involved, and the results obtained in animal neurophysiology. In certain cases, notably in the interpretation of the effects of vibratory stimulations, clinical neurophysiology has preceded animal physiological research (Delwaide, 1969; Gillies et al., 1969).

Owing to the techniques which have now been developed, clinicians have obtained new insights into the neurological syndromes. For example, an important heterogeneity has been demonstrated in the pyramidal syndrome (Castaigne et al., 1972). One may hope that in the near future reflexology will specify, in each patient, the relative contribution of diverse physiopathological mechanisms and provide a logical basis for treatment.

REFERENCES

ASHWORTH, B., GRIMBY, L. and KUGELBERG, E. (1967) Comparison of voluntary and reflex activation of motor units. Functional organization of motorneurones. J. Neurol. Neurosurg. Psychiat., 30, 91—98.

BROCK, L.C., ECCLES, J.C. and RALL, W. (1951) Experimental investigation on the afferent fibers in muscle nerves. Proc. R. Soc. Biol., 138, 453—475.

BRUNE, H.F., DAMMAN, R. and SCHENCK, E. (1960) Chemische Aktivierung der Muskelspindeln beim Menschen: Die Bedeutung der Spindelmechanik für die spinalen Effekte. Pflügers Arch. Ges. Physiol., 181, 484—493.

BURG, D., SZUMSKI, A.J., STRUPPLER, A. and VELHO, F. (1975) Observations on muscle receptor sensitivity in the human. Electromyogr. Clin. Neurophysiol., 15, 15—28.

CASTAIGNE, P., HELD, J.P., CATHALA, H.P., PIERROT-DESEILLIGNY, P., BUSSEL, B. and MORIN, C. (1972) Modifications de l'excitabilité médullaire induites par une stimulation cutanée chez différentes catégories d'hémiplégiques. Rev. Neurol., 126, 393—400.

de GAIL, P., LANCE, J.W. and NEILSON, P.D. (1966) Differential effects on tonic and phasic reflex mechanisms produced by vibration of muscles in man. J. Neurol. Neurosurg. Psychiat., 29, 1—11.

DELWAIDE, P.J. (1969) Approche de la physiopathologie de la spasticité. Réflexe de Hoffmann et vibrations appliquées sur le tendon d'Achille. Rev. Neurol., 121, 72—74.

DELWAIDE, P.J. (1971) Etude expérimentale de l'hyperréflexie tendineuse en clinique neurologique. Editions Arscia S.A. Bruxelles, 324 p.

DELWAIDE, P.J. (1974) Le stimulus vibratoire en neurophysiologie clinique: aspects physiologiques et physiopathologiques. Rev. d'E.E.G. Neurophysiol., 4, 539—553.

ECCLES, J.C. (1964) The physiology of synapses. Springer Verlag, Berlin, G.F.R., 316 p.

ELDRED, E., LINDSLEY, D.F. and BUCHWALD, J.S. (1960) The effects of cooling on mammalian muscle spindles. Exp. Neurol., 2, 144—157.

FORSSBERG, H. and GRILLNER, S. (1973) The locomotion of the acute spinal cat injected with clonidine i.v. Brain Res., 50, 184—186.

GASSEL, M.M. (1973) An objective technique for the analysis of the clinical effectiveness and physiology of action of drugs in man. In (J.E. Desmedt, Ed.) New Developments in Electromyography and Clinical Neurophysiology, Vol. 3, Karger, Basel, pp. 342—359.

GASSEL, M.D. and DIAMANTOPOULOS, E. (1964) The effect of procaine nerve block on neuromuscular reflex regulation in man (an appraisal of the role of the fusimotor system). Brain, 87, 729—742.

GILLIES, D., LANCE, J.W., NEILSON, P.D. and TASSINARI, C.A. (1969) Presynaptic inhibition of the monosynaptic reflex by vibration. J. Physiol. (Lond.), 205, 329—339.

GOODWIN, G.M., Mc CLOSKEY, D.I. and MATTHEWS, P.B.C. (1972) The persistence of appreciable kinesthesia after paralysing joint afferents but preserving muscle afferents. Brain Res., 37, 326—329.

GRANIT, R. and BURKE, R.E. (1973) The control of movement and posture. Brain Res., 53, 1—28.

GRIMBY, L. and HANNERTZ, J. (1968) Recruitment order of motor units on voluntary contraction: changes induced by proprioceptive afferent activity. J. Neurol. Neurosurg. Psychiat., 31, 565—573.

GYBELS, J. and VAN HEES, J. (1972) Unit activity from mechanoreceptors in human peripheral nerve during intensity discrimination of touch. In (G.G. Somjen, Ed.) Neurophysiology Studied in Man. Excerpta Medica, Amsterdam, pp. 198—206.

HAGBARTH, K.E. and VALLBO, A.B. (1968) Discharge characteristics of human muscle afferents during muscle stretch and contraction. Exp. Neurol., 22, 493—503.

HAGBARTH, K.E., HONGELL, A. and WALLIN, B.G. (1970) Parkinson's disease: afferent muscle nerve activity in rigid patients. Acta Soc. Med. Uppsala, 75, 70—76.

HAGBARTH, K.E., WALLIN, G. and LOFSTEDT, L. (1973) Muscle spindle responses to stretch in normal and spastic subjects. Scand. J. Rehab. Med. 32, 18—25.

HENNEMAN, E., SOMJEN, G. and CARPENTER, D.O. (1975) Functional significance of cell size in spinal motoneurons. J. Neurophysiol., 28, 560—580.

HUGON, M. (1967) Réflexes polysynaptiques cutanés et commandes volontaires. Thèse de Doctorat d'Etat des Sciences Naturelles. Fac. Sci. Paris.

HUGON, M. (1973) Methodology of the Hoffmann Reflex in Man. In (J.E. Desmedt, Ed.) New Developments in Electromyography and Clinical Neurophysiology, Vol. 3, Karger, Basel, 277—293.

KNUTSSON, E. and MATTSSON, E. (1969) Effects of local cooling on monosynaptic reflexes in man. Scand. J. Rehabil. Med., 1, 126—132.

KNUTSSON, E., LINDBLOM, U. and MÅRTENSSON, A. (1973) Differences in effects in gamma and alpha spasticity induced by the Gaba derivative Baclofen (Lioresal). Brain, 96, 29—46.

LANCE, J.W., de GAIL, P. and NEILSON, P.D. (1966) Tonic and phasic spinal cord mechanisms in man. J. Neurol. Neurosurg. Psychiat., 29, 535—544.

LAPORTE, Y. and LLOYD, D.P. (1952) Nature and significance of the reflex connections established by large afferent fibers of muscular origin. Am. J. Physiol., 169, 609—621.

LLOYD, D.P. (1943) Conduction and synaptic transmission of reflex response to stretch in spinal cats. J. Neurophysiol., 6, 317—326.

LLOYD, D.P. (1946) Integrative pattern of excitation and inhibition in two-neuron reflex arcs. J. Neurophysiol., 9, 439—444.

LUNDBERG, A. (1964) Supraspinal control of transmission in reflex paths to motorneurones and primary afferents. In (J.C. Eccles and Schade P. Eds) Physiology of Spinal Neurons, Elsevier, Amsterdam; Progr. Brain Res., 12, 197—221.

MATTHEWS, P.B.C. (1972) Mammalian muscle receptors and their central actions. Edward Arnold (Publishers) Ltd., London, 630 p.

MATTHEWS, P.B. and RUSHWORTH, G. (1957) The selective effect of procaine of the stretch reflex and tendon jerk of soleus muscle when applied to its nerve. J. Physiol. (Lond.), 135, 245—262.

PAILLARD, J. (1955) Réflexes et régulations d'origine proprioceptive chez l'homme, Thèse Fac. Sci. Paris (Sér. A nr. 2858-3729) Arnette, Paris, 293 p.

PIERROT-DESEILLIGNY, E. and LACERT, P. (1973) Amplitude and variability of monosynaptic reflexes prior to various voluntary movements in normal and spastic man. In (J.E. Desmedt, Ed.) New Developments in Electromyography and Clinical Neurophysiology, Vol. 3, Karger, Basel, pp. 538—549.

PENDERS, C.A. and DELWAIDE, P.J. (1973) Physiologic approach to the human blink reflex. In (J.E. Desmedt, Ed.) New Developments in EMG and Clinical Neurophysiology, Vol. 3, Karger, Basel, pp. 649—657.

POMPEIANO, O. (1968) Monosynaptic and polysynaptic reflex excitation of motorneurones to plantar muscles in the unrestrained cat. Brain Res., 10, 252—256.

RENSHAW, B. (1940) Activity in the simplest spinal reflex pathways. J. Neurophysiol., 3, 373—387.

RUSHWORTH, G. (1960) Spasticity and rigidity: an experimental study and review. J. Neurol. Neurosurg. Psychiat., 23, 99—117.

SCHMIDT, R.F., VOGEL, M.E. and ZIMMERMAN, M. (1967) Die wirkung von Diazepam auf die präsynaptische Hemmung und andere Rückenmarksreflexe. Arch. Exp. Pathol. Pharmacol., 258, 69—82.

SHAHANI, B.T. and YOUNG, R.R. (1972a) Human orbicularis oculi reflexes. Neurology, 22, 149—154.

SHAHANI, B.T. and YOUNG, R. (1972b) The cutaneous nature of the first component of the monkey's blink reflex. Neurology, 22, 438.

STRUPPLER, A. and ERBEL, F. (1972) Analysis of proprioceptive excitability with special reference to the unloading reflex. In (G.G. Somjen, Ed.) Neurophysiology Studied in Man, Excerpta Medica, Amsterdam, pp. 298—304.

STRUPPLER, A., BURG, D. and ERBEL, F. (1973) The unloading reflex under normal and pathological conditions in man. In (J.E. Desmedt, Ed.) New Developments in Electromyography and Clinical Neurophysiology, Vol. 3, Karger, Basel, pp. 603—617.

YOUNG, R.R. (1973) The clinical significance of exteroceptive reflexes. In (J.E. Desmedt, Ed.) New Developments in Electromyography and Clinical Neurophysiology, Vol. 3, Karger, Basel, pp. 697—712.

5

Effects of vibration on human spinal reflexes

Gyan C. AGARWAL and Gerald L. GOTTLIEB

Vibration applied to the muscle tendon provides an additional mechanism with which to study motor function in man. By means of a specially modified electrical audio speaker system, vibration from 60 to 200 Hz was applied at the Achilles tendon of the gastrocnemius—soleus muscles of normal human subjects. The same device was used to apply a tendon tap to elicit a tendon-jerk reflex. The Hoffmann reflex was elicited by applying a voltage pulse on the tibial nerve in the popliteal fossa.

The tonic vibration reflex is observed mostly at lower frequencies of vibration (up to 120 Hz). At these frequencies, both the tendon-jerk and Hoffmann reflexes are reduced by vibration. At higher frequencies (above 160 Hz) the peak-to-peak amplitude of the synchronized electrical activity of the tendon-jerk reflex increases in some subjects while there is no effect on the Hoffmann reflex.

In 1938, Coermann (referred to by Goldman, 1948) observed that during the operation of a vibrating platform on which a human subject was seated, it was difficult or impossible to obtain the patella reflex. Goldman (1948) studied the effect of mechanical vibration on the patella reflex of the cat. The vibration was applied with a modified permanent magnet loudspeaker at various frequencies (in most experiments at 100 Hz with 1 mm amplitude). He made the following observations:

'When the vibrator was applied directly to the belly of the muscle or to the tendon or the femur, the knee jerk was much reduced or was abolished entirely. The effect appeared immediately upon applying the vibrator and disappeared immediately on removing it. The muscle was often seen to undergo a slight contraction which persisted as long as the vibrator was applied'.

Goldman gave the following interpretation to his findings:

'Vibration produces a periodic, synchronous stretch reflex in which many of the muscle receptors are involved. There is thus a slight continuous contraction of the muscle and tapping the tendon is now ineffective since the reflex arc is in steady use'.

Interest in this vibration effect was renewed by the studies of Hagbarth and Eklund (1966) and De Gail et al. (1966). The tonic vibration reflex and the suppression of both the H-reflex and the tendon-jerk were observed in each of these studies (see Hagbarth, 1973, and Lance et al. 1973, for reviews of the literature).

As shown in recordings from muscle afferents both in cat (Granit and Henatsch, 1956; Brown et al., 1957; Bianconi and Van der Meulen, 1963) and in man (Hagbarth and Vallbo, 1968), the primary endings of the muscle spindles are easily excited by vibration applied to the tendon of muscle. In cats, the upper frequency limit of the spindle primaries can be as high as 800/sec (Von Euler and Peretti, 1966). Little is known about the upper frequency limit of human primary spindle endings, but during weak-to-moderate isometric contraction, frequencies of 75—100/sec have been observed in humans (Vallbo, 1970a,b).

The suppression of the tendon-jerk reflex during muscle vibration may well be due to the fact that the primary endings are so engaged by the vibratory stimulus that they are not able to respond efficiently to a transient superimposed increase in muscle length (Goldman, 1948; De Gail et al., 1966; Hagbarth and Eklund, 1966). This has been termed as the 'busy-line' phenomenon.

It is possible that an afferent busy-line phenomenon contributes to the suppression of the Hoffmann reflex during vibration. There is also evidence that the vibration-induced afferent inflow may cause presynaptic inhibition of the monosynaptic pathway (Lance et al., 1968: Gillies et al., 1969; Delwaide, 1971).

In this paper, we report some preliminary experiments on the effects of vibration on the H-reflex and the tendon-jerk reflex at vibration frequencies of 60, 100, 160 and 200 Hz. We have observed that the tendon-jerk reflex may be enhanced by high frequency vibration which is contrary to what has been reported in the literature so far.

EXPERIMENTAL PROCEDURE

The vibration was applied at the Achilles tendon using a modified Acoustic-Research 12-inch speaker system (see Gottlieb and Agarwal, 1973b for details of the construction) driven by an Inland 100 W dc power amplifier. In all cases the vibrator was driven to the maximum of the linear range of the power amplifier system. The maximum peak-to-peak amplitude of the vibration at 60 Hz was about 1.1 mm. This amplitude fell off at higher frequencies as the square of the frequency, i.e., at 200 Hz the amplitude of vibration was about 0.1 mm.

The vibrators used in experiments by Lance and his associates and by Hagbarth and Eklund were of the physiotherapy type with large surface areas. In our experiment, the vibration applied was localized on the tendon. The tip of the vibrator had a width of 1.2 cm and thickness of 0.5 cm.

A subject was seated normally in a chair with his right leg extended, the knee slightly flexed, and the foot strapped to a fixed plate having four strain gauges in a bridge circuit attached for measuring torque. The experiment was controlled by a digital computer (General Automation SPC-16) which also sampled and recorded five output data channels: (a) foot torque at 250 samples per second; (b) and (c) full wave rectified and filtered EMGs recorded via surface electrodes on the two muscle groups, gastrocnemius—soleus (GSM) and anterior tibial (ATM) at a rate of 500 samples per second; (d) an unfiltered EMG from the GSM at 1000 samples per second for 100 msec following the stimulus for measurement of electrical reflex response, and (e) stimulus at 1000 samples per second for 100 msec.

For the Hoffmann reflex, the electrical stimuli were applied to the subject's tibial nerve by means of cutaneous electrodes located posteriorly in the popliteal fossa and anteriorly above the knee. The stimuli were monophasic, square pulses of 1.5 msec duration provided at 5—7 second intervals by a Grass S-8 stimulator with an SIU5 isolation unit. All electrodes were coated with Sanborn Redux Creme.

The tendon-jerk was elicited by superimposing a 15-msec force pulse on the vibrator. The stimulus force was measured through a strain gauge bridge attached in a U-bend at the head of this electromechanical hammer. The movement of the hammer during tendon taps was recorded via a linear potentiometer. The vibration amplitudes were measured visually using an optical magnifier. For further details of the equipment and procedure, see Gottlieb et al., 1970; Agarwal and Gottlieb, 1972; Gottlieb and Agarwal, 1973a,b.

RESULTS

Vibration at lower frequencies (60 and 100 Hz) produces tonic activity in the muscle, the tonic vibration reflex (TVR), as shown in Fig. 1. No measurable TVR activity was noticed at 160 and 200 Hz. The amplitude of vibration in these experiments is frequency dependent and was about 1.1 mm at 60 Hz and fell off to 0.1 mm at 200 Hz. The peak-to-peak amplitude of the Hoffmann reflex is shown in Fig. 2. At 60 Hz, the H-wave is nearly suppressed. There is no significant effect at 200 Hz.

The effect of vibration on the tendon-jerk reflex at these four frequencies is shown in Fig. 3. This figure shows the peak-to-peak amplitude of the electrical response (equivalent of H-wave) elicited by the tendon jerk. At 60 and 100 Hz, the tendon jerk is inhibited, whereas at 160 and 200 Hz the

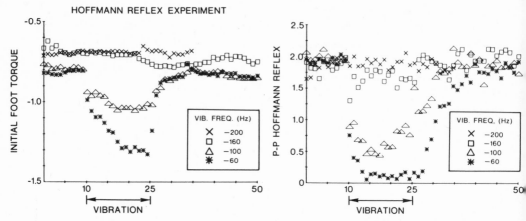

Fig. 1. Dependence of tonic vibration reflex on the vibration frequency. Vibrator is turned on after the 10th stimulus and turned off after the 25th stimulus. The negative torque is in the plantar direction. At 200 Hz only 35 reflexes were recorded.

Fig. 2. Peak-to-peak amplitude of the Hoffmann reflex before, during and after vibration at vibration frequencies of 60, 100, 160, and 200 Hz.

reflex response is increased up to 5 times of the control value without vibration.

This increase of the tendon-jerk reflex at 200 Hz is not due to the synchronization of the motor units. The width of the filtered reflex EMG at 20 percent points is about 34 msec (mean) during vibration at 100, 160, and 200 Hz and about 30 msec (mean) during vibration at 60 Hz. The width of the filtered reflex EMG without vibration is 40 msec (mean). Assuming that

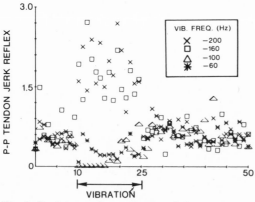

Fig. 3. Peak-to-peak amplitude of the tendon-jerk reflex before, during and after vibration at vibration frequecies of 60, 100, 160 and 200 Hz.

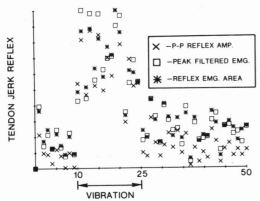

Fig. 4. Tendon-jerk reflex measured by three different methods at vibration frequency of 200 Hz. (a) peak-to-peak reflex amplitude measured as in Fig. 3; (b) peak reflex response of the rectified, filtered EMG, and (c) the area of the rectified, filtered EMG for 30 msec interval from the lower 20 percent point. The Y-axis scales are adjusted to match the maximum and minimum points.

synchronization would increase EMG amplitude by narrowing its width, this indicates some synchronization tendency of the motor units due to vibration, but the degree of synchronization is about the same at all frequencies.

To further analyze this increase in the tendon-jerk reflex, Fig. 4 shows the reflex response measured at 200 Hz vibration frequency by three different methods: (a) the peak-to-peak amplitude of the unfiltered reflex EMG as in Fig. 3, (b) the peak reflex response of the rectified and filtered EMG, and (c) the area of rectified and filtered reflex EMG for the 30 msec interval from

TABLE 1

Peak-to-peak amplitude of Hoffmann reflex (data of Fig. 2).

Vibration frequency (Hz)		200	160	100	60
Range	min.	1.65	1.30	0.445	0.059
	max.	2.06	2.12	2.14	2.03
Before vibration	mean	1.86	1.85	1.99	1.94
points 1—10	S.D.	0.121	0.092	0.063	0.049
During vibration	mean	1.91	1.64	0.685	0.195
points 10—25	S.D.	0.071	0.129	0.173	0.184
After vibration	mean	1.83*	1.95	1.74	1.36
points 26—50	S.D.	0.072	0.138	0.270	0.580
After vibration	mean	—	2.02	1.84	1.79
points 41—50	S.D.	—	0.090	0.116	0.078

* 25—35

TABLE 2

Peak-to-peak amplitude of tendon-jerk reflex (data of Fig. 3).

Vibration frequency (Hz)		200	160	100	60
Range	min.	0.332	0.234	0.022	0.088
	max.	2.66	2.69	1.28	0.949
Before vibration points 1—10	mean	0.507	0.715	0.508	0.521
	S.D.	0.155	0.354	0.115	0.124
During vibration points 11—25	mean	1.84	1.68	0.198	0.301
	S.D.	0.443	0.406	0.237	0.156
After vibration points 26—50	mean	0.639	0.599	0.617	0.582
	S.D.	0.170	0.192	0.211	0.168
After vibration points 41—50	mean	0.613	0.554	0.572	0.582
	S.D.	0.140	0.211	0.262	0.163

the time it exceeds 20 percent its maximum. The correlation between these three measurements is exceedingly good.

The mean and the standard deviation of the data in Fig. 2 and 3 are shown in Tables 1 and 2, respectively, for the peak-to-peak Hoffmann reflex and tendon-jerk reflex.

DISCUSSION

The TVR as seen in Fig. 1, builds up and decays rather slowly. This slowness of the vibration-induced responses suggests that they depend only in part upon simple monosynaptic excitation of motoneurones and in part upon polysynaptic spinal and supraspinal pathways involving higher centers. In some spasticity states it is not unusual to find that the TVR is weak or absent even though tendon jerks are exaggerated (De Gail et al., 1966; Lance et al., 1966). This is a strong indication that the TVR utilizes central or polysynaptic spinal pathways.

Considering the hypothesis that TVR is actuated via the long loop pathways, such pathways are likely to act as low-pass filters due to transmission and synaptic delays. This could explain why TVR is not observed at higher frequencies. It must be added here that the vibratory stimulus is not selective for the primary endings and thus absence of TVR at high frequency may well be due to an abnormal release of vibration-induced autogenetic inhibitory reflexes that oppose or conceal the TVR. In our experiments the amplitude of vibration fell off as a square of the frequency. It is therefore also possible that the stimulus became sub-threshold to the Ia fibers at higher frequencies. This could explain the lack of vibration influence on the H-reflex at 160 and 200 Hz as seen in Fig. 2.

The facilitatory effect of vibration at 160 and 200 Hz on the tendon jerk is unexpected. We have not observed a similar effect on the H reflex. However, Hagbarth and Eklund (1966) report that, according to Yamanaka, facilitation of the H-reflex is promoted by high frequency vibration (about 300 Hz) of the calf muscles, whereas inhibition is promoted by vibration at lower frequencies (below 50 Hz). They further report that the excitatory effects are obtained only when the vibrator is applied to the Achilles tendon.

The excitatory effects on the tendon jerks by high-frequency vibration could be due to several alternative mechanisms: (a) changes in the spindle sensitivity produced by small generator potentials at sub-threshold vibration levels, (b) changes in the spindle sensitivity via long loops and the gamma motor system, and (c) frequency-dependent behavior of the peripheral receptors (spindles, Golgi tendon organ, cutaneous receptors) and their complex interaction at the spinal cord. These questions may be answered by a more extensive investigation applying vibration inputs at many amplitudes and frequencies.

ACKNOWLEDGEMENT

This work was supported in part by the National Science Foundation.

REFERENCES

AGARWAL, G.C. and GOTTLIEB, G.L. (1972) Computer controlled human motor system experimentation. In (C.V. Freiman, Ed.) Information Processing-71, North Holland Publishing Co., Amsterdam, pp. 1174—1178.

BIANCONI, R. and VAN DER MEULEN, J.P. (1963) The response to vibration of the end-organs of mammalian muscle spindles. J. Neurophysiol., 26, 177—190.

BROWN, M.C., ENGBERG, I. and MATTHEWS, P.B.C. (1967) The relative sensitivity to vibration of muscle receptors of the cat. J. Physiol., 192, 773—800.

DELWAIDE, P.J. (1971) Etude experimentale de l'hyperreflexie tendineuse en clinique neurologique. Arscia, Bruxelles.

DE GAIL, P., LANCE, J.W. and NEILSON, P.D. (1966) Differential effects on tonic and phasic reflex mechanisms produced by vibration of muscles in man. J. Neurol. Neurosurg. Psychiat., 29, 1—11.

EULER, C. VON and PERETTI, C. (1966) Dynamic and static contributions to the rhythmic gamma activation of primary and secondary spindle endings in external intercostal muscle. J. Physiol., 187, 501—516.

GILLIES, D., LANCE, J.W., NEILSON, P.D. and TASSINARI, C.A. (1969) Presynaptic inhibition of the monosynaptic reflex by vibration. J. Physiol., 205, 329—339.

GOLDMAN, D.E. (1948) Effect of mechanical vibration on the patella reflex in the cat. Am. J. Physiol., 155, 78—81.

GOTTLIEB, G.L. and AGARWAL, G.C. (1973a) Modulation of postural reflexes by voluntary movement: modulation of the active limb. J. Neurol. Neurosurg. Psychiat., 36, 529—539.

GOTTLIEB, G.L. and AGARWAL, G.C. (1973b) Modulation of postural reflexes by voluntary movement: modulation at an inactive joint. J. Neurol. Neurosurg. Psychiat., 36, 540—546.

GOTTLIEB, G.L., AGARWAL, G.C. and STARK, L. (1970) Interactions between voluntary and postural mechanisms of the human motor system. J. Neurophysiol., 33, 365—381.

GRANIT, R. and HENATSCH, H.D. (1956) Gamma control of dynamic properties of muscle spindles. J. Neurophysiol., 19, 356—366.

HAGBARTH, K.E. (1973) The effect of muscle vibration in normal man and in patients with motor disorders. In (J.E. Desmedt, Ed.) New Developments in Electromyography and Clinical Neurophysiology, Vol. 3, Karger, Basel, pp. 428—443.

HAGBARTH, K.E. and EKLUND, G. (1966) Motor effects of vibratory muscle stimuli in man. In (R. Granit, Ed.) Nobel Symposium I- Muscular afferents and motor control, Almquist and Wiksell, Stockholm, pp. 177—186.

HAGBARTH, K.E. and VALLBO, A.B. (1968) Discharge characteristics of human muscle afferents during muscle stretch and contraction. Exp. Neurol., 22, 674—694.

LANCE, J.W., BURKE, D. and ANDREWS, C.J. (1973) The reflex effects of muscle vibration. In (J.E. Desmedt, Ed.) New Developments in Electromyography and Clinical Neurophysiology, Vol. 3, Karger, Basel, pp. 444—462.

LANCE, J.W., NEILSON, P.D. and TASSINARI, C.A. (1968) Suppression of the H-reflex by peripheral vibration. Proc. Aust. Assoc. Neurol., 5, 45—49.

VALLBO, A.B. (1970a) Slowly adapting muscle receptors in man. Acta Physiol. Scand., 78, 315—333.

VALLBO, A.B. (1970b) Discharge patterns in human muscle spindle afferents during isometric voluntary contraction. Acta Physiol. Scand., 80, 552—566.

6

Effect of vibration on the F response

B.T. SHAHANI and R.R. YOUNG

Primary endings of muscle spindles are extremely sensitive to vibration both in cat (Granit and Henatsch, 1956; Bianconi and Van der Meulen, 1963; Brown et al., 1967) and in man (Hagbarth and Vallbo, 1968). When applied to the belly or tendon of a muscle, vibration normally induces a tonic reflex contraction of the muscle. Since vibration-induced Ia discharge imitates that produced by static fusimotor activation of the primary endings (Hagbarth and Vallbo, 1968), the tonic vibration reflex (TVR) has been used as a model for the study of tonic stretch reflexes in man. The observation that vibration of a muscle also produces suppression of phasic stretch reflexes, such as the tendon jerk and the H reflex in that muscle in normal man, has received great attention in recent years (Yamanaka, 1964; Lance et al., 1966; Hagbarth and Eklund, 1966; Rushworth and Young, 1966). It has been postulated that the principal physiological mechanism responsible for the suppression of these phasic reflexes is spinal 'presynaptic inhibition' (Lance et al., 1967; Gillies et al., 1969; Delwaide, 1971). In favor of this hypothesis, Lance and colleagues (Gillies et al., 1969) suggest that the excitability of motoneurones is substantially unchanged during vibration, since they found no influence of vibratory stimuli on the F response in the cat.

In human studies (Thorne, 1965; Mayer and Feldman, 1967), it has been established that the F response arises from the centrifugal discharge of a small percentage of motoneurones initiated by antidromic volleys in their axons. Although its latency is similar to that of the H reflex, the F response can be differentiated from this reflex response by certain specific characteristics which include: (1) appearance at a higher threshold than that required for the H reflex and the direct muscle (M) response (i.e., the evoked compound muscle action potential), (2) an amplitude of less than 5% of the M response, (3) impersistence of the F response, (4) fluctuations in latency and amplitude of the F response under constant conditions, (5) failure of supramaximal stimulation for the M response to block the F response, and (6) appearance of the F response in many muscles including small muscles of hands and feet in contrast to the H reflex which is normally present only in some of the large postural muscles in adults. Because F responses have been shown to occur in the absence of dorsal root input (Mayer and Feldman, 1967; McLeod and Wray, 1966), their initiation must be independent, at least under those circumstances, of segmental afferent input. Since F responses can arise from purely antidromic activation of motoneurones, our hypothesis is that an effect of vibration on the F response would be mediated elsewhere than presynaptically prior to the first Ia synapse. If vibration of a limb were to affect the F response in it, that would imply that vibration produces changes in the excitability of the spinal motoneurone pool itself, in addition to its presumed 'presynaptic' actions. The purpose of the present study was to determine whether it is possible or probable that vibration has other physiological actions besides pure presynaptic inhibition. It was therefore decided to study effects of vibration on the behavior of antidromically induced F responses in man.

METHODS

Studies were performed in 3 healthy volunteer subjects, 23 to 33 years of age, who lay supine on a comfortable couch in a warm room (24—27° C). Electromyographic activity was recorded from the abductor pollicis brevis muscle by means of surface electrodes (TECA 6030) applied with tape over the belly of the muscle, inter-electrode distance being approximately 2 cm. The hand was fixed in a specially designed splint. Single electric shocks (0.1 msec, square wave pulses) were delivered via surface bipolar-stimulating electrodes to the median nerve at the wrist at a rate of one every 2 seconds. In order to record F responses, stimulus intensity (voltage) was adjusted to be supramaximal for the direct muscle (M) response (i.e., approximately 20% more than the intensity required to produce a maximal M response). Vibration at approximately 150 Hz was applied to the lateral aspect of the thumb over the insertion of the abductor pollicis brevis muscle by means of the TVR vibrator 1a (F.A. Keydon, Uppsala, Sweden), which consists of a dc motor with an eccentric disc. The recording electrodes were connected to a TECA TE-4 EMG system, and F responses were recorded on 100 mm wide photographic paper with the fiber-optic graphic recorder in the sweep mode. Some 5—10 responses were recorded before, during, and after the application of vibratory stimuli, and experiments were repeated several times in these subjects.

RESULTS

With low-intensity stimuli, only the direct M response was seen in the

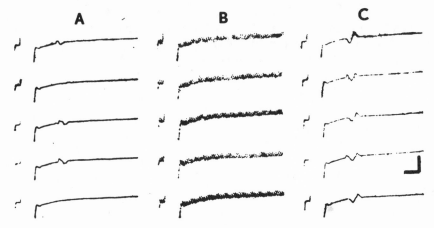

Fig. 1. Effects of vibration on the F response. Five sequential sweeps are recorded (A) before, (B) during, (C) immediately after vibratory stimulation. Note the artifact of vibration in (B) and the post-vibratory facilitation of the F response in (C). There is no change at any time in the M response. Calibrations are 15 msec and 500 μV.

abductor pollicis brevis muscle. Increases in the intensity of stimulation produced, in addition to an increase in amplitude of the direct M response, a 'late response' — the F response — which appeared at a latency of 26—28 msec. In different experiments, the persistence of the F response ranged from 3—5 F responses out of any 5 sequential trials in 2 subjects and 0—3

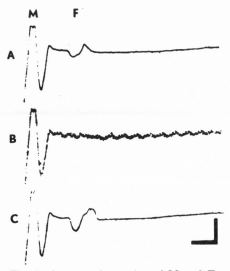

Fig. 2. A successive series of M and F responses at 2-sec intervals before (A), during (B), and immediately after (C) vibration. Note the vibratory artifact and depression of F response during (B). After vibration, the F response is large and more persistent (C). Calibrations are 10 msec and 500 μV.

out of 5 in one subject. In the first 2 subjects (F persistence 3—5/5), vibration produced not only suppression in the amplitude of the F response (Fig.
1B) but also a significant reduction in its persistence so that, during vibration, F responses were seen only 0—3 times out of 5 (Fig. 2B). In the other
subject who initially had a relatively impersistent F response (F persistence
0—3/5), vibration caused a marked increase in both amplitude and persistence of the F response. In all 3 subjects, there was post-vibratory facilitation — both the amplitude and the persistence of the F response was greater
in the immediate post-vibration phase than it was during the control records
(Figs. 1C; 2C). Indeed, in most experiments, the F response persistence was
5/5 in the post-vibratory phase. There was no evidence of voluntary background contraction or tonic reflex activity in the abductor pollicis brevis
muscle during these studies.

DISCUSSION

Several hypotheses have been put forward to explain the suppression by
vibration of H reflexes and tendon jerks in man. One of these is termed the
afferent busy-line theory — that is, most or all of the primary endings on (or
Ia fibers from) muscle splindles might be so engaged by the continuous
vibratory stimuli that they would be unable to respond to the transient
superimposed muscle stretch produced by a tap on the muscle's tendon. In
fact, in multi-unit recordings from human muscle nerves, the afferent response to a tendon tap (which normally appears as a fairly discrete shower of
impulses) is barely recognizable against the continuous background barrage
of Ia impulses produced by vibration (Hagbarth, 1973). However, by recording the more synchronous afferent volleys during H reflexes from the human
sciatic nerve with needle electrodes, Lance and his colleagues (Lance et al.,
1968; Gillies et al., 1970) found that the reduction in amplitude of the
afferent volley caused by Ia fibers being engaged by vibration-induced impulses appeared insufficient to account for the observed suppression of H
reflex. Because this 'occlusion' of the peripheral receptor was judged insufficient, it was necessary to postulate a central inhibiting process to account for
the phasic reflex suppression. This second hypothesis is usually formulated
in terms of presynaptic inhibition.

In recent years, it has been shown that vibratory stimulation, applied to
the tendon of an extensor muscle in the cat, causes appreciable presynaptic
inhibition of Ia fibers arising from the same muscle (Gillies et al., 1969;
Barnes and Pompeiano, 1970). The central effects of vibration, even when it
is applied to an isolated muscle in the animal laboratory, are complex, and
indeed, it has also been demonstrated that high-frequency longitudinal vibration of the lateral gastrocnemius-soleus muscles can produce facilitation of
the monosynaptic reflex recorded from medial gastrocnemius. This facilita-

tion disappears at the end of stimulation and is replaced by prolonged inhibition (Magherini et al., 1972). It would not be possible to separate these conflicting effects in human studies. In the clinical situation, where vibrators are applied to intact limbs, the vibration affects muscles other than those ending in the tendon immediately beneath the vibrator. It also affects receptors in skin, subcutaneous tissue, joints and so forth. Gillies et al., (1969) found no influence of vibratory stimuli on the F response in the cat at a time when there was profound suppression of the monosynaptic reflex in the same motoneurone pool, and therefore concluded that the excitability of the spinal motoneurones themselves was substantially unchanged. On the basis of this finding, they suggested that the inhibitory process must be acting at a presynaptic level.

In our present study on human volunteer subjects, we have been unable to confirm the findings they reported from studies on cats. On the contrary, our findings suggest that there are significant changes in the excitability of motoneurones, not only during vibration but also during the period immediately following cessation of vibratory stimuli. Since F responses were evoked by supramaximal stimuli for the M response, there was no possibility of any contamination of these late responses by a reflex component (H reflex) which, under these circumstances, would have been blocked by antidromic impulses set up in motor fibers of the mixed nerve. The effects of vibration, therefore, must be on the antidromically induced F response. Furthermore, since there was neither any evidence of a 'tonic vibration reflex' nor background voluntary activity in the abductor pollicis brevis muscle, the changes seen in the amplitude and persistence of the F response could not easily be attributed to either of these phenomena which are known to increase the excitability of the motoneurone pool. Vibration, as it is applied in man, must stimulate, in addition to the primary endings of the muscle being vibrated, similar endings in antagonist and other nearby muscles and a large number of cutaneous, joint and other receptors. It is, therefore, not surprising that vibration, in addition to any presynaptic inhibition it may produce, has significant post-synaptic effects on interneurones and the motoneurone pool in man.

The most convincing evidence to support the hypothesis that presynaptic inhibition accounts for the vibratory suppression of phasic reflexes in man has come from the work of Delwaide and his associates (Delwaide, 1969, 1973; Delwaide and Bonnet, 1969). He demonstrated differential effects of vibration on the activity in soleus motoneurones by showing that vibratory stimuli applied to the Achilles tendon can produce suppression of monosynaptic reflexes at a time when the amplitude of a polysynaptic reflex in the same muscle is enhanced (Delwaide, 1973). On the basis of this finding, he concluded that vibratory inhibition must selectively affect the myotatic arc upstream from the motoneurones since there was no evidence of post-synaptic inhibition of the motoneurones. On the basis of these studies, interaction of vibration with monosynaptic reflexes has been used as a model for the study of presynaptic inhibition in man, and some investigators have gone to the extent of using this model to evaluate the mode of action of certain pharmacological agents (Ashby and White, 1973; Ashby et al., 1974). If, indeed, the suppression of phasic reflexes by vibration in man were an example of pure presynaptic inhibition, one might justify using the interaction as a tool to study such phenomena. However, our preliminary studies have clearly demonstrated that vibration, as it is applied in man, has complex effects on the motoneurone pool and that there is a need for further systematic studies of actions of vibration on F responses. Suffice it to say that vibration, in addition to any presynaptic actions, also has post-synaptic (polysynaptic) inhibitory and other effects. It would, therefore, be an over-simplification either to use vibration clinically in physiological studies as a method to demonstrate pure presynaptic inhibition or to draw, from such studies, conclusions about basic mechanisms underlying the pathophysiology of spasticity in man.

REFERENCES

ASHBY, P. and WHITE, D.G. (1973) Presynaptic inhibition in spasticity and the effect of β-(4-chlorophenyl)-GABA. J. Neurol. Sci., 20, 329—338.
ASHBY, P., VERRIER, M. and LIGHTFOOT, E. (1974) Segmental reflex pathways in spinal shock and spinal spasticity in man. J. Neurol. Neurosurg. Psychiat., 37, 1352—1360.
BARNES, C.D. and POMPEIANO, O. (1970) Inhibition of monosynaptic extensor reflex attributable to presynaptic depolarization of the group I A afferent fibres produced by vibration of flexor muscle. Arch. Ital. Biol., 108, 233—258.
BIANCONI, R. and VAN DER MEULEN, J.P. (1963) The response to vibration of the end-organs of mammalian muscle spindles. J. Neurophysiol., 26, 177—190.
BROWN, M.C., ENGBERG, I. and MATTHEWS P.B.C. (1967) The relative sensitivity to vibration of muscle receptors of the cat. J. Physiol., 192, 773—800.
DELWAIDE, P.J. (1969) Approche de la physiopathologie de la spasticité: réflexe de Hoffmann et vibrations appliquées sur le tendon d'Achille. Rev. Neurol., 121, 72—74.
DELWAIDE, P.J. (1973) Human monosynaptic reflexes and presynaptic inhibition In (J.E. Desmedt, Ed.) New Developments in Electromyography and Clinical Neurophysiology, Vol. 3, Karger, Basel pp. 508—522.
DELWAIDE, P.J. and BONNET, M. (1969) Nouveau mécanisme à considérer dans l'inhibition du réflexe de Hoffmann. J. Physiol. (Paris), 61, 119.
GILLIES, J.D., LANCE, J.W., NEILSON, P.D. and TASSINARI, C.A. (1969) Presynaptic inhibition of the monosynaptic reflex by vibration. J. Physiol. (Lond.), 205, 329—339.
GILLIES, J.D., LANCE, J.W. and TASSINARI, C.A. (1970) The mechanism of the suppression of the monosynaptic reflex by vibration. Proc. Austr. Assoc. Neurol., 7, 97—102.
GRANIT, R. and HENATSCH, H.-D. (1956) Gamma control of dynamic properties of muscle spindles. J. Neurophysiol., 19, 356—366.
HAGBARTH, K.-E. (1973) The effect of muscle vibration in normal man and in patients with motor disorders. In (J.E. Desmedt, Ed.) New Developments in Electromyography and Clinical Neurophysiology, Vol. 3, Karger, Basel, pp. 428—443.

HAGBARTH, K.-E. and EKLUND, G. (1966) Motor effects of vibratory stimuli in man. In (R. Granit, Ed.) Muscular Afferents and Motor Control, Almquist and Wiksell, Stockholm, pp. 177—186.

HAGBARTH, K.-E. and VALLBO, A.B. (1968) Discharge characteristics of human muscle afferents during muscle stretch and contraction. Exp. Neurol., 22, 674—694.

LANCE, J.W., DE GAIL, P. and NELSON, P.D. (1966) Tonic and phasic spinal cord mechanisms in man. J. Neurol. Neurosurg. Psychiat., 29, 535—544.

LANCE, J.W., NEILSON, P.D. and TASSINARI, C.A. (1968) Suppression of the H-reflex by peripheral vibration. Proc. Austr. Assoc. Neurol., 5, 45—49.

MAGHERINI, P.D., POMPEIANO, O. and THODEN, U. (1972) The relative significance of presynaptic and postsynaptic effects on monosynaptic extensor reflexes during vibration of synergic muscles. Arch. Ital. Biol., 110, 70—89.

MAYER, R.F. and FELDMAN, R.G. (1967) Observations on the nature of the F wave in man. Neurology, 17, 147—156.

McLEOD, J.G. and WRAY, S.H. (1966) An experimental study of the F wave in the baboon. J. Neurol. Neurosurg. Psychiat., 29, 196—200.

RUSHWORTH, G. and YOUNG, R.R. (1966) The effect of vibration on tonic and phasic reflexes in man. J. Physiol. (Lond.), 185, 63—64P.

THORNE, J. (1965) Central responses to electrical activation of the peripheral nerves supplying the intrinsic hand muscles. J. Neurol. Neurosurg. Psychiat., 28, 482—495.

YAMANAKA, T. (1964) Effect of high frequency vibration on muscle spindles in the human body. J. Chiba Med. Soc., 40, 338—346.

7

Single muscle spindle afferent recordings in human flexor reflex

A. STRUPPLER and F. VELHO

Percutaneous recording of single muscle spindle afferents of the anterior tibial muscle has shown that a special type of muscle spindle ending can be activiated by skin afferents. These spindles show clear differences with respect to the primary endings and can be identified as group II afferents, according to the results of animal experiments. They can also facilitate a flexor reflex response. The role of skin afferents in human motor control is discussed.

Skin afferents act upon the motor system e.g. spinal (flexor reflex), cerebellar and cortical pathways. In the spinal cord the following possibilities exist:

(a) skin afferents activate alpha motoneurones,

(b) skin afferents activate gamma motoneurones, or

(c) skin afferents activate both alpha and gamma motoneurones (co-activation).

In order to investigate the role of skin afferents in motor control in humans, we decided to analyse an exteroceptive reflex because, in this case, a skin stimulus provokes the reflex response. The most appropriate model seems to be the flexor reflex for several reasons: anatomically, in the deep peroneal nerve almost all afferent fibres originate from muscle receptors, (except for a few joint and fascia afferents and a few skin afferents coming from the interosseal area of the foot). Functionally, the activity of muscle spindle afferents in such a flexor muscle can be investigated via proprioceptive (stretch), exteroceptive (skin stimulation of dorsum and plantar pedis) and voluntary innervation (dorsal flexion).

METHODS

In 23 experiments on 17 subjects in a supine position we recorded muscle spindle afferent activity and the flexor reflex response (EMG) simultaneous-

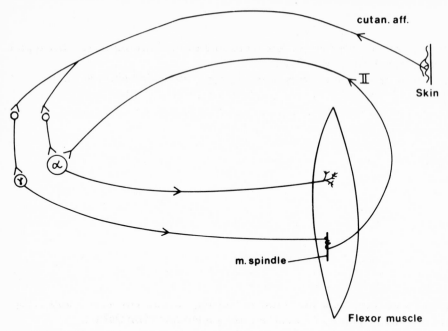

Fig. 1. Possible pathways mediating the flexor reflex on a spinal level.

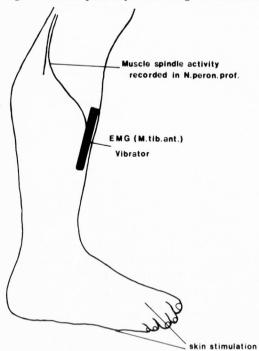

Fig. 2. Stimulation and recording points for analysis of the flexor reflex.

ly, following various stimuli. Muscle spindle afferents were detected according to the technique of Hagbarth and Vallbo (1968) in the deep peroneal branch (Fig. 2) and were identified according to our own methods (Struppler and Erbel, 1971; Burg et al., 1973).

The muscle spindle receptors were isolated, identified and recorded in the deep peroneal nerve of an unanesthetized human subject using tungsten semi-micro-electrodes. The electrode impedance was about 100—150 kOhm measured at 1000 Hz.

Single units were isolated in the nerve by minute manual manipulations of the electrode and the receptor was identified by criteria which included passive stretch, mechanical stimuli (muscle and tendon tap, ramp stretches, vibration) as well as spontaneous activity, voluntary activation and reinforcement (Jendrassik maneuvre). The ramp- and vibration-stimuli applied to the muscle were elicited by an electromagnetic transducer with an tip diameter of 1.5 mm. The deformations of the muscle ranged from microns to 2 mm and the slope, plateau, duration and frequency of the ramp stretches could be varied. In order to discriminate between Golgi- and muscle-spindle afferents we applied electrically induced twitch contraction of muscle fibres. Other types of receptors, like joint receptors, Paccini corpuscles and receptors of deep fascias, could be avoided using adequate stimulation.

In order to see whether skin stimuli could activate muscle receptors we applied slight skin stimuli (scratching with a needle or with a needle wheel) in the area of the N. suralis or saphenus, respectively (i.e. in the receptive field of the flexor reflex). The flexor response was recorded by means of EMG. The EMG electrodes were placed on the area of the tibial anterior muscle or flexor digitorum profundus muscle in which the muscle spindle could be activated by local tapping.

RESULTS

Multifibre recording — effect of slight skin stimulation on the foot

Multifibre recordings in a muscle fascicle supplying the tibial anterior muscle showed an increased background activity following slight skin stimulation (Fig. 3). In order to concentrate on the main point we selected amplitudes of more than 50 μV (2. line). The firing frequency is shown in the 3. line. The bar under the 2. line indicates skin stimulation eliciting increased afferent activity. The skin stimuli were sufficiently low so as not to evoke a reflex response, either in the muscle of the leg, or in the foot. Note that the afferent activity outlasted the skin stimulation by many seconds.

Single-fibre recording — identification of secondary endings

In some experiments we succeeded in recording single units, which we interpreted to be secondary spindle endings. Our evidence came from the

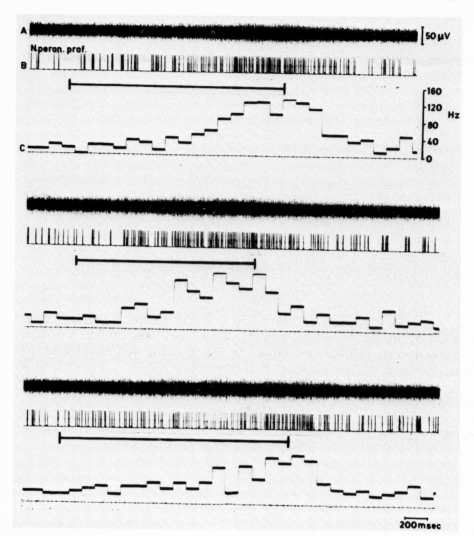

Fig. 3. Muscle spindle activity (multifibre recording) of m. tib. ant. following skin stimulation of the foot. A — multifibre recording of nerve fibre activity within the n. peroneus. B — electrically selected potentials with amplitudes higher than 50 μV (bar: skin stimulation). C — firing rate of selected potentials.

following observations:

   To elicit activity of this muscle spindle ending we usually had to apply a slight constant local pressure over the muscle area in which the receptor was probably located. No reinforcement effect by Jendrassik maneuvre could be detected on this type of receptor, suggesting that it could not be a Ia receptor. For further analysis, especially of the dynamic or static activity and the rate of frequency, we used passive stretch and unloading, ramp stimuli and

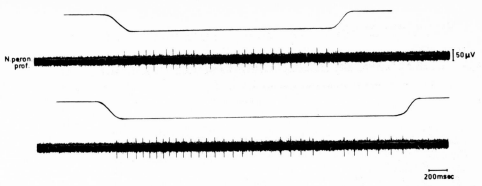

Fig. 4. Muscle spindle activity (secondary endings) of m. tib. ant. following passive stretch. Upper myogram of the ankle joint. Lower trace: single unit potentials recorded from the deep branch of the peroneal nerve.

vibration. The ramp and vibration stimuli were elicited by a vibrator and applied to the muscle in the area of the receptor. Following passive stretch the same unit showed a pronounced static sensitivity (Fig. 4). This was particularly evident following various ramp stretches (Fig. 5). No dynamic discharge was seen. Note in the lower line that the receptor could regularly follow vibration up to approximately 5/sec, but was unable to follow higher frequencies (25/sec and 80/sec in Fig. 5). It is well established that primary afferent endings respond in an approximately 1 : 1 relationship to vibratory stimuli up to 400 Hz (Brown et al., 1967; Fig. 6). Slight isometric voluntary contraction of the tibial anterior muscle could activate the same receptor. Note the relatively regular firing frequency of the afferent activity (Fig. 7). Furthermore, there is no increase of activity during the phase of muscle relaxation, as is seen in primary endings (Vallbo, 1970).

The activation of secondary endings by skin stimulation via gamma loop in a reflex arc

Recording single afferent activity we could also show that the secondaries were activated in a reflex fashion by skin stimuli. Following slight stimulation of the skin in different areas of the dorsum pedis with a steel needle, a sustained increase in the recruitment and firing frequencies of isolated receptors was noted (Fig. 8). The same effect can be evoked by slight stimulation of the plantar pedis, especially of the heel which is innervated from the tibial nerve (Fig. 9). Because the spindle activity followed the skin stimulation very constantly and regularly, without variation in latency or amount of activity, we can assume that this activity is evoked in a reflex arc and not by a voluntary reaction. The secondary endings of muscle spindles could be activated in a completely relaxed muscle by skin stimulation (Fig. 10). This was tested by monitoring subclinical muscle contractions in leg muscles and

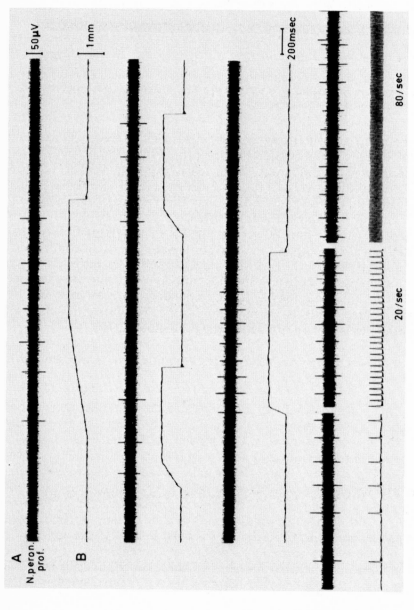

Fig. 5. Muscle spindle activity (secondary endings) of m. tib. ant. following ramp stretches. A — single unit potentials recorded from the deep branch of the peroneal nerve. B — ramp stretches applied on the receptor area of the muscle.

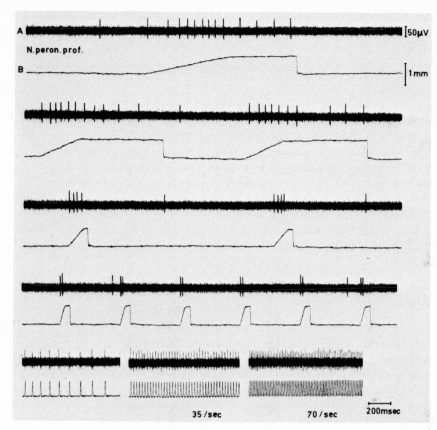

Fig. 6. Muscle spindle activity (primary endings) of m. tib. ant. following various ramp stretches. A — single unit potentials recorded from the deep branch of the peroneal nerve. B — ramp stretches applied on the receptor area of the muscle.

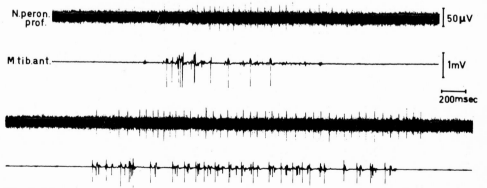

Fig. 7. Muscle spindle activity (secondary endings) of m. tib. ant. during slight isometric contraction. Upper trace: single unit potentials recorded from the deep branch of the peroneal nerve. Lower trace: m. tib. ant. EMG.

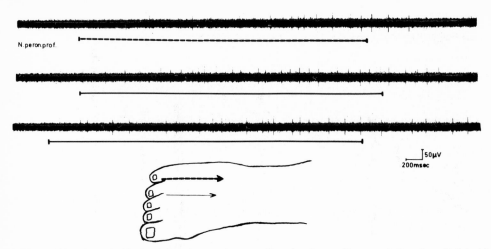

Fig. 8. Muscle spindle activity (secondary endings) of m. tib. ant. following slight skin stimulation.

small foot muscles using EMG. Primary endings, on the other hand, reveal another feature: they are not activated by skin stimulation, and only when the tibialis anterior muscle was activated in the flexor reflex could we detect an increased frequency of the primary endings during the relaxation phase of the muscle at the end of contraction.

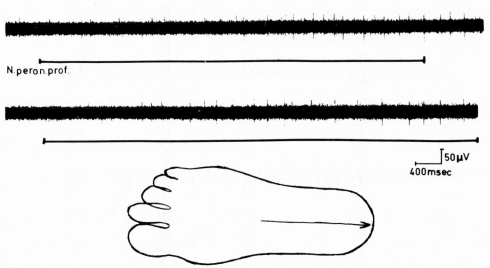

Fig. 9. As Fig. 8 (Struppler, 1974).

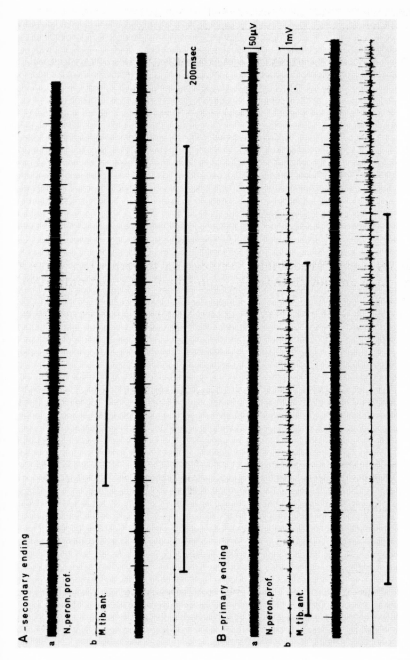

Fig. 10. Muscle spindle activity of secondary (A) and primary (B) endings of the m. tib. ant. following skin stimulation (bar). a — single unit potentials recorded from deep branch of peroneal nerve. b — m. tib. ant. EMG.

DISCUSSION

We have been able to record muscle spindle afferents in the deep peroneal branch which could be activated in a reflex fashion via skin stimuli on the receptive field of the flexor reflex (Struppler, 1974), and we shall now discuss the nature of this receptor. According to the results of experiment performed in animals (Cooper, 1961; Mathews, 1962; Bessou and Laporte, 1962; Hunt and Ottoson, 1973) the receptors could be interpreted as secondary endings; in contrast to the primary endings they showed a static sensitivity only, they only followed a low vibration frequency, the discharge outlasted the skin stimuli and there was no reinforcement effect. Following voluntary innervation the spindles were more regularly activated and did not show any unloading effect following muscle relaxation. Finally, they could be activated in a reflex fashion by skin stimulation without any alpha activation.

As a result of these findings a question arises as to the role of skin afferents in human motor control. Hagbarth (1952) has shown that skin stimulation activates the muscle underlying the skin, probably via gamma and alpha drive. In cats, Lloyd (1943, 1946, 1952) showed that the activity of secondary endings can activate the flexor response. Blocking the skin afferents by local anesthesia in man changes the unloading effect during a voluntary innervation (Marsden et al., 1971). In animals it could be demonstrated, however, that the excitation of flexor motor neurones by group II muscle afferents is much weaker and usually manifest only as facilitation of monosynaptic test reflex or the accompanying synaptic depolarisation recorded by intracellular micro-electrodes (McIntyre, 1974). These findings on experimental animals are in good agreement with our finding in man that secondary endings can be activated in a reflex arc by skin stimuli. The afferent activity in a muscle fascicle of a flexor muscle following slight skin stimulation of the foot provokes a facilitatory effect and seems to precede the alpha-motoneurone flexor activity.

ACKNOWLEDGEMENT

This work was supported by the Deutsche Forschungsgemeinschaft.

REFERENCES

BESSOU, P. and LAPORTE, Y. (1962) Responses from primary and secondary endings of the same neuromuscular spindle of the tenuissimus muscle of the cat. In (Barker, D., Ed.) Symposium on Muscle Receptors. Hong Kong Univ. Press.
BROWN, M.C., ENGBERG, I. and MATTHEWS, P.B.C. (1967) The relative sensitivity to vibration of muscle receptors of the cat. J. Physiol., 192, 773—800.

BURG, D., SZUMSKI, A., STRUPPLER, A. and VELHO, F. (1973) Afferent and efferent activation of human muscle receptors involved in reflex and voluntary contraction. Exp. Neurol., 41, 754—768.

COOPER, S. (1961) The responses of the primary and secondary endings of muscle spindles with intact motor innervation during applied stretch. J. Exp. Physiol., 46, 389—398.

HAGBARTH, K.-E. and VALLBO, A.B. (1968) Discharge characteristics of human muscle afferents during muscle stretch and contraction. Exp. Neurol., 22, 674—694.

HUNT, C.C. and OTTOSON, D. (1973) Receptor potentials and impulse activity in isolated mammalian spindles. J. Physiol., 230, 49.

LLOYD, D.P.C. (1943) Neuron patterns controlling transmission of ipsilateral hind limb reflexes in cat. J. Neurophysiol., 6, 293—315.

LLOYD, D.P.C. (1946) Integrative patterns of excitation and inhibition in two-neuron reflex arcs. J. Neurophysiol., 9, 439—444.

LLOYD, D.P.C. (1952) On reflex actions of muscular origin. Res. Publ. Assoc. Nerv. Ment. Dis., 30, 48—67.

MARSDEN, C.H., MERTON, P.A. and MORTON, H.B. (1971) Servo action and stretch reflex in human muscle and its apparent dependence on peripheral sensation. J. Physiol., 216, 21.

MATTHEWS, P.B.C. (1962) The differentiation of two types of fusimotor fibres by their effects on the dynamic response of muscle spindle primary endings. Quart. J. Exp. Physiol., 47, 324—333.

McINTYRE, A.K. (1974) Central actions of impulses in muscle afferent fibres. In (C.C. Hunt, Ed.) Handbook of Sensory Physiology, Vol. III/2, Ch. 3, 262.

STRUPPLER, A. and ERBEL, F. (1971) Analysis of proprioceptive reflex excitability with special reference to the unloading reflex. Satell. Symp. XXV Int. Congr. Physiol. Paris, Excerpta Medica Int. Congr. Series 253.

STRUPPLER, A. (1974) Données actuelles de microneurographie chez l'homme. Rev. EEG Neurophysiol., 4, 525—538.

VALLBO, A.B. (1970) Slowly adapting muscle receptors in man. Acta Physiol. Scand., 78, 315—333.

Central control of movement

1. Supraspinal mechanisms on a spinal level
   by P.G. Kostuyk   211

2. Functional organization of the primate oculomotor system
   by G. Westheimer and S.M. Blair   237

3. The spatial distribution of climbing fibre suppression of Purkinje
   cell activity
   by F.J. Rubia and W. Lange   247

4. Visual input and its influence on motor and sensory systems in man
   by M. Shahani   261

5. The effects of tonic, isometric contraction on the evoked EMG
   by G.C. Agarwal and G.L. Gottlieb   283

6. The EMG analysis of certain negative symptoms caused by lesions
   of the central nervous system
   by B.T. Shahani and R.R. Young   293

7. Asterixis — a disorder of the neural mechanisms underlying sustained muscle contraction
   by B.T. Shahani and R.R. Young   301

8. A review of physiological and pharmacological studies of human
   tremor
   by B.T. Shahani and R.R. Young   307

1

Supraspinal mechanisms on a spinal level

P.G. KOSTYUK

Descending signals coming to the spinal cord from supraspinal structures are transmitted directly to motoneurones only in certain cases. Monosynaptic connections with the latter are established by the medial descending system (vestibulo- and fast reticulo-spinal pathways). The lateral system (cortico- and rubro-spinal pathways) is connected almost exclusively to the spinal interneuronal apparatus, and only in primates some of its fibers terminate directly on motoneurones innervating distal limb muscles.

A quantitative study of the terminal distribution of different descending pathways in the spinal gray matter indicates the existence of specialized interneuronal groups connected to separate pathways. Both morphological and electrophysiological data prove that most interneurones in these specialized groups can be classified as proprio-spinal. Their axons enter the lateral or ventral funiculi where they pass over several segments and, after re-entering the gray matter, establish connections with motoneurones or other interneurones. Such proprio-spinal neurones often have no synaptic inputs from peripheral afferents. They may serve in transmission of specialized descending signals to motoneurones. A certain transformation of the internal structure of the signal takes place here on the basis of post-activation and synaptic inhibition.

Micro-electrode recordings from segmental interneurones connected to primary afferents show that the synaptic action of descending pathways upon such neurones is comparatively weak and not very specific. The lateral descending system exerts a general facilitatory effect upon spinal reflex mechanisms, which is to some extent antagonistic to the general depression of spinal reflex activity mediated through ventral and lateral reticulo-spinal pathways. A more specific facilitatory effect is observed only from the medial descending system in interneurones mediating reciprocal inhibition to flexor motoneurones.

A special type of descending action upon segmental interneurones can be described as a releasing one. In this case the descending volley releases the activity of a whole interneuronal network which may produce complex patterned motor activity (stepping, scratching etc.), without affecting the pattern itself. Monoaminergic descending pathways may be responsible for this action.

Present electrophysiological data indicate that the supraspinal centers can exert their action upon motoneurones through different spinal mechanisms. Lundberg (1972) has classified them schematically as follows:

(1) monosynaptic excitation by descending fibers,

(2) polysynaptic excitation through 'private' interneurones not connected to spinal primary afferents,

(3) polysynaptic excitation (or inhibition) through interneurones of spinal reflex arcs.

Descending action on complex interneuronal systems capable of producing patterned motor activity has also to be considered. The peripheral feedback loop formed by gamma motoneurones and stretch receptors evidently also plays an important role in the realization of supraspinal motor commands, but this topic needs a special presentation.

MONOSYNAPTIC DESCENDING ACTION ON MOTONEURONES

The extent of descending monosynaptic action upon motoneurones is relatively limited. In mammals, such monosynaptic connections are established mainly by the medial descending system (vestibulo-spinal and medial reticulo-spinal pathways). The vestibulo-spinal fibers produce monosynaptic EPSPs in extensor, and the fast reticulo-spinal in flexor motoneurones of lumbar and thoracic spinal segments (Lund and Pompeiano, 1965, 1968; Grillner and Lund, 1966; Grillner et al., 1966; Shapovalov, 1966; Shapovalov et al., 1966; Shapovalov et al., 1967; Shapovalov and Grantyn, 1968; Preobrazhensky et al., 1969). An example of such action is presented in Fig. 1. Monosynaptic EPSPs were only recorded in the upper cervical segments of the same motoneurone after stimulation of both Deiters' nucleus and reticular formation (Wilson and Yoshida, 1969a). These motoneurones control head movements and cannot be classified as flexors or extensors.

A quite unique monosynaptic inhibitory action is produced in cervical motoneurones by vestibulo-spinal fibers coming from the medial vestibular nucleus. This is the only known example of descending inhibitory neurones sending their axons from the brainstem into the spinal cord. In all other cases the primary action of descending fibers is excitatory, and inhibition may be produced only by additional spinal interneurones (Wilson and Yoshida, 1969b).

The monosynaptic action of medial descending pathways on spinal motoneurones is important for the adjustment of their excitability during postural, rightening and kinetic tonic reflexes.

Contrary to the medial descending system, the lateral descending system (which includes cortico- and rubro-spinal pathways) is connected almost exclusively to the spinal interneuronal apparatus (Lloyd, 1941; Lundberg and Voorhoeve, 1962; Agnew et al., 1963; Corazza et al., 1963; Kato et al.,

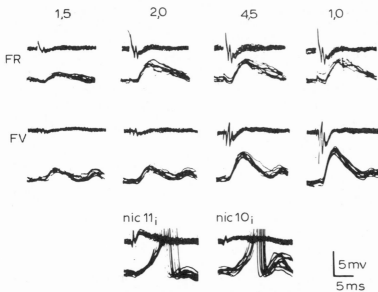

Fig. 1. Monosynaptic reticular responses in a thoracic motoneurone. Stimulated structures: reticular formation (FR), ipsi-lateral ventral funiculus (FV) and intercostal nerves (NIC). The relative strength of stimulation is indicated near each record. Upper trace in this and other figures — potential of the cord dorsal surface; lower trace — micro-electrode recording.

1964; Vasilenko and Vučo, 1966; Kostuyk and Pilyavski, 1967; Hongo et al., 1969; Bayev, 1971).

Only in primates do some fast cortico-spinal fibers excite motoneurones innervating distal limb muscles directly (Bernhard et al., 1953; Preston and Whitlock, 1960, 1961; Landgren et al., 1962; Uemura and Preston, 1965; Kernell and Wu, 1967).

Monosynaptic EPSPs in cat spinal motoneurones were observed after stimulation of the red nucleus (Shapovalov and Shapovalova, 1966; Shapovalov and Karamyan, 1968), but such findings have not been confirmed by other authors (Kostuyk and Pilyavsky, 1967; Hongo et al., 1969). In primates monosynaptic action on motoneurones from the red nucleus is a regular finding (Shapovalov et al., 1971).

Such direct connections of the lateral descending system are important for the control of fine voluntary phalangeal movements; according to morphological data, they may be present also in some carnivores capable of producing these movements, such as the racoon (Petras and Lehman, 1966; Buxton and Goodman, 1967).

The effectiveness of monosynaptic descending action upon motoneurones depends, of course, on the background synaptic activity produced in them by all other synaptic inputs. This action may select those cells in the motor nucleus which have already been brought close to the firing threshold.

SPECIALIZATION OF SPINAL INTERNEURONES WITH RESPECT TO
DESCENDING AND PRIMARY AFFERENT INPUTS

As direct connections of descending pathways to motoneurones are limited, it is obvious that the main stream of supraspinal signals is directed to
spinal interneurones.

Electrophysiological data show the existence of considerable specialization between spinal interneurones with respect to their main synaptic inputs.
There is also a spatial heterogeneity in the distribution of such interneurones. The location of spinal interneurones receving synaptic inputs from
different types of primary afferents was studied by several authors using
micro-electrode recordings. These neurones are located mainly in the base of
the dorsal horn, and their functional and topographic separation corresponds
to a certain extent to the division of the gray matter into Rexed's laminae
(Eccles et al., 1960; Wall, 1960, 1967; Pomeranz et al., 1968; Gokin, 1970).

The spatial separation of interneurones receiving different descending projections was shown morphologically using the experimental degeneration
technique (Szentágothai-Schimert, 1941; Nyberg-Hansen, 1966, and others).
To have a systematic picture of the topography of the synaptic connections
formed by different descending pathways comparable to the topography of
the synaptic connections of primary afferents, a quantitative analysis of the
distribution of axon terminals in the gray matter of various segments of the
cat spinal cord was made using Fink-Heimer's technique. This technique
stains the pre-terminals as well as the terminals of degenerating fibers and
thus gives reliable data about the location of their synaptic junctions. The
30-μm thick transverse sections of the spinal cord were systematically
scanned, and the density of degenerating elements was measured in 100 ×
100 μm squares. The diagrams obtained from animals with different experimental lesions could be easily compared in this way.

The results of this analysis are in general agreement with the previously
obtained results. The terminals of the cortico-spinal (pyramidal) fibers are
located mainly in the lateral parts of Rexed's laminae V and VI (Kostyuk et
al., 1972). The density of distribution increases in the direction from the
upper to lower cervical segments, and in the 8th cervical segment they are
distributed also in more ventro-lateral parts of the gray matter (lateral parts
of lamina VII). Some terminals can be traced in the medial parts of the base
of the dorsal horn. In the lumbar segments the relative density of pyramidal
tract terminals is considerably lower compared to the cervical ones (Fig. 2A).
The rubro-spinal fiber terminals are also located in the lateral part of the
intermediate gray matter. This region corresponds to the lateral parts of
Rexed's laminae VI and VII, partially overlapping with a region occupied by
terminals of the cortico-spinal system (Kostyuk and Skibo, 1974; see Fig.
2B). The difference in the topographic distribution of primary terminals and
terminals of the lateral descending systems is quite obvious; the primary

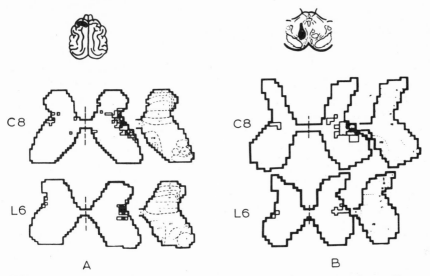

Fig. 2. Diagrams showing the terminal distribution of the lateral descending system in the gray matter of different segments of spinal cord. The terminals were revealed by the Fink-Heimer's technique after distribution of the contra-lateral sensorimotor cortex (A) and red nucleus (B). White squares indicate 5—10 degenerating elements, hatched squares 10—15 and black squares above 15.

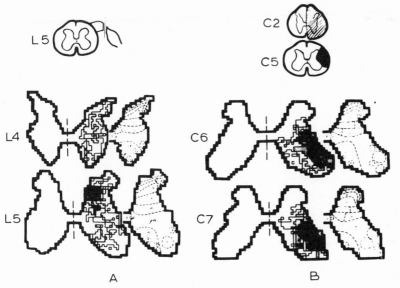

Fig. 3. Diagrams showing the terminal distribution of the primary afferents (A) and the proprio-spinal fibers (B) of the lateral funiculus in different spinal segments. Indications similar to Fig. 2.

afferent terminals are practically absent in the lateral parts of laminae V—VI—VII (Pogorelaya, 1973; see Fig. 3A).

The lack of primary afferent terminals in the lateral parts of the intermediate gray matter is compensated for here by abundant terminals of proprio-spinal neurones. The axons of such neurones enter the lateral column, pass over several segments and re-enter the gray matter. Their terminals can be revealed separately in experiments with a preliminary (several months before) hemisection of the spinal cord in the more cranial (lower thoracic) segments which causes the degeneration and consequent removal of all the long descending fibers. A subsequent local lesion of the lateral funiculus results in the degeneration of terminals of the proprio-spinal fibers cut during this lesion. The main quantity of such terminals is located just in the lateral parts of Rexed's laminae V—VI—VII, and in the region close to the lateral and dorso-lateral motor nuclei (Fig. 3B). They are less numerous in the Cajal's intermediate nucleus (central parts of laminae VI—VII) and rare in the dorsal part of lamina VIII. Proprio-spinal fiber terminals are absent in the dorsal, ventro-medial and more ventral parts of the gray matter. Terminals can be tracted at a distance of up to 5 segments from the level of lesion in the caudal direction; in the oral direction they extend over a shorter distance. The distribution of proprio-spinal fiber terminals is generally similar both in cervical and lumbar segments (Sterling and Kuypers, 1968; Kostyuk and Maisky, 1972; Pogorelaya and Tarusina, 1974). Retrograde degenerative changes after a lesion of the lateral funiculus can be found in the cells located in the same region of the gray matter where most of their axons terminate (i.e. in the lateral parts of Rexed's laminae V—VI—VII).

The presented morphological data support the suggestion that the lateral descending system is connected mainly with specialized groups of interneurones located in the most lateral parts of the intermediate gray matter. The 'specialized' neurones may interconnect several spinal segments and terminate on other interneurones as well as on motoneurones.

The medial descending system (vestibulo- and medial reticulo-spinal pathways) terminate mostly in the Rexed's lamina VIII and in the ventro-medial parts of lamina VII. Some terminals of this system are located also in the Cajal's intermediate nucleus, and can be traced up to the lateral border of the base of the dorsal horn. The latter projections are seen better in the lower thoracic segments. Medial system terminals are found also in the motor nuclei (lamina IX); here they are distributed irregularly, occurring mostly in the ventro-medial nuclei, being absent in the dorso-lateral ones (Kostyuk and Skibo, 1972; see Fig. 4A).

Using the technique of two subsequent spinal cord sections, the termination of proprio-spinal fibers passing in the ventral funiculus can be followed in the same way as is shown above for the lateral funiculus. The terminals of these fibers are distributed in the same region as those of long descending pathways (Skibo, 1974, see Fig. 4B). The somata of proprio-spinal neurones

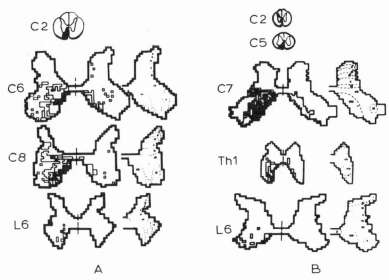

Fig. 4. Diagrams showing the terminal distribution of the medial descending system in the gray matter of different spinal segments. The whole ventral funiculus was sectioned in the 1st cervical segment (A). The terminal distribution of the proprio-spinal fibers of the ventral funiculus is shown in B. Indications similar to Fig. 2.

are located in lamina VIII and the adjacent part of lamina VII, and terminals of their axons are distributed over several segments in the caudal direction.

The region receiving predominantly terminals of the medial descending and proprio-spinal pathways contains only few terminals of the primary afferents (compare Fig. 3A).

In the same experiments the relative amount of degenerating terminals belonging to a certain descending pathway in the region under investigation was determined electron-microscopically by counting a sufficiently large number of all axon terminals. About 10% of these in the lateral parts of laminae V—VI were found to belong to the cortico-spinal fibers (from 2000 terminals counted). About 10% of terminals in the lateral parts of laminae VI—VII belong to the rubro-spinal fibers. The whole remaining mass of terminals in this region does not belong either to the descending or to the primary afferent fibers as, after transection of the dorsal roots, the amount of degenrating terminals here does not exceed 0.4%. Obviously they are formed by the axons of proprio-spinal neurones. In fact, a considerable number of them undergo degenerative changes after transection of the lateral funiculus. But many terminals still remain unchanged even after this lesion; they have to be considered as terminals of local short-axon neurones. After the transection of the ventral funiculus at the level of upper cervical segments, degenerative features are found in about 16% of terminals of the latter; the remaining ones belong probably to proprio-spinal fibers of ventral funiculus and to short-axon cells.

SYNAPTIC PROCESSES IN INTERNEURONES 'PRIVATE' FOR THE DESCENDING SYSTEMS

In accordance with morphological data, the interneurones located in different parts of the gray matter reveal different types of synaptic activity in response to stimulation of descending and afferent inputs.

Interneurones responding with a short latency to stimulation of the lateral descending system are regularly found in the lateral parts of Rexed's laminae V—VI—VII. They either do not respond to stimulation of peripheral nerves and dorsal funiculus or produce weak and long latent responses (Vasilenko and Kostyuk, 1966). Many of these neurones can be identified as propriospinal neurones: they generate antidromic spikes after direct stimulation of the dorsolateral funiculus 19—36 mm caudally to the recording level (Fig. 5). The antidromic spikes appear after a short and constant latent period and follow high-frequency stimulation of the funiculus (Vasilenko et al., 1967). On the basis of measurement of conduction distances and latencies of antidromic excitation, the conduction velocities have been calculated for many lumbar proprio-spinal neurones; they range from 15 to 55 m/sec (mean value about 35 m/sec).

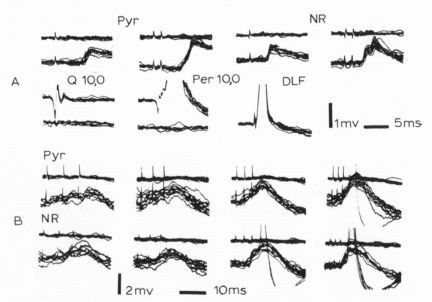

Fig. 5. Synaptic and antidromic responses in two proprio-spinal neurones (A,B) projecting into the lumbar dorso-lateral funiculus. Stimulated structures: pyramidal tract (Pyr), red nucleus (NR), dorso-lateral funiculus (DLF), nerves quadriceps (Q) and peroneal (Per).

Intracellular recording from such neurones reveal the presence of EPSPs in response to stimulation of pyramids and (or) red nucleus. The synaptic effects produced by these two structures in different neurones vary in relative amplitude and latency. Single stimuli evoke in both cases low-amplitude responses (rarely exceeding 0.4—0.8 mV). When a high-frequency series of stimuli is applied, an increase of the synaptic response is observed due to potentiation of separate EPSPs and their superposition (Fig. 5). Potentiation of the synaptic responses is observed during stimulation of both the pyramidal and rubro-spinal fibers, but during pyramidal stimulation it is more prominent. It should be noted that an increase in the number of stimuli usually evokes the appearance of late (obviously polysynaptic) reactions; this prolongs the whole duration of the EPSP up to 30—45 msec (Vasilenko et al., 1972).

A constant property of proprio-spinal neurones in the lateral funiculus is the development of a considerable hyperpolarization after the spike discharge; its amplitude reaches 3—5 mV. In some cases hyperpolarization can be evoked by stimulation of the dorso-lateral funiculus without a preceding antidromic spike (Fig. 6); this indicates that it may represent an IPSP (possibly of recurrent nature). This hyperpolarization establishes a limit for the transmission through proprio-spinal neurones of rhythmic descending volleys under repetitive stimulation. The maximal frequency of the evoked discharge does not exceed 25—30 imp/sec (see Fig. 7), and only short bursts of higher frequency may occur in response to high-frequency stimulation (Kostyukov, 1973).

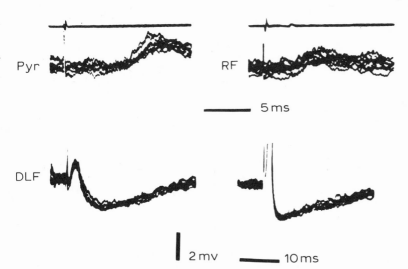

Fig. 6. Synaptic excitation and inhibition in a proprio-spinal neurone projecting into the lumbar dorso-lateral funiculus. Stimulated structures: pyramidal tract (Pyr), reticular formation (RF), dorso-lateral funiculus (DLF, different strength of stimulation).

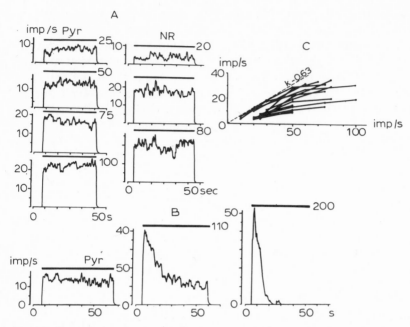

Fig. 7. The relation between the frequency of stimulation of the suprasegmental structures and the mean discharge frequency of 'private' interneurones in the lateral part of
the gray matter. (A,B) Mean frequency recordings of the discharge of two interneurones
in response to the stimulation of the pyramidal tract (Pyr) and red nucleus (NR). Frequency of stimulation is indicated near each record. (C) Relation between the frequency
of stimulation of the more effective suprasegmental structure and mean discharge frequency for 13 neurones.

Intracellular recordings confirm the conclusion that proprio-spinal neurones in the lateral funiculus are free of direct synaptic inputs from primary
afferents. In some neurones synaptic responses could be produced by stimulation of peripheral nerves but they were of polysynaptic nature. On the
other hand, in some neurones short-latency EPSPs appeared after stimulation
of the brain stem reticular formation (nucl. gigantocellularis). Such EPSPs
are connected with the activation of fast reticulo-spinal fibers (Anastasievich
et al., 1973). The convergence of pyramidal and rubro-spinal inputs in the
absence of direct primary afferent inputs is characteristic also for many
interneurones in the lateral part of dorsal horn of cervical cord (Bayev and
Kostyuk, 1973). A transection of the dorso-lateral funiculus in the cervical
and lumbar cord does not abolish di-synaptic EPSP in motoneurones evoked
by pyramidal stimulation, thus confirming the presence of proprio-spinal
neurones activated by cortico-spinal fibers (Stewart et al., 1968; Illert et al.,
1974).

To understand the functional role of proprio-spinal neurones receiving descending signals from the lateral system, it is important to know the projections of these neurones and the nature of synaptic processes produced by them in the following neuronal elements. This can be done to a certain extent by recording synaptic processes in motoneurones and interneurones after direct stimulation of the lateral funiculus in conditions when the long descending pathways are eliminated by preceding spinal cord hemisection in more cranial segments. Such stimulation evokes in the lateral funiculus a synchronized volley which can be recorded at a distance up to 60—65 mm (4—5 segments). The mean conduction velocity of this volley is about 38 m/sec in the lumbar segments and 44.5 m/sec in the cervical ones. These properties indicate that the volley represents the activation of relatively rapidly conducting proprio-spinal fibers of the lateral funiculus. If the strength of stimulation is increased, additional late components appear in the response, representing probably the activation of slowly conducting proprio-spinal fibers or the transsynaptic activation of other groups of spinal inter-neurones (Bayev et al., 1973b).

Similarities in the properties of the mass response produced by direct stimulation of the lateral funiculus and of the antidromic potentials recorded from unitary proprio-spinal neurones in the lateral parts of the inter-mediate gray matter justify the conclusion that both events are produced by the same structures.

The direct stimulation of the lateral funiculus deprived of long descending pathways produces characteristic post-synaptic responses in the motoneu-rones and interneurones of the corresponding segments. In the lumbar seg-ments monosynaptic EPSPs are observed predominantly in motoneurones innervating distal flexor muscles and monosynaptic IPSPs, and mixed reac-tions are observed in extensor cells (Fig. 8). Monosynaptic and polysynaptic EPSPs are also observed in interneurones, but somewhat stronger stimuli are necessary to evoke them comparing with PSPs in motoneurones (Kostyuk et al., 1971). In cervical segments similar stimulation also produces mono- and polysynaptic excitation of motoneurones but, contrary to what happens in the lumbar region, no distinct reciprocal pattern of PSP is observed. A more effective activation of interneurones is also characteristic for the cervical region compared to the lumbar one. Probably even the most rapidly con-ducting proprio-spinal fibers in the cervical cord establish synaptic contacts not only with motoneurones but also with interneurones (Bayev et al., 1973). The presented data seem to give indirect but reliable evidence for the suggestion that the proprio-spinal neurones located in the lateral parts of the gray matter and capable of transmitting descending signals from the cortico- and rubro-spinal fibers, form a direct pathway to motoneurones and, addi-tionally, sideways to other spinal neurones.

Stimulation of the medial descending system produces monosynaptic responses in many interneurones located in the medial part of the ventral

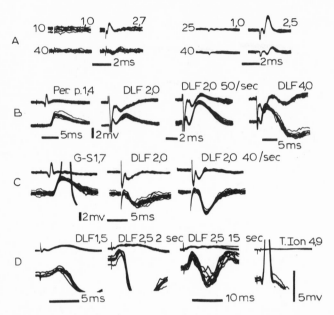

Fig. 8. Synaptic responses produced by separate stimulation of the proprio-spinal pathways in the lateral funiculus. The long descending pathways were eliminated by a preliminary hemisection of the spinal cord in the lower thoracic region. (A) Recording of the propagated volley in the proprio-spinal pathways of dorso-lateral funiculus (DLF) in the cervical (1) and lumbar (2) segments. The distance between the stimulation and recording sites and the relative strength of stimulation are indicated near each record. (B) Intracellular recording from a posterior biceps—semitendinosus motoneurone. (C) Intracellular recording from a gastrocnemius—soleus motoneurone. (D) Intracellular recording from a triceps—Longus motoneurone. Frequency of stimulation of the dorso-lateral funiculus (DLF) and its relative strength are indicated near each record.

horn (Rexed's lamina VIII). Micro-electrode recordings from the lower thoracic segments reveal that some of these neurones belong to segmental interneuronal pathways, while others cannot be activated by primary afferents and may be also considered as 'private' interneurones (Bezhenaru et al., 1972; see Fig. 9).

Selective stimulation of the proprio-spinal pathways in the ventral funiculus was performed by a technique similar to that already described for the lateral funiculus — after a preliminary section of the spinal cord that eliminates the long descending fibers in this part of the white matter. In this case a more cranial level of section is preferable because long proprio-spinal fibers connecting cervical and lumbar enlargements are present in the ventral funiculus and absent in the lateral one. Under such experimental conditions a proprio-spinal volley is also recorded when the ventral surface of the spinal cord is stimulated. The mean conduction velocity of this volley is higher

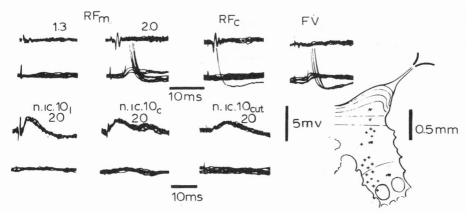

Fig. 9. Synaptic responses of an interneurone in the medial part of the ventral horn of the lower thoracic cord activated predominantly by medial descending system. Stimulated strcutures: ipsi-lateral medial reticular formation (RFm), contra-lateral medial reticular formation (FR_c), ipsi-lateral ventral funiculus (FV), ipsi-lateral internal intercostal nerve (nic IO_i), contra-lateral internal intercostal nerve (nic IO_{ic}), ipsi-lateral cutaneous intercostal nerve (nic IO_{cut}). The diagram shows the location of the recorded interneurones of this type.

when the stimulation point is in the thoracic segments than when it is in the lower lumbar region (corresponding values 50—70 and 38—45 m/sec; Vasilenko and Manzhelo, 1974). The most probable explanation of this phenomenon is that long proprio-spinal fibers in the ventral funiculus are fast-conducting while the shorter ones which are added to them in lumbar segments have lower conduction velocities.

Excitation of proprio-spinal pathways in the ventral funiculus exerts an intensive synaptic action upon lumbo-sacral motoneuronal pools. This action substantially differs from the effects of the stimulation of lateral pathways in two aspects:

(1) Reciprocity in action upon flexor and extensor motoneurones is not observed. Excitatory PSPs are recorded in many cells of both groups but mixed effects are also frequent. IPSPs are found in few motoneurones.

(2) Synaptic action from ventral proprio-spinal pathways upon motoneurones of proximal muscles is more intense than upon 'distal' motoneurones. Synaptic action is evoked in the majority of motoneurones of the first group when stimulation intensity is about threshold for producing the 'propriospinal volley' in the ventral funiculus. The amplitude of PSPs in motoneurones of distal muscles is less and more intensive stimulation of propriospinal pathways is usually required to evoke this action (Vasilenko, 1974). Examples of synaptic reactions in different motoneurones produced by stimulation of the proprio-spinal fibers in the ventral funiculus are shown in Fig. 10. It was claimed that the majority of lumbo-sacral motoneurones of

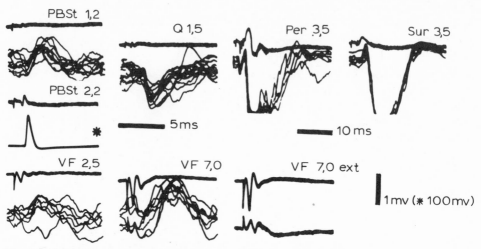

Fig. 10. Synaptic responses produced by separate stimulation of the proprio-spinal pathways in the ventral funiculus. The long descending pathways were eliminated by a preliminary ventral hemisection of the spinal cord in the cervical region. Intracellular recording from a posterior biceps—semitendinosus motoneurone. Stimulated structures: posterior biceps—semitendinosous (PBSt), quadriceps(Q), peroneal (Per), sural (Sur) nerves, ventral funiculus (VF), Extracellular field during funiculus stimulation (VFext). The relative strength of stimulation is marked near each record.

the cat have monosynaptic connections with ventral proprio-spinal pathways (Kozhanov, 1974). Perhaps it is true only for relatively short proprio-spinal fibers connecting neighbouring segments. When long ventral proprio-spinal pathways are stimulated, di- and polysynaptic effects are observed in neurones. It seems also that proprio-spinal fibers establishing monosynaptic contacts with motoneurones are thinner than the longer ones. Even when the conduction distance is short, the initial effects in motoneurones are usually di-synaptic, and monosynaptic PSP is only added when the stimulus is increased.

Direct stimulation of the ventral funiculus in cats with a normal spinal cord produces antidromic excitation of interneurones located in the medial part of the ventral horn of more cranial lumbar segments. Some of these neurones can be monosynaptically excited by reticulo-spinal pathways, but usually do not reveal synaptic responses to the stimulation of the primary afferents (Vasilenko, 1974; see Fig. 11).

The functional role of 'private' interneuronal pathways transmitting signals from both lateral and medial descending systems to motoneurones can be suggested on the basis of the described properties of their synaptic activation and connections.

(1) Most 'private' interneurones are in fact proprio-spinal neurones that send axons into the lateral or ventral funiculus where they pass over several

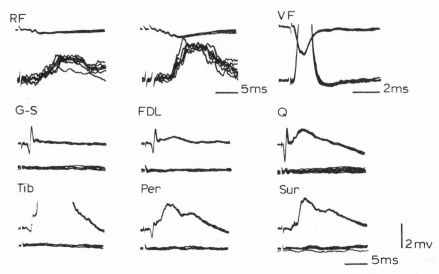

Fig. 11. Synaptic and antidromic reponses of a proprio-spinal neurone in the medial part of the lumbar spinal cord. Stimulated structures: reticular formation (RF), ventral funiculus caudal to the recording site (VF), gastrocnemius—soleus (GS), flexor digitorum longus (FDL), quadriceps (Q), tibial (Tib), peroneal (Per), sural (Sur) nerves.

segments before termination. Therefore, such interneurones may serve as spatial distributers of descending signals, producing synchronous synaptic action on many motoneurones and interneurones.

(2) 'Private' interneurones may integrate signals arriving through different descending pathways before transmitting them to other cells.

(3) 'Private' interneurones may serve as filters which facilitate the transmission to motoneurones of a certain form of descending signals and eliminating background noise.

SYNAPTIC PROCESSES IN INTERNEURONES OF SEGMENTAL REFLEX ARCS

Interneurones located in the central and medial parts of the base of the dorsal horn usually receive strong mono- and oligosynaptic excitatory action from primary afferents. On the basis of the PSP pattern a functional differentiation of interneurones can be made according to their preferential connection to a certain type of primary afferents, (see Eccles et al., 1960; Hongo et al., 1966).

Synaptic effects produced in these neurones by volleys from the lateral descending system are usually of polysynaptic nature. This has already been shown in the first investigation of pyramidal influences upon spinal interneurones (Lundberg et al., 1962). There is not much specificity in the effect of lateral descending systems upon segmental interneurones: facilitation of the transmission of volleys from group Ia and Ib muscle afferents is observed (in some cases inhibition of the transmission from high-threshold afferents was observed after stimulation of the red nucleus, but this may be an effect of concomitant involvement of reticulo-spinal pathways).

The facilitation of segmental interneuronal transmission produced from the red nucleus has a very short latency, indicating the possibility that it is produced at the last-order interneurone in the spinal neuronal chain (Hongo et al., 1969). The same conclusion can be drawn from the facilitatory effects of the cutaneous afferent volley upon di-synaptic rubro-motoneuronal responses (Baldissera et al., 1969, 1971).

Intracellular recording from segmental interneurones in cat lumbar cord shows that synaptic effects produced here by volleys from the lateral descending system have a relatively long latency, small amplitude and variable time-course (Fig. 12). They are more pronounced in interneurones transmitting signals from high-threshold afferents than in those connected to group I muscle or low-threshold cutaneous fibers (Zadorozhny et al., 1970). In the cervical cord the effectiveness of descending activation is probably higher; in some interneurones directly connected to primary afferents, monosynaptic EPSPs could be evoked also by pyramidal and (or) rubral volleys (Bayev and Kostyuk, 1972; see Fig. 13).

All these features of the lateral descending control of segmental interneurones are consistent with the idea of a general facilatatory action upon spinal reflex mechanisms, preserving the existing spinal coordinations (as the facilitation encompasses not only the excitatory but also the inhibitory neurones producing reciprocal inhibition of antagonistic muscles). Such general facili-

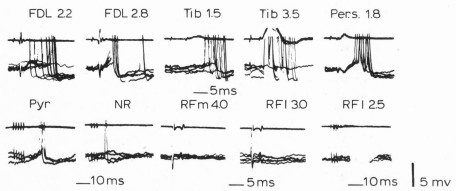

Fig. 12. Synaptic responses of an interneurone in the central part of the gray matter of the cat lumbar cord, monosynaptically activated by group Ia muscle afferents. The stimulation of pyramids (Pyr) resulted in variable long-latency PSPs. The stimulation of the dorso-lateral funiculus (DLF) produced no response. Stimulated nerves: gastrocnemius-soleus, flexor digitorum longus, suralis.

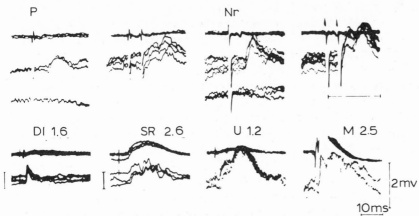

Fig. 13. Synaptic responses in an interneurone of cat cervical spinal cord. Stimulated structures: pyramidal tract (P), red nucleus (Nr), dorsal interosseus (DI), superficial radial (SR), ulnar (U) and median (M) nerves. Third trace in the upper oscillograms — extracellular field. Calibration 2 mV, 10 msec.

tation is to some extent antogonistic to the general depression of spinal reflex activity mediated through the ventral and lateral reticulo-spinal pathways and manifest at the level of both interneurones and motoneurones (Llinas and Terzuolo, 1964, 1965; Jankowska et al., 1964, 1968; Engberg et al., 1965, 1968; Kostyuk and Preobrazhensky, 1966). Probably, these opposite general descending actions regulate the transition of the spinal neuronal apparatus from a highly active state during performance into a damped one during rest.

Contrary to the lateral descending system, the medial system seems to produce a more specific effect upon the segmental interneurones. Stimulation of the vestibulo-spinal tract produces monosynaptic excitation of interneurones connected to group Ia muscle afferents (mediating reciprocal inhibition of flexor motoneurones) without affecting interneurones transmitting signals from cutaneous or high-threshold afferents (Grillner et al., 1966). Some facilitation is observed only in the transmission of influences from the contra-lateral high-threshold afferents (Bruggencate et al., 1969). Both the ipsi-lateral group Ia and contra-lateral high-threshold afferents produce similar effects in motoneurones, corresponding to the effects of the vestibulo-spinal volley: they inhibit flexor motoneurones and help to maintain tonic excitation of extensor muscles. Monosynaptic EPSPs in interneurones of this type can also be evoked by the stimulation of the medial reticular formation (Bezhenaru et al., 1972).

All described effects in segmental interneurones, contrary to the effects in direct and 'private' interneuronal pathways, do not bring quantitatively new features into the spinal reflex activity. They can be considered as more or less specific forms of descending regulatory action.

A most advanced type of descending action upon segmental spinal interneurones can be described as a releasing one. In this case the descending
volley releases the activity of a whole interneuronal network which otherwise is out of action. This network may produce complex alternating or
simultaneous activity of many functionally different motoneurones. The pattern of the activity is determined by spinal mechanisms, and the descending
signal only switches them on or off.

An example of this kind of action is the supraspinal control of stepping.
Stepping can be observed in acute spinal animals (Brown, 1911), but not in
chronic spinal conditions. In a decerebrated animal fixed over a moving
tread-mill it is regularly evoked by stimulation of the nucleus cuneiformis in
the midbrain (Shik et al., 1966b, 1967; see Fig. 14). Optimum stimulation
frequency is 30—60/sec, bearing no relation to the stepping rhythm. Deafferentation of the hind limbs does not abolish stepping in these conditions,
but preservation of the afferent inflow from the forelimbs is important (Shik
et al., 1966a).

Obviously the spinal cord has an intrinsic mechanism producing patterned
motor activity. The function of this mechanism is facilitated by afferent
inflow, but it can manifest itself only if a certain releasing signal reaches the
spinal cord from the brainstem. Stepping in acute spinal animals is obvious-

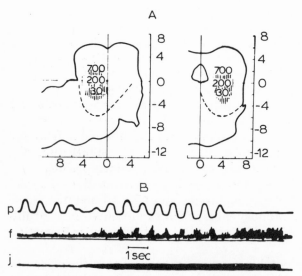

Fig. 14. Diagrams of sections through the 'locomotor' region in cat midbrain (A) and
discharges in ventral root filaments produced by its stimulation. Recordings of leg movement (P), discharge (F) and midbrain stimulation (J).

ly evoked by direct stimulation of the corresponding descending pathways; they may be of monoaminergic nature, as the injection of Dopa (a precursor of monoamines) can evoke stepping in a spinal animal (Grillner, 1969; Budakova, 1971).

Data about the action of Dopa on the spinal reflex pathways are important for the understanding of the mechanism of this releasing action. In spinal cats Dopa inhibits the usual short-latent post-synaptic effects produced by high-threshold afferents in spinal neurones; they are replaced by late long-lasting excitation of ipsi-lateral flexor and contra-lateral extensor motoneurones. Activity of contra-lateral flexor motoneurones is inhibited without post-synaptic hyperpolarization, obviously by blocking the interneuronal transmission (Jankowska et al., 1967). Long-lasting presynaptic depolarization of group I afferents is also observed (Anden, et al., 1966).

It is suggested that monoaminergic descending pathways stimulated by the injection of Dopa tonically inhibit the interneurones in the short latency path which in turn are inhibitory to the neurones of long-lasting action; consequently the action of the latter is released. Their reciprocal bilateral interaction can be a suitable mechanism for the rhythmic alternation of flexor and extensor movements during stepping. Interneurones which receive long-lasting reciprocal influences from high-threshold afferents of both sides can be traced in the dorso-lateral part of the ventral horn; possibly it is only these neurones that are carrying, in their connections, the spinal program for stepping.

A similar type of descending action probably releases such activities as scratching but no experimental data are yet available on this question.

The differentiation of spinal pathways into 'private' and 'common' ones is, to a certain extent, schematic. As has already been mentioned, the descending action upon segmental interneurones can be mediated primarily through specialized proprio-spinal interneurones as the direct stimulation of the latter produces synaptic effects not only in the motoneurones but also in other interneurones. But the close relations between the two forms of interneuronal activity still remain to be studied.

The interaction between different groups of interneurones can be characterized to a certain extent by direct recordings of motoneuronal PSPs produced by combined stimulation of descending and afferent systems. The occurrence of mutual facilitation of polysynaptic PSPs in motoneurones during near-threshold stimulation of descending and peripheral afferent systems, as was first stated by Lundberg et al., (1963), reflects with certainty the presence of a common interneurone in the spinal pathway transmitting the signals from these systems. For instance, the application of this technique for combined stimulation of the pyramidal and rubro-spinal systems always results in marked facilitation of the produced polysynaptic PSPs (Bayev and Kostuyk, 1973), thus confirming the presence of a common interneuronal pathway in the spinal cord (Fig. 15). At the same time facilita-

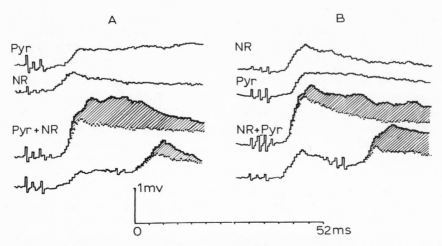

Fig. 15. Interaction of pyramidal and rubral PSPs in two flexor motoneurones (A,B) of the cat lumbar spinal cord (averaged recordings). The pyramids (Pyr) and the red nucleus (NR) were stimulated by successive 3 shocks. The difference between the PSPs produced by combined stimulation of both structures and the algebraic sum of separate responses is dashed.

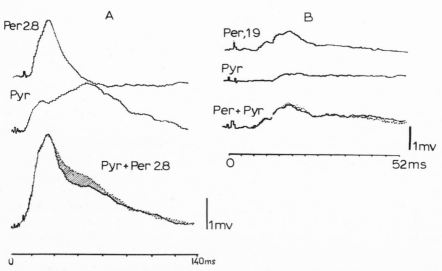

Fig. 16. Interaction of pyramidal and peripheral PSPs in two flexor motoneurones (A,B) of the cat lumbar spinal cord (averaged recordings). The pyramids (Pyr) were stimulated by 2 successive shocks, the peroneal nerve (Per), by a single stimulus. The relative strength of peroneal stimulation is indicated near the records.

tion of polysynaptic PSPs during combined stimulation of one of these descending systems and the peripheral afferents is a common but no universal finding; such facilitation usually involves only the late components of the response (Fig. 16). In some motoneurones descending and peripheral PSPs are summed up in a linear manner. This finding has to be expected from the data about the existence of relatively independent interneuronal pathways for the transmission of descending and afferent signals to motoneurones.

REFERENCES

AGNEW R.F., PRESTON J.B. and WHITLOCK D.G. (1963) Patterns of motor cortex effects on ankle flexor and extensor interneurones in the 'pyramidal' cat preparation. Exp. Neurol. 8, 248—263.

ANASTASIEVIĆ R., VASILENKO D.A., KOSTYUKOV A. I. and PREOBRAZHENSKY N.N. (1973) Reticulofugal activation of interneurons in the lateral region of the spinal grey matter in the cat. Neurophysiology (Kiev) 5, 525—536.

ANDÉN N.-E., JUKES M.G.M., LUNDBERG A. and VYKLICKY L. (1966) The effect of Dopa on the spinal cord. I. Influences on transmission from primary afferents. Acta Physiol. Scand., 67, 373—386.

BALDISSERA F., BRUGGENCATE G. TEN and LUNDBERG A. (1969) Monosynaptic action from the rubro-spinal tract on last order interneurons of segmental reflex pathways to motoneurones. Pflügers Arch., 313, 107R.

BALDISSERA F., BRUGGENCATE G. TEN and LUNDBERG A. (1971) Rubro-spinal monosynaptic connexions with last-order interneurones of polysynaptic reflex paths. Brain Res., 27, 390—392.

BAYEV K.V. (1971) Convergence of cortico- and rubro-spinal influences on cervical motoneurons. Neurophysiology (Kiev), 3, 599—608.

BAYEV K.V. and KOSTYUK P.G. (1972) Investigation of the modes of connections of cortico- and rubro-spinal tracts with neuronal elements of the cervical spinal cord in the cat. Neurophysiology (Kiev), 4, 158—167.

BAYEV K.V. and KOSTYUK P.G. (1973) Convergence of cortico- and rubro-spinal influences on interneurones of cat cervical spinal cord. Brain Res., 52, 159—171.

BAYEV K.V., VASILENKO D.A. and KOSTYUK P.G. (1973a) Synaptic processes in cervical motoneurons and interneurons evoked by stimulation of propriospinal pathways in the dorsolateral funiculus of cat spinal cord. Neurophysiology (Kiev), 5, 61—69.

BAYEV K.V., VASILENKO D.A. and MANZHELO L.I. (1973b) Functional properties of propriospinal pathways in the dorsolateral funiculus of the cat spinal cord. Neurophysiology (Kiev), 5, 54—60.

BERNHARD C.G., BOHM E. and PETERSEN I. (1953) Investigation on the organization of the corticospinal system in monkeys. Acta Physiol. Scand., 29, suppl. 106, 79—105.

BEZHENARU I.S., GOKIN A.P., ZADOROZHNY A.G. and PREOBRAZHENSKY N.N. (1972) Synaptic activation of thoracic interneurones by reticulospinal pathways. Neurophysiology (Kiev), 4, 566—578.

BUDAKOVA N.N. (1971) Stepping movement produced by rhythmic stimulation of dorsal roots in mesencephalic cat. Fiziol. Zh. SSSR (USSR), 57, 1632—1640.

BROWN T.G. (1911) The intrinsic factors in the act of progression in the mammal. Proc. R. Soc. B, 84, 308—319.

BRUGGENCATE G. TEN, BURKE R., LUNDBERG A. and UDO M. (1969) Interaction between the vestibulo-spinal tract, contralateral flexor reflex afferents and Ia afferents. Brain Res., 14, 529—532.

BUXTON D.F. and GOODMAN D.G. (1967) Motor function and the corticospinal tracts in the dog and raccon. J. Comp. Neurol., 129, 341—360.

CORAZZA R., FADIGA E. and PARMEGGIANI P.L. (1963) Pathways of pyramidal activation of cat's motoneurones. Arch. Ital. Biol., 101, 337—364.

ECCLES J.C., ECCLES R.M. and LUNDBERG A. (1960) Types of neurones in and around the intermediate nucleus of the lumbo-sacral cord. J. Physiol. (Lond.), 154, 89—114.

ENGBERG I., LUNDBERG A. and RYALL R.W. (1965) Reticulo-spinal inhibition of transmission through interneurones of spinal reflex pathways. Experientia, 21, 612—613.

ENGBERG I., LUNDBERG A. and RYALL R.W. (1968) Reticulospinal inhibition of transmission in reflex pathways. J. Physiol. (Lond.), 194, 201—223.

GOKIN A.P. (1970) Synaptic activation of interneurons in the thoracic spinal cord by cutaneous, muscle and visceral afferents. Neurophysiology (Kiev), 2, 563—572.

GRILLNER S. (1969) Supraspinal and segmental control of static and dynamic gamma-motoneurones in the cat. Acta Physiol. Scand., suppl. 327.

GRILLNER S., HONGO T. and LUND S. (1966) Interaction between the inhibitory pathways from the Deiters' nucleus and Ia afferents to flexor motoneurones. Acta Physiol. Scand., 68, suppl. 277.

GRILLNER S. and LUND S. (1966) A descending pathway with monosynaptic action in flexor motoneurones. Experientia, 22, 390.

HONGO T., JANKOWSKA E. and LUNDBERG A. (1966) Convergence of excitatory and inhibitory action on interneurones in the lumbo-sacral cord. Exp. Brain Res., I, 338—358.

HONGO T., JANKOWSKA E. and LUNDBERG A. (1969) The rubrospinal tract. II. Facilitation of interneuronal transmission in reflex path to motoneurones. Exp. Brain Res., 7, 365—391.

ILLERT M., LUNDBERG A. and TANAKA R. (1974) Disynaptic corticospinal effects in forelimb motoneurones in the cat. Brain Res., 75, 312—315.

JANKOWSKA E., JUKES M.G.M., LUND S. and LUNDBERG A. (1967) The effects of DOPA on the spinal cord. V. Reciprocal organization of pathways transmitting excitatory action to alpha motoneurones of flexors and extensors. Acta Physiol. Scand., 70, 369—388.

JANKOWSKA E., LUND S., LUNDBERG A. and POMPEIANO O. (1964) Postsynaptic inhibition in motoneurones evoked from the lower reticular formation. Experientia, 20, 701—702.

JANKOWSKA E., LUND S., LUNDBERG A. and POMPEIANO O. (1968) Inhibitory effects evoked through ventral reticulo-spinal pathways. Arch. Ital. Biol., 106, 124—140.

KATO M., TAKAMURA H. and FUJIMORI B. (1964) Studies on effects of pyramid stimulation upon flexor and extensor motoneurones and gamma motoneurones. Jap. J. Physiol., 14, 34—44.

KERNELL D. and WU C.-P. (1967) Post-synaptic effects of cortical stimulation of fore-limb motoneurones in the baboon. J. Physiol. (Lond.), 191, 673—690.

KOSTYUK P.G. and MAISKY V.A. (1972) Propriospinal projections in the lumbar spinal cord of the cat. Brain Res., 39, 530—535.

KOSTYUK P.G. and PILYAVSKY A.I. (1967) Postsynaptic potentials in spinal moto-neurons under rubro-spinal influences. Zh. Vyssh. Nervn. Dyat. (Moskva), 17 497—504.

KOSTYUK P.G., POGORELAYA N.Ch. and DYACHKOVA L.N. (1972) Structural features of cortico-spinal connections in the cat. Neurophysiology (Kiev), 4, 480—488.

KOSTYUK P.G. and PREOBRAZHENSKY N.N. (1966) Differentiation of reciprocal and unspecific descending synaptic influences during stimulation of the bulbar reticular formation. Fiziol. Zh. (Kiev), 12 712—720.

KOSTUYK P.G. and SKIBO G.G. (1972) Structural characteristics of the connections of the medial descending systems with spinal cord neurons. Neurophysiology (Kiev), 4, 579—586.

KOSTUYK P.G. and SKIBO G.G. (1974) Investigation of synaptic connections of the rubrospinal tract fibers in the spinal cord of the cat. Neurophysiology (Kiev), 6, in press.

KOSTYUK P.G., VASILENKO D.A. and LANG E. (1971) Propriospinal pathways in the dorsolateral funicle and their effects on lumbosacral motoneuronal pools. Brain Res., 28, 233—249.

KOSTYUKOV A.I. (1973) Transformation of descending activity evoked by prolonged stimulation of pyramids and red nucleus by some groups of spinal neurons. Neurophysiology (Kiev), 5, 644—653.

KOZHANOV M.V. (1974) Propriospinal monosynaptic influences from the ventral descending pathways on lumbar motoneurones in the cat. Fiziol. Zh. SSSR (USSR), 60, 171—178.

LANDGREN S., PHILLIPS C.G. and PORTER R. (1962) Minimal synaptic actions of pyramidal impulses of soma alpha motoneurones of the baboon's hand and forearm. J. Physiol. (Lond.), 161, 91—111.

LLINAS R. and TERZUOLO C.A. (1964) Mechanisms of supraspinal actions upon spinal cord activities. Reticular inhibitory mechanisms in alpha extensor motoneurones. J. Neurophysiol., 27, 579—590.

LLINAS R. and TERZUOLO, C.A. (1965) Mechanisms of supraspinal actions upon spinal cord activities. Reticular inhibitory mechanisms upon flexor motoneurones. J. Neurophysiol., 28, 413—422.

LLOYD D. (1941) The spinal mechanism of the pyramidal system in cats. J. Neurophysiol., 4, 525—546.

LUND S. and POMPEIANO O. (1965) Descending pathways with monosynaptic action on motoneurones. Experientia, 21, 602—603.

LUND S. and POMPEIANO O. (1968) Monosynaptic excitation of alpha motoneurones from supraspinal structures in the cat. Acta Physiol. Scand., 73, 1—21.

LUNDBERG A. (1972) The significance of segmental spinal mechanisms in motor control. Symposial paper 4th Internatl. Biophys. Congress, Moscow, pp. 1—13.

LUNDBERG A., NORRSELL U. and VOORHOEVE P. (1962) Pyramidal effects on lumbosacral interneurones activated by somatic afferents. Acta Physiol. Scand., 56, 220—229.

LUNDBERG A., NORRSELL U. and VOORHOEVE P. (1963) Effects from the sensorimotor cortex on ascending spinal pathways. Acta Physiol. Scand., 59, 462—473.

LUNDBERG A. and VOORHOEVE P. (1962) Effects from the pyramidal tract on spinal reflex arcs. Acta Physiol. Scand., 56, 201—219.

NYBERG-HANSEN R. (1966) Functional organization of descending supraspinal fibre systems to the spinal cord. Anatomical observations and physiological correlations. Ergeb. Anat. Entwickl.-Gesch., 39, 1—48.

PETRAS J.M. and LEHMAN R.A.W. (1966) Corticospinal fibers in the racoon. Brain Res., 3, 195—197.

POGORELAYA N.Kh. (1973) Experimental-morphological study of primary afferent terminals in the base of dorsal horn of the cat spinal cord. Neurophysiology (Kiev), 5, 406—414.

POGORELAYA N.Kh. and TARUSINA V.N. (1974) Experimental-morphological study of lateral funiculus propriospinal fibre terminals in cat cervical spinal cord. Neurophysiology (Kiev), 6, 44—51.

POMERANZ B., WALL P.D. and WEBER W.V. (1968) Cord cells responding to fine myelinated afferents from visceral muscle and skin. J. Physiol. (Lond.), 199, 511—532.

PREOBRAZHENSKY, N.N., BEZHENARU, I.S., and GOKIN, A.P. (1969) Monosynaptic EPSP in thoracic motoneurons under reticulo-spinal effect. Neurophysiology (Kiev), 1, 243—252.

PRESTON J.B. and WHITLOCK D. (1960) Precentral facilitation and inhibition of motoneurones. J. Neurophysiol., 23, 154—170.

PRESTON J.B. and WHITLOCK D. (1961) Intracellular potentials recorded from motoneurones following precentral gyrus stimulation in primate. J. Neurophysiol., 24, 91—100.

SHAPOVALOV A.I. (1966) Excitation and inhibition of spinal neurones during supraspinal stimulation. In: Muscular afferents and motor control. (R. Granit, Ed.), Almqvist and Wiskell, Stockholm, pp. 331—348.

SHAPOVALOV A.I. and GRANTYN A.A. (1968) Suprasegmentary synaptic influences on chromatolized motoneurones. Biofizika (Moskva), 12, 260—269.

SHAPOVALOV A.I., GRANTYN A.A. and KURCHAVYI G.G. (1967) Short-latency reticulo-spinal synaptic projections to alpha-motoneurons. Bull. Exp. Biol. Med. (Moskva), 64 (7), 3—9.

SHAPOVALOV A.I. and KARAMYAN O.A. (1968) Short-latency interstitiospinal and rubrospinal synaptic influences on alpha-motoneurons. Bull. Exp. Biol. Med. (Moskva), 66 (12), 3—7.

SHAPOVALOV A.I., KURCHAVYI G.G., KARAMYAN O.A., and REPINA Z.A. (1971) Extrapyramidal pathways with monosynaptic effects upon primate alpha-motoneurons. Experientia, 27, 522—524.

SHAPOVALOV A.I., KURCHAVYI G.G., and STROGONOVA M.N. (1966) Synaptic mechanisms of vestibulo-spinal influences on alpha-motoneurons, Fiziol. Zh. SSSR (U.S.S.R.), 52, 1401—1409.

SHAPOVALOV A.I. and SHAPOVALOVA K.B. (1966) Activity of alpha-motoneurones under rhythmical stimulation of red nucleus and influence of strychnine on rubrospinal responses. Dokl. Akad. Nauk SSSR (Moskva), 168, 1430—1433.

SHIK M.L., ORLOVSKY G.N. and SEVERIN F.V. (1966a) Organization of locomotor synergy. Biofizika (Moskva), 11, 879—886.

SHIK M.L., SEVERIN F.V. and ORLOVSKY G.N. (1966b) Control of stepping and running by electric stimulation of the midbrain. Biofizika (Moskva), 11, 659—666.

SHIK M.L., SEVERIN F.V. and ORLOVSKY G.N. (1967) Structures of the brain stem responsible for evoked locomotion. Fiziol. Zh. SSSR (USSR), 53, 1125—1132.

SKIBO G.G. (1974) Propriospinal pathways in the cat ventral funiculus. Neurophysiology (Kiev), 6, in press.

STERLING P. and KUYPERS H.G.J.M. (1968) Anatomical organization of the brachial spinal cord of the cat. III. The propriospinal connections. Brain Res., 7, 419—443.

STEWART D.H., PRESTON J.B. and WHITLOCK D. (1968) Spinal pathways mediating motor cortex evoked excitability changes in segmental motoneurones in pyramidal cats. J. Neurophysiol., 31, 928—937.

SZENTÁGOTHAI-SCHIMERT J. (1941) Endigungsweise der absteigenden Rückenmarksbahnen. Z. Anat. Ent. Gesch., 111, 322—330.

UEMURA K. and PRESTON J.B. (1965) Comparison of motor cortex influences upon various hind-limb motoneurones in pyramidal cats and primates. J. Neurophysiol., 28, 398—412.

VASILENKO D.A. (1974) Synaptic action on lumbar motoneurones evoked by stimulation of propriospinal pathways in the ventral funiculus of cat cord. Neurophysiology (Kiev), in press.

VASILENKO D.A. and KOSTUYK P.G. (1966) Functional Properties of interneurones activated monosynaptically by the pyramidal tract. Zhurn. Vyssh. Nervn. Deyat. (Moskva), 16, 1046—1054.

VASILENKO D.A., KOSTYUKOV A.I. and PILYAVSKY A.I. (1972) Cortico- and rubrofugal activation of propriospinal interneurones sending axons into the dorsolateral funiculus of the cat spinal cord. Neurophysiology (Kiev), 4, 489—500.

VASILENKO D.A. and MANZHELO L.I. (1974) Transmission through propriospinal pathways of different length in the ventral funiculus of the cat spinal cord. Neurophysiology (Kiev), in press.

VASILENKO D.A. and VUCO J. (1966) Synaptic processes in lumbar motoneurons induced by stimulation of the sensorimotor area of the cerebral cortex. Zhurn. Vyssh. Nervn. Deyat. (Moskva), 16, 52—61.

VASILENKO D.A., ZADOROZHNY A.G. and KOSTUYK P.G. (1967) Synaptic processes in the spinal neurons, monosynaptically activated by the pyramidal tract. Bull. Exper. Biol. Med. (Moskva), 64, (II), 20—25.

WALL P.D. (1960) Cord cells responding to touch, damage, and temperature of skin. J. Neurophysiol., 23, 197—210.

WALL P.D. (1967) The laminar organization of dorsal horn and effects of descending impulses. J. Physiol. (Lond.), 188, 403—423.

WILSON V.J. and YOSHIDA M. (1969a) Comparison of effects of stimulation of Deiters' nucleus and medial longitudinal fasciculus on neck, forelimb and handlimb motoneurones. J. Neurophysiol., 32, 743—758.

WILSON V.J. and YOSHIDA M. (1969b) Monosynaptic inhibition of neck motoneurones by the medial vestibular nucleus. Exp. Brain Res., 9, 365—380.

ZADOROZHNY A.G., VASILENKO D.A. and KOSTYUK P.G. (1970) Pyramidal influences on interneurons of spinal reflex arcs in cat. Neurophysiology (Kiev), 2, 17—25.

2

Functional organization of the primate oculomotor system

Gerald WESTHEIMER and S.M. BLAIR

If one considers the magnitude of the task of giving a full description in neurophysiologically acceptable terms of, say, a mammal walking, one is filled with despair. So one looks for a more manageable task, usually one involving single cells. When the single cell is representative of an important class of cells, we learn a lot. This is especially true when the class of cells thus investigated, such as the motoneurone or the retinal ganglion cell, constitutes an obligatory component in a channel; one is then studying the cellular basis of behavior.

But the answer is really not yet at hand unless there is a biunique relationship between the cell's behavior and the animal's behavior. We need only remind ourselves of the reason why muscle spindles and their connections are so important: an analysis of motoneurone firing rates in terms of limb position leads nowhere unless load is taken into consideration.

Neural control of motor activity above the motoneurone has been elucidated principally by the older techniques of lesion making and electrical stimulation. The experimental situation is complicated by the need to avoid anesthesia. Even where — in ideally designed and executed experiments on single cells in awake monkeys — attempts are made to get a closer grip on the relationship between cell firing and motor behavior, a directness of results is not yet at hand. In part, the reason lies in the multiplicity of possible pathways — a monkey who wants to touch a target in three-space with his fingertips, can do so by a very large number of contraction patterns involving a variety of limb positions and muscle groups. In the end it may not be entirely fortuitous that specific coding is so much more easily demonstrated by focal stimulation than by single-cell recording.

No wonder, then, that a neurophysiologist interested in the organization of motor behavior is tempted by a subsystem that seems less encumbered by

* Supported by Grant EY-00592 from the National Eye Institute, U.S. Public Health Service

the difficulties just enumerated. In the primate oculomotor system we do not need to worry much about the spindles, the muscles operate under a constant load, and there is direct coupling of the muscles to the skull on one end and the target organ on the other end. In many ways we may, therefore, expect the simplicity of an open-loop kind of system. There are even some additional constraints, known in the ophthalmological literature for over a century, but only recently resurrected as providing outlines for neurophysiological organization.

From the days of Hering we have known that, barring gross pathology in the orbit, the two eyes of the primate always move in parallel, except during a deliberate attempt to converge their lines of sight. Considering that each orbit contains six muscles in a peculiar anatomic arrangement, and that the two orbits are mirror-symmetrical rather than identical, this parallelism of ocular movements of the two eyes betrays no mean feat of neural organization. Similarly, we know that while the orbits act beautifully as ball and socket joints, the eye balls do not ordinarily utilize their full facility of movement with three rotational degrees of freedom. In inter-saccadic intervals, the human eyes occupy positions that are describable by only two instead of the available three parameters. In particular, there is one and only one torsional position occupied by the eye for a given direction of the line of sight, regardless of the motion that brought the line of sight into this direction. Since rotations are not commutative, this indicates that neural coding for the eyes in inter-saccadic intervals is in terms of position occupied by the eye as a solid body in three-space rather than in terms of movement changing the position. We will return later to the consequence of this fact.

Finally there is the observation, made at the turn of this century, that there are only a few, rather well-defined modes of eye movement. Though Dodge talked about five, there are probably only four distinct kinds of oculomotor behavior: saccadic movements, smooth pursuit movements, vestibular responses and convergence movements.

Here then is a summary of the features that should make a neurophysiological attack on the primate oculomotor system more than usually rewarding:

(1) Direct coupling of muscles to skull and target organ and unchanging external load allow operation at the muscular level to approach open-loop conditions; the relative insignificance of the muscle spindle system bears witness to this;

(2) Very few patterns of muscular activity exist and each is well defined;

(3) Careful behavioral observations have laid down laws — Hering's law, Donders' law, Listing's law — which are in reality overt demonstrations of principles of neural organization at the supranuclear level.

With such a background, what has been achieved in the present neurophysiological generation to elucidate this particular motor system? Let us examine one difficulty at the outset: significant differences occur in major aspects of oculomotor organization between species. Not only is this evident where phyla lack, say, an established cerebral cortex, but we even have to reckon with major differences among mammals. The result is that findings in such commonly used laboratory animals as the rabbit and the cat cannot be accepted automatically as holding also for the primate. This essay is directed towards a synthesis of neurophysiological findings with behavioral observations, but the latter are quite sketchy in the lower animals. As a result, the synthesis will have to rely strongly on monkey data, and since we are particularly interested in the supranuclear area, the alert, behaving monkey at that. Work in progress in several laboratories may achieve a similar synthesis in the rabbit and goldfish, and it will be interesting to see eventually how much overlap there is. As regards the rabbit, one has to recognize that, starting from the way its retina processes information, its visual system seems to be different. There is serious doubt whether it can ever be regarded as paradigmatic for the primate.

A discussion of the functional organization of the oculomotor system may well take its departure from the observation, now a century old, that stimulation of the frontal cortex in the dog causes a contra-lateral eye movement, an observation confirmed by Sherrington and Leighton in the ape, and by Vogt, Vogt and Barany in the monkey. To put this finding into perspective, we need, however, also to keep in mind the following findings: such stimulation causes an eye movement only in the alert monkey, not the sleeping or anesthetized monkey and this says something about the nature of the synaptic connection. Ablation of both frontal eye-fields causes marked reduction in number of saccadic and smooth pursuit movements. Nevertheless, while the distribution of eye movement types may no longer be normal, all movements can still be executed. Finally, such single-unit recording as has been collected from the monkey, does not at all give this area the look of one initiating eye movement: almost all of the unit discharge comes after the onset of a movement. At this stage, then, we have to conclude that, as far as the organization of eye movement patterns is concerned, the frontal eye-fields of the cerebral cortex do not play a necessary role. When the relationship between a visual stimulus and the eye movement it evokes is considered, the story may be totally different, but here we are talking about neural pathways concerned with the execution of an eye movement.

Perhaps it is unreasonable to expect to find a strict neuronal analogue to motor behavior in the cerebral cortex, so we will turn to a much lower level, the motoneurone. We are in better luck here. Single-unit recordings of neurones in the III, IV and VI nuclei show impulse rates that are excellent correlates of steady eye position. We may, therefore, start to investigate the supranuclear connections with the viewpoint that the latter deliver signals to the motoneurones that are translated by the motoneurones into eye-position-coded impulse rates. While the monkey is alert and fixing his gaze, his ocular motoneurones fire steadily at rates up to 200 or 300 Hz, depending

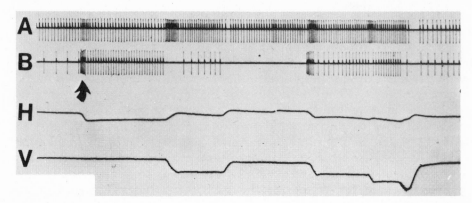

Fig. 1. Simultaneous record of two ocular motoneurones in an alert macaque. (A) left inferior oblique, (B) Right abducens, (H) Horizontal EOG ↑ = Left, (V) Vertical EOG ↑ = Down. The units show the saccadic transients and position-coded inter-saccadic impulse rate characteristic of ocular motoneurones. Arrow indicates horizontal saccade with transient involvement of vertically acting muscle. (Reprinted with permission from Eckmiller, R., Blair, S.M. and Westheimer, G. (1974) Exp. Brain Res., 21, 241—250.)

on the pull of the particular eye muscle for that particular direction of gaze (Fig. 1). For the straight-ahead position of gaze, the impulse rate is usually of the order of 50 Hz. What is the origin of the impulse rate? We are here talking of a postural input, and not of a dynamic response to a specific movement signal. The first thought would be to postulate an inherent rhythmicity of oculomotoneurones such that, when they are left alone, they steadily send impulses along their axons. Intracellular exploration of these neurones has, however, revealed that they are not much different from ordinary motoneurones and certainly require synaptic input to initiate and sustain firing. One can think of a positive feedback system, that depends on axonal collaterals, or muscle spindles. But axonal collaterals do not exist in primate oculomotoneurones, and spindle action can also be effectively ruled out. This steady postural oculomotor impulse rate exists in labyrinthectomized monkeys, in cerebellectomized monkeys, and even in monkeys with brainstem lesions giving them paralysis of lateral gaze. The impulse rate, however, becomes slower and less uniform in sleep and anesthesia. An appealing view is to suppose the existence of an alertness-dependent pacemaker which gives ocular motoneurones a synaptic input to make them fire more or less regularly at a rate that keeps the eyes more or less parallel and straight ahead. Withdrawal of this input slackens the muscles, which then let the eyes go to their position of rest. Eye movement and eccentric gaze-holding then result from transient and sustained modulation, respectively, of this pacemaker-generated activity.

What support can be drawn for this view from recordings of single units other than lower motor units in the oculomotor system in the monkey? As is

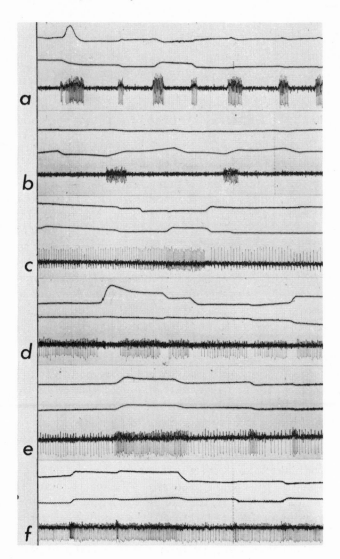

Fig. 2. Single-unit discharges in the brain stem of alert macaque monkeys. The units are not in the extra-ocular motor nuclei, yet are tightly coupled to eye movements, and may be involved in supranuclear oculomotor control. In each record: upper trace = vertical electro-oculogram (↑ up, ↓ down); middle trace = horizontal electro-oculogram (↑ left, ↓ right); lower trace = unit discharge. Duration of each record = 2 sec. (a) Omnidirectional saccade-burst unit; (b) unidirectional (right) saccade-burst unit; (c) tonic position code unit; (d) unit with tonic position coded, as well as omnidirectional saccade-stop characteristics; (e) unit with tonic position coded, as well as omnidirectional saccade-burst characteristics; (f) unit with tonic position coded, as well as unidirectional (up) saccade-burst characteristics. (Reprinted with permission from Westheimer, G. and Blair, S.M. (1972) Bibliotheca Ophthalmol., 82, 28—35.)

shown in Fig. 2 there are several classes of such cells. All classes have good temporal correlation with eye movements but, on the whole, attempts to find signal patterns that could code for amplitude and direction of movement have been disappointing. Perhaps the reason is that we are as yet naive in our expectation of the code that is being used. It is here that the behaviorally established laws alluded to earlier can profitably be applied.

For example, the laws relating to constancy of torsion teach that the code is for final eye position, and not for movement. If this is the case, it follows that, if one seeks constancy of firing pattern for a given amplitude and direction of movement, one is bound to be disappointed, because the firing pattern may depend also on the position that is being reached. The universality of conjugacy in eye movements makes it mandatory that there be a nerve network that accepts the command signals reaching the midbrain, which are undoubtedly coded for coordinates related to the mid-sagittal plane of the head, and recodes them into excitation patterns appropriate to the 12 individual muscles. Excitation and inhibition are involved, but the story is not that of simple reciprocity, because the vertical and oblique eye muscles act not even approximately as antagonistic pairs. There is evidence that this is a hardwired network. It comes from the observation that patients with partial paralysis of one muscle continue to see double for years even though the affected eye is capable of reaching the eye position which would allow single vision. It is also evident that there is a fixed relation between the impulse patterns in the muscles brought into play by eye-movement instructions, regardless of whether they are issued by the vestibular system or by one of the other authorities in the brain that have access to the eye-movement system. Because the circuitry for such a translating network is of necessity fairly complex, one would be surprised if more than one such network exists. Since the vestibulo-ocular connections are very old and quite direct, it may well be that the place to look is right there.

One of the major problems of this whole research is facing us here. It appears that all the components involved in the immediate supra- and internuclear circuitry of eye movements are concentrated in a small area of the brainstem between the superior colliculi and the vestibular centers. They are not laid out uniformly, or sequentially, but are intertwined and distributed so that physical position is no clear guide. Even right and left position is not a guarantee of functional connection, witness the crossing-over of the fourth nerves. All we can report is that several laboratories are trying to classify neuronal firing patterns and correlate them with eye position, eye movement, muscle action, difference in action of muscles, differences in velocities, duration of movements, and so forth. The situation is made more difficult by the need to concentrate on comparable species, and by the fact that most firing patterns are disrupted when alertness fails (Fig. 3). Correlated neuro-anatomical work is promising but slow. Extracellular or, preferably, intracellular, identification before staining and display of connectivity, while

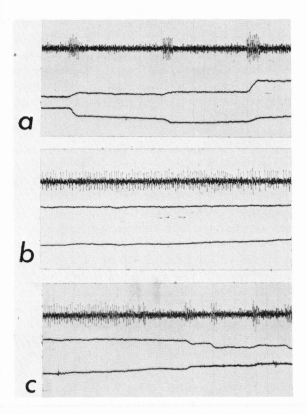

Fig. 3. Single-unit recording from the vicinity of the ocular motor nuclei in an unmedi-
cated monkey: (a) Alert with visual stimulation, (b) during light sleep, (c) transition from
light sleep to alertness. In each record, upper trace: unit discharge; middle trace: vertical
electro-oculogram ($\uparrow$ = down, $\downarrow$ = up; lower trace horizontal electro-oculogram ($\uparrow$ = left,
$\downarrow$ = right). Duration of each record = 1.4 sec. The unit shows a burst of discharges during
each active eye movement and irregular tonic activity during sleep. This is the type of
unit characterized as an omnidirectional burst saccade unit. (Reprinted with permission
from Westheimer, G. and Blair, S.M. Vision Res. (1973) 13, 1035—1040.)

a difficult and costly procedure, is now frequently attempted. The more
standard neuro-anatomical tracing techniques depend on accurate and
functionally restricted lesions, which only seldom reach the needed specificity.

Indirect evidence, largely from patients with oculomotor defects, points
to the pontine reticular formation as the place from which important supranuclear connections originate, and, in the cat, some monosynaptic pathways
to the ocular motoneurones have been traced from there. Much more evidence is available for the three-neurone pathway between the vestibular
afferents and the motoneurones. Here there are also inhibitory connections,

just as one would like to have it for reciprocal innervation. The major questions are whether the direct vestibulo-ocular connection, so far studied in intra- and extracellular detail, constitutes the only such pathway, and the extent to which this pathway contains the switching circuits necessary to translate three spatial dimensions into the complex excitatory—inhibitory inter-relationships required for the proper operation of the 12 extra-ocular muscles. Elucidation of this will go a long way to a full understanding of all supranuclear oculomotor connectivity.

In the above, little has been said about the cerebellum. This is not for lack of theories of cerebellar influence on eye movement — almost every function has at some time or other been ascribed to the cerebellum — nor for lack of factual material — ever since Flourens, experiments (usually with mutually contradictory results) have implicated the cerebellum with nystagmus. These multiple theories and contradictory results have demanded a new look.

Perhaps the most decisive approach to the role of the cerebellum is to see what happens when it is totally removed without damage to other structures. For functions remaining normal, the cerebellum is not an obligatory component. To begin with, monkeys without cerebellum have perfectly normal saccades and excellent vestibulo-ocular reflexes. They do have, however, a peculiar syndrome in that they cannot track smoothly, nor can they maintain their eyes in eccentric gaze (Fig. 4). This permanent syndrome can be largely prevented in a young monkey by the precaution of taking out only half the cerebellum, letting recovery supervene (it will be almost complete), and then removing the other half of the cerebellum. There will be considerable recovery and a young monkey after total cerebellectomy (albeit performed as two hemi-cerebellectomies done seriatim) will have no defects in

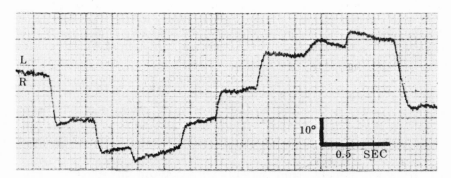

Fig. 4. Eye movements of cerebellectomized monkey when presented with a visual target moving sinusoidally in the horizontal plane. Record shows horizontal d.c. electro-oculogram. Saccades are normal, pursuit pattern is saccadé, there is absence of smooth pursuit movements (pursuit failure), and inability to maintain eccentric gaze (gaze-holding failure). (Reprinted with permission from Westheimer, G. and Blair, S.M. (1973) Invest. Ophthalmol. 12(8), 618-621.)

saccades, some tracking, some gaze holding, and full vestibulo-ocular responses. This speaks against the cerebellum being an obligatory constituent of these functions, though it seems to play some major supporting role in them. In fact, its role in vestibular reflexes is being made clear by a series of interesting experiments on their habituation. It has long been known that vestibulo-ocular reflexes, while nicely describable by transfer functions and such, are not immutable and in 1935 their habituability was ascribed by Halstead to the cerebellum. It now seems that he was indeed right, for cats without cerebellum have much less capability of changing the gain of their vestibulo-ocular reflexes than normal ones.

The most definite thing learned from cerebellectomy, however, is that it has been wrong to put too literal an interpretation on the concept of eye movement. It appears that it requires a special input to keep the eye steadily fixating on a target that is not straight ahead, and that this input is identical, or at any rate closely related, to the input required to give a smooth pursuit movement, for these two functions come and go together in the syndromes of complete and partial cerebellectomy in the primate.

We can now attempt to outline the organizational features of the primate oculomotor system. It is based, first of all, on a pacemaker acting as a source of steady synaptic input to all the twelve extra-ocular muscles. Normally the neuronal output to all the muscles is fairly high and balanced to keep the eyes parallel and straight ahead. There is a saccadic input, which supplies properly distributed excitation and inhibition to all the extra-ocular motoneurones in a specific fashion and this serves to move both eyes, again in parallel, to an eccentric position of gaze. To hold the eyes there, it is necessary to provide an input proportional to the eccentricity of gaze, otherwise the eyes drift back to the midline. This gaze-holding innervation is of the same kind as the innervation used to make smooth tracking movements.

While this scheme is based in part on ablation and behavioral data, we would have no trouble to provide you with all the cellular recordings necessary to prove it. The difficulty is that there is at present no way of distinguishing cellular firings that give correlative input to other systems or are merely reverberations, from those that are an essential constituent of the cellular substrate of this system. We are still faced with the difficulty of separating the necessary patterns of neuronal discharges from those that would be sufficient.

It is hoped, however, that continued neurophysiological analyses, together with new neuro-anatomical work and insights from lesion and behavioral studies, will in the foreseeable future provide a picture of the organization of the oculomotor system that is reasonably complete yet compact.

3

The spatial distribution of climbing fibre suppression of Purkinje cell activity *

F.J. RUBIA and W. LANGE

Stimulation of high-threshold afferents of the splanchnic nerve in the nembutalized cat produces a para-sagittal band of activity in the vermian part of the anterior lobe of the cerebellum. Purkinje cells in this band responded in two ways to the climbing fiber input. ON-cells gave the characteristic climbing fiber burst, which was followed by a suppression of spontaneous activity. OFF-cells showed similar suppressions, without the climbing fiber burst. ON-cells were found in a broad central portion of the band of climbing fiber evoked activity, while OFF-cells were recorded at the edges. Some cells near the edges of the band changed from one response type to the other with changes in stimulus parameters. These results suggest a lateral inhibitory mechanism mediated by inhibitory interneurones activated by climbing fiber collaterals and/or recurrent effects from Purkinje cell axon collaterals. Variations in the pattern of suppression of Purkinje cell activity following climbing fiber input suggest that more than one circuit is involved. Functional implications of the crossing patterns of lateral inhibition from mossy and climbing fibers are discussed.

INTRODUCTION

Langhof et al. (1973) showed that activity of high-threshold afferents of the splanchnic nerve in the nembutalized cat was transmitted to the Purkinje cell of the cerebellar cortex via the climbing fibers. Even at the surface of the anterior lobe, the field potentials evoked by stimulation of these afferents showed a discrete distribution in the para-sagittal plane. This distribution was very similar to that of the ventral funiculus spino-olivo-cerebellar pathway of Oscarsson (1968). Field potential analysis within the different lobules of the anterior lobe confirmed the narrow sagittality of the climbing

* Supported by the Deutsche Forschungsgemeinschaft. Correspondence should be addressed to F.J. Rubia.

fiber responses in the depths of all lobules (II through V) studied (Langhof et al., 1973). Thus, the stimulation of the splanchnic nerve provides a means of studying the spatial distribution of Purkinje cell responses to climbing fiber activation.

An indispensable condition for this analysis is the absence of evoked mossy fiber influence of the Purkinje cell. The well-known action of barbiturate anesthesia on the reticular formation probably reduces the level of background excitatory drive on the granular cells from the spino-reticulo-cerebellar pathway (Latham and Paul, 1971a). This excitatory background has been assumed to be necessary for the normal functioning of the mossy fiber-granule cell synapses (Gordon et al., 1973). This would explain the complete suppression of mossy fiber-evoked activity in the Purkinje cell in the nembutalized cat. In our experimental conditions, we never observed mossy fiber field potentials in the cerebellar cortex evoked by stimulation of the splanchnic afferents. All of the field potentials recorded were produced by the climbing fiber afferents, according to the conventional criteria of the latency and configuration of these potentials in the different layers of the cortex. We assume therefore that the observed effects of stimulation were due exclusively to climbing fiber activation.

An analysis of the Purkinje cell discharge within the sagittal band of climbing fiber responses in the anterior lobe showed both ON- and OFF-type responses (Rubia et al., 1974). The ON-response consisted of a repetitive discharge or complex spike followed immediately by a period of suppression of spontaneous activity. The OFF-response was simply a cessation of ongoing single-spike activity. Both the OFF-response and the later part of the ON-response were assumed to be mediated by the action of climbing fiber collaterals, which either inhibit the Purkinje cell by way of the inhibitory interneurones (basket and stellate cells) or disfacilitate them via inhibitory action of the Golgi cells on the granule cells (Bell and Grimm, 1969; Murphy and Sabah, 1970, 1971; Bloedel and Roberts, 1971; Latham and Paul, 1971b; Burg and Rubia, 1972; Harrison and Paul, 1973).

It was observed that the occurrence of ON- or OFF-responses was related to the location of the Purkinje cell within the para-sagittal band on the anterior lobe. ON-type discharges were recorded in the middle of the band and OFF-type near the borders. This suggested that lateral inhibition of Purkinje cell responses in the para-sagittal plane via climbing fiber is similar to that found in the transversal plane from the mossy fiber system (Anderson et al., 1964).

The present paper presents further evidence that the Purkinje cell discharge patterns evoked by climbing fiber activation from splanchnic stimulation depends on the location of the Purkinje cell within the excited sagittal band. Possible mechanisms underlying the various sequences of activity in Purkinje cell following climbing fiber activation will be discussed. A preliminary report of these results has been presented (Rubia and Lange, 1974).

METHODS

The 30 adult cats (2.2—3.0 kg) used were anesthetized initially with 40 mg/kg of Nembutal (Abbot), intraperitoneally injected. The femoral artery and vein were cannulated. Supplemental doses of anesthetic (8 mg/kg/h) were given intravenously. After the skull was opened, the left occipital lobe was removed by aspiration and the bony tentorium was opened. The dura was dissected and the left anterior cerebellar lobe was exposed. The left splanchnic nerve was approached retro-peritoneally. It was cut distally, placed on stimulating electrodes, and covered with warm paraffin oil. The animal was paralyzed with Pancuronium (Organon) and artificially venti-lated. Pneumothorax was sometimes performed. Arterial blood pressure and expired CO_2 were continuously monitored. Body temperature was automati-cally maintained at $37 \pm 1°C$.

Splanchnic stimulation was applied at a frequency of 0.33 Hz. The intensi-ty was 10 times the threshold for the $A\delta$ fibers and the duration was 0.1—0.3 msec. The area of greatest representation of the splanchnic afferents was localized with a surface electrode 0.5 mm in diameter. Glass micro-elec-trodes (3 M NaCl, resistance 3—7 MΩ) were used to record extracellular activity of Purkinje cell units. This activity was filtered and amplified con-ventionally. A window discriminator was used as necessary. Peri-stimulus time histograms (PSTH) of the unit activity were constructed, as well as averaged field potentials from the same recording site.

RESULTS

Purkinje cell units were identified by the presence of the characteristic climbing fiber response (Granit and Phillips, 1956; Eccles et al., 1966a). The responses of 79 such units to splanchnic nerve stimulation were analyzed. All were within the sagittal band of evoked potentials produced by such stimula-tion. ON-type responses occurred in 54 cells (68.4%). The form of the ON-response appeared to be related to level of anesthesia. With deep anesthesia the rate of spontaneous activity was usually low, and the ON-response con-sisted simply of a climbing fiber burst (latency 20—25 msec) followed by a 'post-climbing fiber-pause' (Latham and Paul, 1971b) of varying duration (as long as 100 or more msec). With lighter anesthesia, spontaneous rates were higher, and the post-climbing fiber-pause was sometimes replaced by a 're-bound' increase in firing rate.

OFF-responses occurred in 25 cells (31.6%). This response resembled the post-climbing fiber-pause seen in the ON-cells, but no burst preceded the pause. Again, the duration of the pause was variable, and it was sometimes followed by a rebound, i.e., an increase in firing frequency above the sponta-neous rate.

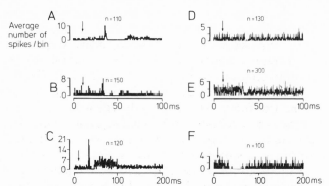

Fig. 1. Peri-stimulus time histograms (PSTH) of several different Purkinje cell responses to splanchnic stimulation. Arrows indicate the time of stimulation (always at 10 msec on the time scale). A, B, and C: ON-responses. D, E and F: OFF-responses. Bin widths: A, B, D and E, 100 μsec; C and F, 200 μsec.

.   Figures 1 and 2 demonstrate the PSTHs associated with these response types. Figs 1A—C and 2A—D show responses of seven different ON-cells. Arrows indicate the time of stimulation which is always at 10 msec on the time scale. Latency of the climbing fiber burst was 20—25 msec. The pattern of activity following the burst varied considerably from cell to cell. The post-climbing fiber-pause varied in duration from about 10 msec to more than 60 msec. This initial pause was followed by a variable pattern of partial recoveries (or sometimes rebounds) with subsequent depressions in firing rate. OFF-responses were similarly variable in the duration of the initial pause and pattern of subsequent activity (Figs 1D—F). The latency of the initial pause (25—30 msec) corresponds closely to that of the post-climbing fiber-pause in the ON-cells.

It should be noted that the ON- and OFF-cells were not always perfectly consistent in their responses. Some ON-cells (2.5%) sometimes lacked the climbing fiber burst but still gave the characteristic pause. That is, some

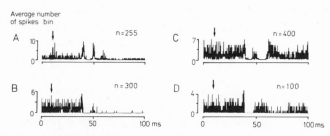

Fig. 2. PSTHs of different Purkinje cell ON-responses, showing various subsequent suppressions of spike firing as described in text. Bin widths: 100 μsec.

ON-cells occasionally gave OFF-responses. In a corresponding fashion, some OFF-cells (6.4%) occasionally showed a climbing fiber burst at the typical latency (an ON-response). Thus the classification of Purkinje cell units into ON- and OFF-types is not absolute, but rather refers to the pattern of response which is predominant in each cell.

As was noted in previous papers (Rubia and Lange, 1974; Rubia et al., 1974) the ON-response is found most frequently in the center of the sagittal band of activity evoked by splanchnic stimulation, while OFF-cells are more common near the edges of this band. Field potentials recorded from the same site as the unit activity show a clear relationship to the response type. At recording sites where ON-responses were seen, the field potentials were large (typically greater than 500 μV), and usually had a small initial negativity followed by a large positive deflection. OFF-responses were associated with small field potentials (less than 300 μV) and the deflections were frequently negative.

Some cells were found to change response type with changes in stimulus intensity. In these cases, corresponding changes in the field potentials were always seen. Fig. 3 shows two examples of such changes in response with the associated changes in average field potential (n = 16). In Figs 3A—C, a cell

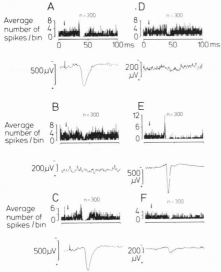

Fig. 3. Response of a single ON-cell (A—C) and a single OFF-cell (D—F) to changes in stimulus parameters. Reduction of intensity from 10 times the threshold for Aδ-fibers (in A) to threshold (in B) changes the ON-responses to an OFF-response. A return to original stimulus conditions (in C) restored the original response. The inverse effect is shown in D—F. An OFF-response to the standard stimulus (D and F) was changed to an ON-response by the application of a train of three stimuli at a frequency of 600/sec. The averaged field potentials (n = 16) associated with each PSTH were recorded at the same site as the Purkinje cell responses. Bin widths: 100 μsec.

which gave a typical ON-response to the standard stimulus (Fig. 3A) changed to an OFF-response when stimulus intensity was reduced to just above threshold (Fig. 3B). A return to the original stimulus conditions reproduced the original ON—pause—rebound response (Fig. 3C) Figs 3D—F show the inverse change in pattern. This cell gave a typical OFF-response to the standard stimulus. When a train of three such stimuli was given at 600 Hz, the response and accompanying field potential (Fig. 3E) changed to the ON-type. An OFF-response similar to the original was produced by a return to the standard stimulus (Fig. 3F). In two cases, changing the OFF-response to an ON-response by increasing stimulation resulted in a facilitatory effect. In order to restore the original response, stimulus intensity had to be reduced below the initial value.

DISCUSSION

Previous experiments (Langhof et al., 1973; Rubia and Lange, 1974; Rubia et al., 1974) have demonstrated that stimulation of high-threshold afferents in the splanchnic nerve of the nembutalized cat results in the activation of a narrow para-sagittal band of climbing fibers in the cortex of the anterior cerebellar lobe. The band of activation is about 1.5 mm wide; its center is 2.5 to 3.0 mm from the midline. Activation of the climbing fiber in this band has two effects on the Purkinje cell in the band: direct excitation with the characteristic climbing fiber burst, and suppression of ongoing Purkinje cell activity. In a broad central portion of the band, both the excitation and the suppression are observed, i.e., the cells respond with a climbing fiber burst followed by a suppression. At the edges of the band, cells show only the suppression of ongoing activity (OFF-response). A few cells near the edges of the band sometimes show ON- and sometimes OFF-responses. Evidence presented in Fig. 3 is consistent with the notion that the width of the band varied with stimulus intensity. Cells in the OFF-fringe can be converted to ON-cells by increasing the intensity of stimulation. Also, ON-cells near this fringe can be changed to OFF-cells by reduction in stimulation. Bloedel and Roberts (1971) also reported such variations in response with varying amounts of climbing fiber input evoked by stimulation of the inferior olivary nucleus.

The excitatory and inhibitory effects of climbing fiber activation differ in their spatial and temporal properties. Direct excitation of Purkinje cells which receive synapses from the active climbing fiber occurs for a brief period in the central portion of the band of evoked activity. Indirect suppression of Purkinje cell activity follows this excitation in nearly all of the activated Purkinje cells. A similar suppression is also observed in a fringe of neighboring Purkinje cells which are not directly excited by the active climbing fiber. The more extensive spread of suppression produces a sort of lateral inhibition in the para-sagittal dimension of the folium. This long-lasting suppression may play an important role in cerebellar function, since it would correspond to a disinhibition of the target cells on which the Purkinje cells synapse (Ito and Yoshida, 1964, 1966; Ito et al., 1964). Andersen et al., (1964) described a similar lateral inhibitory phenomenon on the transversal plane of the folium resulting from mossy fiber activation.

The climbing fiber-produced suppression of Purkinje cell activity varies considerably in both strength and duration. Several mechanisms may be involved in this suppression: (1) Direct inhibition of Purkinje cells by basket and stellate cells activated by climbing fiber collaterals, (2) disfacilitation produced by inhibition of granule cells by Golgi cells excited by climbing fiber collaterals; and (3) inhibition produced by recurrent axon collaterals of the Purkinje cells which are excited by the climbing fiber volley. Physiological and anatomical evidence related to each of these possible mechanisms will be discussed in turn.

Direct inhibition of Purkinje cells by interneurones excited by climbing fiber collaterals

One feature of our results which suggests this mechanism is the frequently seen inversion of the field potential recorded at the Purkinje cell level near OFF-cells. This could well be the extracellular sign of an IPSP occurring far from the electrode tip, for example at the synapses of basket and/or stellate cells in the Purkinje cell dendritic tree. The activation of these interneurones by climbing fibers was first demonstrated by Eccles et al. (1966c) who stimulated the inferior olivary nucleus and saw a weak excitatory effect on the stellate, basket and Golgi cells. The intracellular recordings of Bloedel and Roberts (1971) showed hyperpolarization of the Purkinje cell membrane from stimulation of the inferior olivary nucleus that produced reductions in Purkinje cell firing rate.

Bloedel and Roberts also demonstrated that antidromic invasion of the Purkinje cell could be prevented during the pause in cell firing produced by inferior olivary nucleus stimulation too weak to evoke the complex spike. This is clear evidence for active inhibition of the Purkinje cell as a consequence of climbing fiber activity. It was interpreted as being the result of climbing fiber collateral activation of inhibitory cerebellar interneurones. This inhibition was graded with stimulus strengths. The graded nature of effects in this pathway is also indicated in our results by variability in the duration of pauses in Purkinje cell activity following splanchnic stimulation. This graded response can be interpreted in terms of variation in the number of excited interneurones from which inhibitory effects converge on the Purkinje cell.

A clear anatomical basis for this mechanism is known to exist. Scheibel and Scheibel (1954) first demonstrated climbing fiber collaterals terminating in the granular layer, using the Golgi method. This finding was confirmed by Szentágothai and Rajkovits (1959), using degeneration techniques, and by Fox et al. (1969) with Golgi preparations. By electron microscopy, Lemkey-Johnston and Larramendi (1968) showed climbing fiber collaterals ending on basket cells, and Chan-Palay and Palay (1971) demonstrated endings of these collaterals on all of the interneurones of the cerebellar cortex. The fact that these climbing fiber collaterals spread in the transversal plane along the folium, along with the spread of the axons of the cells excited by them, provides an anatomical basis for the lateral spread of Purkinje cell suppression noted above.

It is also clear from the anatomy that activation of these interneurones by climbing fibers (Eccles et al., 1964a, 1966b) could exert a considerable range of inhibitory effects on the Purkinje cell. Palkovits et al. (1971) calculated that there were about six basket cells for each Purkinje cell, and that since each basket cell has terminals on about nine Purkinje cells, a typical Purkinje cell would receive inhibitory inputs from about sixty basket cells. Although the axonal spread of the stellate cells is not as great as that of the basket cells, there are roughly 20 stellates for each Purkinje cell (Palkovits et al., 1971), so convergence of inhibition from these cells onto the Purkinje cell is likely to be at least as great as from the basket cells.

Disfacilitation of Purkinje cell by Golgi cell inhibition of granular cells

Some of the histological evidence just discussed suggests another mechanism which may underly prolonged suppression of Purkinje cell activity following climbing fiber input: reduction in the excitatory drive from the granular cells or disfacilitation. This would result from an inhibition of the granular cells by Golgi cells excited by climbing fiber axon collaterals. Although this effect has not been conclusively demonstrated, there is much physiological data consistent with its existence. As mentioned earlier, Eccles et al. (1966c) showed at least a weak excitatory effect of climbing fiber stimulation on Golgi cells. In another paper (1964b) they showed a suppression of granule cell activity following stimulation of the inferior olivary nucleus.

The fact that more than one pause is frequently seen following climbing fiber activation (see Fig. 2), and that pauses of varying duration (up to 500 msec and more) can occur with or without the firing of a complex climbing fiber burst, would seem to indicate that more than a single mechanism is involved in producing the pauses. Some of the pauses last far longer than any observable changes in the polarization or excitability of the Purkinje cell membrane (Bell and Grimm, 1969; Murphy and Sabah, 1970, 1971; Bloedel and Roberts, 1971; Latham and Paul, 1971b; Burg and Rubia, 1972; Harrison and Paul, 1973). Disfacilitation produced by Golgi cell action on the granule cells could also account for at least the later part of the long-lasting suppression of Purkinje cell activity which follows climbing fiber inputs.

Recurrent inhibition via Purkinje cell axon collaterals.

These collaterals were first described by Golgi (1874) one hundred years ago. His observations were confirmed and extended by Ramón y Cajal (1888, 1889, 1890a,b, 1907, 1911, 1912) but localization of the terminals of these collaterals had to await much more recent electron-microscopic work (Fox et al., 1964; Larramendi and Victor, 1967; Hámori and Szentágothai, 1968; Lemkey-Johnston and Larramendi, 1968; Larramendi and Lemkey-Johnston, 1970; Chan-Palay, 1971). Since the activation of Purkinje cell axon terminals is known to produce post-synaptic inhibition (Ito and Yoshida, 1964, 1966; Ito et al., 1964), the collateral terminals on Purkinje cells would clearly be expected to play a role in the suppression which follows activation of Purkinje cells by climbing fiber input. Indeed, Eccles et al. (1966b) and Llinás and Precht (1969) have demonstrated such an inhibitory effect in the chronically de-afferented cerebellum. However, since the climbing fiber input produces only a brief burst of Purkinje cell activity (the complex spike), this recurrent pathway probably cannot explain the long-lasting suppressions that are commonly seen.

The possible functional significance of Purkinje cell axon collateral terminals on Golgi and basket cells is enigmatic. These pathways would act as positive feedback loops by disinhibiting the granule and Purkinje cells, thus producing a slightly delayed Purkinje cell activation which would spread beyond the Purkinje cell directly activated by the climbing fiber input. We have observed exactly the opposite effect, a spreading delayed suppression. Clearly, the precise timing and balance of these multiple antagonistic effects is critical. In terms of closed feedback loops, it is difficult to understand the significance of such antagonistic effects (Bloedel and Roberts, 1971). But if the loops are open, as would be the case if recurrent effects are distributed to Purkinje cells other than those in which they originate, such feedback may have clearer functional significance. For this to be the case, the spatial distribution of the recurrent collateral effects must be organized in a very precise fashion (Szentágothai, personal communication, 1974). These effects could well be involved in the oscillations in firing rate which frequently follow climbing fiber activation of Purkinje cells (cf. Figs 2A—D).

Cross-correlation of cerebellar inputs

Purkinje cells are excited both by climbing fibers and (via the granular cells) by mossy fibers. Each of these input pathways also produces a suppression of Purkinje cell activity by its actions on the interneurones of the cerebellar cortex. Since these suppressions have longer duration and greater spatial extent than the excitatory effects, they seem likely to play an important role in the integrative functions of the cerebellum (Bloedel and Roberts, 1971; Murphy and Sabah, 1971; Rubia and Lange, 1974; Rubia et al., 1974).

Localized input via the mossy fibers tends to excite a group of Purkinje cells lying in a transverse plane (i.e., parallel to the longitudinal axis of the folium). After a brief delay, these Purkinje cells are inhibited, and the inhibition spreads laterally to Purkinje cells adjacent to the plane of excited cells. Our results show that the situation with a restricted climbing fiber input is similar, except that the plane of excitation and the direction of the lateral spread of inhibition are both functionally orthogonal to those produced by mossy fiber input, even though the same cells can be excited by both input pathways. This difference in the spatial organization of effects of the two inputs would contribute to the kind of cross-correlation mechanism proposed by Oscarsson and Uddenberg (1966).

Herrick (1924) suggested that the phylogenetic development of the cerebellum arose from the necessity to integrate polysensory information in the control of movement. Many Purkinje cells in various parts of the cerebellum receive inputs from more than one modality, (Dow and Anderson, 1942; Snider and Stowell, 1944; Bremer and Bonnet, 1951; Takahira and Nacimento, 1962; Talbot et al., 1967; Freeman, 1970) and the different modalities of input may frequently arrive via different input channels. For example, visual inputs via climbing fibers and vestibular inputs via mossy fibers have been shown to converge on the same cells in some parts of the cerebellum (Maeka-

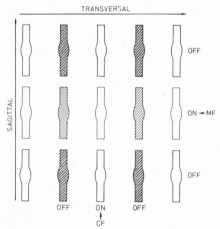

Fig. 4. Schematic representation of the actions of nearly simultaneous inputs to Purkinje cell from a mossy and a climbing fiber. Purkinje cell dendritic trees are represented as seen from above the folium. The parallel fibers activated by the mossy fiber input excite a row of Purkinje cells from right to left, and inhibit the adjacent rows shown in grey shadow. The climbing fiber input is assumed here to excite only the Purkinje cell in the middle of the figure and inhibit two adjacent rows of Purkinje cell lying in a para-sagittal plane (diagonal hatching). Important interactions between the effects of the two inputs seem likely to occur in the cells which are inhibited by both as a result of their long-lasting effects on the inhibitory interneurones.

wa and Simpson, 1972, 1973; Simpson et al., in press). When the two inputs are stimulated simultaneously, as would normally occur when the head moves, slight differences in conduction time between the two pathways prevent the excitatory effects of the two inputs from interacting. The parallel fiber volley arrives slightly before the climbing fibers fire, so the climbing fiber burst cannot influence the initial excitatory effects of the mossy fiber volley. Conversely, the extremely powerful excitatory effect of the climbing fiber—Purkinje cell synapses is not very much affected by the mossy fiber activity about 10 msec earlier (Eccles et al., 1964a, 1966d). However, the long-lasting inhibitory effects of the two inputs which spread spatially in orthogonal directions would produce a pattern of interaction something like that shown in Fig. 4. This crossing pattern of Purkinje cell suppression would of course produce patterned changes in the activity of disinhibited target cells of the Purkinje cell. It remains for further experiments to show whether such increases in Purkinje cell target cell activity play an important part in the integrative functions of the cerebellar cortex.

REFERENCES

ANDERSON, P., ECCLES, J.C. and VOORHOEVE, P.E. (1964) Postsynaptic inhibition of cerebellar Purkinje cells, J. Neurophysiol., 27, 1138—1153.
BELL, C.C. and GRIMM, R.J. (1969) Discharge properties of Purkinje cells recorded on single and double microelectrodes, J. Neurophysiol., 32, 1044—1055.
BLOEDEL, J.R. and ROBERTS, W.J. (1971) Action of climbing fibers in cerebellar cortex of the cat, J. Neurophysiol., 34, 17—31.
BREMER, F. and BONNET, V. (1951) Convergence et interaction des influx afférents dans l'écorce cérébelleuse, principe fonctionel du cervelet, J. Physiol. (Paris), 43, 665—667.
BURG, D. and RUBIA, F.J. (1972) Inhibition of cerebellar Purkinje cells by climbing fiber input, Pflügers Arch. Ges. Physiol., 337, 367—372.
CHAN-PALAY, V. (1971) The recurrent collaterals of Purkinje cell axons: A correlated study of the rat's cerebellar cortex with electron microscopy and the Golgi method, Z. Anat. Entwickl.-Gesch., 134, 200—234.
CHAN-PALAY, V. and PALAY, S.L. (1971) Tendril and glomerular collaterals of climbing fibers in the granular layer of the rat's cerebellar cortex, Z. Anat. Entwickl.-Gesch., 133, 247—273.
DOW, R.S. and ANDERSON, R. (1942) Cerebellar action potentials in response to stimulation of proprioceptors and exteroceptors in the rat. J. Neurophysiol., 5, 363—371.
ECCLES, J.C., LLINÁS, R. and SASAKI, K. (1964a) Excitation of cerebellar Purkinje cells by the climbing fibers, Nature, 203, 245—246.
ECCLES, J.C., LLINÁS, R. and SASAKI, K. (1964b) Golgi cell inhibition in the cerebellar cortex, Nature, 204, 1265—1266.
ECCLES, J.C., LLINÁS, R. and SASAKI, K. (1966a) The excitatory synaptic action of climbing fibers on the Purkinje cells of the cerebellum, J. Physiol. (Lond.), 182, 268—296.

ECCLES, J.C., LLINÁS, R. and SASAKI, K. (1966b) The action of antidromic impulses on the cerebellar Purkinje cells, J. Physiol. (Lond.), 182, 316—345.

ECCLES, J.C., LLINÁS, R. and SASAKI, K. (1966c) The inhibitory interneurons within the cerebellar cortex, Exp. Brain Res., 1, 1—16.

ECCLES, J.C., LLINÁS, R., SASAKI, K. and VOORHOEVE, P.E. (1966d) Interaction experiments on the responses evoked in Purkinje cells by climbing fibers, J. Physiol. (Lond.), 182, 297—315.

FOX, C.A., ANDRADE, A. and SCHWYN, R.C. (1969) Climbing fiber branching in the granular layer. In (R. Llinás, Ed.) Neurobiology of Cerebellar Evolution and Development, AMA-ERF Institute for Biomedical Research, Chicago, pp. 603—611.

FOX, C.A., SIEGESMUND, K.A. and DUTTA, C.R. (1964) The Purkinje cell dendritic branchlets and their relation with the parallel fibers: light and electron microscopic observations. In (M.M. Cohen and R.S. Snider, Eds.) Morphological and Biochemical Correlates of Neural Activity, Hoeber-Harper and Row, New York, pp. 112—141.

FREEMAN, J.A. (1970) Responses of cat cerebellar Purkinje cells to convergent inputs from cerebral cortex and peripheral sensory systems, J. Neurophysiol., 33, 697—712.

GOLGI, C. (1903) Sulla fina anatomia del cervelletto umano. Lecture, Istituto Lombardo di Sci. e Lett., 8. Jan. 1874. In Opera Omnia, vol. I. Istologia Normale, 1870—1883, Ulrico Hoepli, Milan, pp. 99—111.

GORDON, M., RUBIA, F.J. and STRATA, P. (1973) The effect of pentothal on the activity evoked in the cerebellar cortex, Exp. Brain Res., 17, 50—62.

GRANIT, R. and PHILLIPS, C.G. (1956) Excitatory and inhibitory processes acting upon individual Purkinje cells of the cerebellum in cats, J. Physiol. (Lond.), 133, 520—547.

HÁMORI, J. and SZENTÁGOTHAI, J. (1968) Identification of synapses formed in the cerebellar cortex by Purkinje axon collaterals: an electron microscope study, Exp. Brain Res., 5, 118—128.

HARRISON, M.T. and PAUL, D.H. (1973) The block of spontaneous spike discharges in cerebellar Purkinje cells. J. Physiol. (Lond.), 234, 56—57P.

HERRICK, C.J. (1924) Origin and evolution of the cerebellum, Arch. Neurol. Psychiatr., 11, 621—652.

ITO, M. and YOSHIDA, M. (1964) The cerebellar-evoked monosynaptic inhibition of Deiters neurones. Experientia, 20, 515—516.

ITO, M. and YOSHIDA, M. (1966) The origin of cerebellar-induced inhibition of Deiters neurones. I. Monosynaptic initiation of the inhibitory postsynaptic potentials. Exp. Brain Res., 2, 330—349.

ITO, M., YOSHIDA, M. and OBATA, K. (1964) Monosynaptic inhibition of the intracerebellar nuclei induced from the cerebellar cortex. Experientia, 20, 575—576.

LANGHOF, H., HÖPPENER, U. and RUBIA, F.J. (1973) Climbing fiber responses to splanchnic nerve stimulation. Brain Res., 53, 232—236.

LARRAMENDI, L.M.H. and LEMKEY-JOHNSTON, N.J. (1970) The distribution of recurrent Purkinje collateral synapses in the mouse cerebellar cortex: an electron microscopic study. J. Comp. Neurol., 138, 451—482.

LARRAMENDI, L.M.H. and VICTOR, T. (1967) Synapses on the Purkinje cell spines in the mouse. An electronmicroscopic study. Brain Res., 5, 15—30.

LATHAM, A. and PAUL, D.H. (1971a) Effects of sodium thiopentone on cerebellar neurone activity. Brain Res., 25, 212—215.

LATHAM, A. and PAUL, D.H. (1971b) Spontaneous activity of cerebellar Purkinje cells and their responses to impulses in climbing fibers. J. Physiol. (Lond.), 213, 135—156.

LEMKEY-JOHNSTON, N.J. and LARRAMENDI, L.M.H. (1968) Types and distribution of synapses upon basket and stellate cells of the mouse cerebellum. J. Comp. Neurol., 134, 73—112.

LLINÁS, R. and PRECHT, W. (1969) Recurrent facilitation by disinhibition in Purkinje cells of the cat cerebellum. In (Llinás, R., Ed.) Neurobiology of Cerebellar Evolution and Development, AMA-ERF Institute for Biomedical Research, Chicago, pp. 619—628.

MAEKAWA, K. and SIMPSON, J.I. (1972) Climbing fiber activation of Purkinje cells in the flocculus by impulses transferred through the visual pathway. Brain Res., 39, 245—251.

MAEKAWA, K. and SIMPSON, J.I. (1973) Climbing fiber responses evoked in vestibulo-cerebellum of rabbit from visual system. J. Neurophysiol., 36, 649—666.

MURPHY, J.T. and SABAH, N.H. (1970) The inhibitory effect of climbing fiber activation on cerebellar Purkinje cells. Brain Res., 19, 486—490.

MURPHY, J.T. and SABAH, N.H. (1971) Cerebellar Purkinje cell responses to afferent inputs. I. Climbing fiber activation. Brain Res., 25, 449—467.

OSCARSSON, O. (1968) Termination and functional organization of the ventral spino-olivocerebellar path. J. Physiol. (Lond.), 196, 453—478.

OSCARSSON, O. and UDDENBERG, N. (1966) Somatotopic termination of spino-olivo-cerebellar path. Brain Res., 3, 204—207.

PALKOVITS, M., MAGYAR, R. and SZENTAGOTHAI, J. (1971) Quantitative histological analysis of the cerebellar cortex in the cat. III. Structural organization of the molecular layer. Brain Res., 34, 1—18.

RAMÓN Y CAJAL, S. (1888) Estructura de los centros nerviosos de las aves, Rev. Trimestr. Histol., No. 1 (May), 1—10.

RAMÓN Y CAJAL, S. (1889) Sobre las fibras nerviosas de la capa granulosa del cerebelo. Rev. Trimestr. Histol., No. 4 (March), 107—118.

RAMÓN Y CAJAL, S. (1890a) Sur les fibres nerveuses de la couche granuleuse du cervelet et sur l'évolution des éléments cérébelleux. Int. Mschr. Anat. Physiol., 7, 12—30.

RAMÓN Y CAJAL, S. (1890b) Á propos de certains éléments bipolaires du cervelet avec quelques détails nouveau sur l'évolution des fibres cérébelleuses. Int. Mschr. Anat. Physiol., 7, 447—468.

RAMÓN Y CAJAL, S. (1911) Histologie du Système Nerveux de l'Homme et des Vertébrés. Vols. I and II, Maloine, Paris.

RAMÓN Y CAJAL, S. (1912) Sobre ciertos plexos pericelulares de la capa de los granos del cerebelo. Trab. Lab. Invest. Biol. (Madrid), 10, 273—276.

RAMÓN Y CAJAL, S. and ILLERA, R. (1907) Quelques nouveaux détails sur la structure de l'écorce cérébelleuse, Trav. Lab. Invest. Biol. (Madrid), 5, 1—22.

RUBIA, F.J. and LANGE, W. (1974) Lateral inhibition of Purkinje cells via climbing fibers, Pflügers Arch., suppl. 347, R 51.

RUBIA, F.J., HÖPPENER, U. and LANGHOF, H. (1974) Lateral inhibition of Purkinje cells through climbing fiber afferents? Brain Res., 70, 153—156.

SCHEIBEL, M.W. and SCHEIBEL, A.B. (1954) Observations on the intracortical relations of the climbing fibers of the cerebellum. J. Comp. Neurol., 101, 733—763.

SIMPSON, J.I., PRECHT, W. and LLINÁS, R. (1975) Sensory separation in climbing and mossy fiber input to cat vestibulo-cerebellum. Pflügers Arch., in press.

SNIDER, R.S. and STOWELL, A. (1944) Receiving areas of the tactile, auditory and visual systems in the cerebellum. J. Neurophysiol., 7, 331—357.

SZENTÁGOTHAI, J. and RAJKOVITS, U. (1959) Über den Ursprung der Kletterfasern des Kleinhirns. Z. Anat. Entwickl.-Gesch., 121, 130—141.

TAKAHIRA, H. and NACIMIENTO, A.C. (1962) Afferent convergence upon a single cerebellar cell in the cat. 22nd Internatl. Congr. Physiol. Sci., Leiden, p. 1147.

TALBOTT, R.E., TOWE, A.L. and KENNEDY, T.T. (1967) Physiological and histological classification of cerebellar neurones in chloralose-anesthetized cats. Exp. Neurol., 19, 46—64.

4

Visual input and its influence on motor and sensory systems in man

Manik SHAHANI

Since the monumental work of Sherrington (1898) on eliciting the resistance of a limb to passive displacement in a decerebrate animal, the interest of many neurophysiologists all over the world has been focussed on the importance of the spindle afferents in the study of the motor system. Granit and co-workers (1955, 1956), Lundberg (1970, 1972) and others have also added to the great fund of knowledge available on the behaviour and excitation of motor neurones. The enormous quantity of data on muscle spindle gathered by many physiologists for nearly a century has been meticulously reviewed and discussed by Mathews (1972); Vallbo (1970) has successfully launched into the recording of spindle afferents in man, which has given further impetus to other workers around the globe (see Burg 1974; Struppler and Velho, 1974). The work on the effect of other inputs and how they exert their influence on motor neurones appears to be scanty when compared to the fund of knowledge so painstakingly accumulated on spindle afferents, and the gamma system. In man it has been realized by observation of his activities and skills that the possible role of visual input is likely to be greater than that of other inputs. With evolution, man has probably begun to rely more and more on visual information. Interestingly, however, there have been hardly any reports in literature as to how the visual input affects the motor neurone pool. In 1971, pioneering work was started by the author to study the effect of visual input on alpha-pool in the performance of learnt activities (Shahani, 1973). Anderson et al. (1972) were perhaps the first to report the tectal and tegmental influences on cat forelimb and hindlimb motoneurones, thus indirectly showing the involvement of visual input and excitability of spinal motor neurones, although the same group had reported earlier (1971) on the influence of the superior colliculus on neck motoneurones in cat, finding this to be essentially the same as a reflex function. It may be added at this stage that there have been some reports on the influence of other inputs, excluding spindle and visual, on the motoneurone pool; Eldred and Hagbarth (1954) in the case of exteroceptors from skin and

Lundberg (1972), Grillner (1972), Delwaide et al. (this volume, Section IV, Ch. 3) and Shapovolov (1966) in the case of vestibulor influences.

In order to study in detail the influences of visual input on the motor system in man various simple experiments were devised by the author. In all these experiments the recording of different parameters was carried out with the eyes of the subject open and blindfolded, both in situations in which the subject was asked to perform, and also in situations where specific responses were elicited from him as a result of precise stimulation. These experiments were performed in normal men and also in a number of pathophysiological conditions. The following experiments were designed to study the influence of visual input in man:

  (1) Visual input and learnt movements in patients with upper motor neurone lesions
  (2) Visual input and firing rate of motor units in purposeful isometric contraction
  (3) Visual input and 'M' response at threshold stimulus
  (4) Visual input and monosynaptic and polysynaptic reflexes
  (5) Visual input and sensory potentials

VISUAL INPUT AND LEARNT MOVEMENTS IN PATIENTS WITH UPPER MOTOR NEURONE LESIONS

Two patients (hemiplegics) were made to sit on a couch with their legs outstretched and the back-rest raised to support the back. On a 16-channel Grass EEG machine, electrodes for 8 channels were fixed on the scalp for EEG recordings, while the other 8 channels were utilized for the muscles of neck and shoulder (4 channels on each side). Two surface electrodes at a distance of 2.5—4 cms were used on each channel to pick up from the following muscles: upper fibres of trapezius, pectoralis major, latisimus dorsi and deltoid. The patients were made to perform such common activities as picking up blocks, tearing papers, raising a glass of water to the mouth, etc. These activities were carried out first with the eyes open, and then eyes shut, while the trace was running to record the activity.

Fig. 1. Tearing papers with both hands. Significant decrease in the EMG activity is noticed both in the proximal and axial muscles (trapezius) bilaterally, that is in both the affected (right) and unaffected sides of a patient with hemiplegia. Notice the maximum reduction in axial muscles.

Fig. 2. Patient 1: drinking a glass of water (affected side). Slight reduction is seen in the proximal muscles like pectoralis major and latisimus dorsi. Almost no change is seen in the axial muscle (right trapezius).

Fig. 3. Picking up blocks (affected side). Reduction in activity is noticed on the affected side both in axial and proximal muscle. Interestingly, the EMG seems to have increased on blindfolding in the axial muscle (left trapezius of the unaffected side).

TEARING PAPER WITH BOTH HANDS

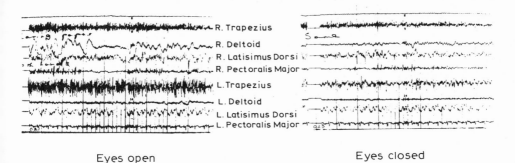

R. Trapezius

R. Deltoid

R. Latisimus Dorsi

R. Pectoralis Major

L. Trapezius

L. Deltoid

L. Latisimus Dorsi

L. Pectoralis Major

Eyes open   Eyes closed

Fig. 1. Tearing paper with both hands.

PATIENT 1:   DRINKING GLASS OF WATER

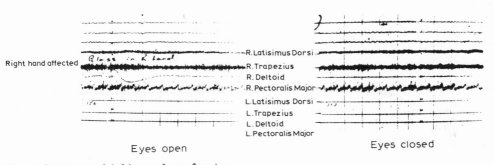

Right hand affected

R. Latisimus Dorsi

R. Trapezius

R. Deltoid

R. Pectoralis Major

L. Latisimus Dorsi

L. Trapezius

L. Deltoid

L. Pectoralis Major

Eyes open   Eyes closed

Fig. 2. Patient 1: drinking a glass of water.

PATIENT 2: PICKING UP BLOCKS

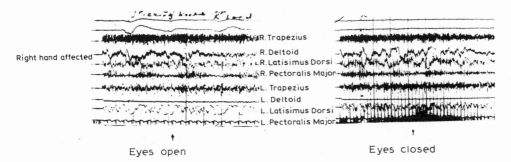

Right hand affected

R. Trapezius

R. Deltoid

R. Latisimus Dorsi

R. Pectoralis Major

L. Trapezius

L. Deltoid

L. Latisimus Dorsi

L. Pectoralis Major

Eyes open   Eyes closed

Fig. 3. Patient 2: picking up blocks.

TEARING UP PAPER WITH BOTH HANDS

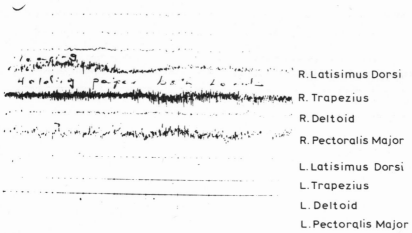

R. Latisimus Dorsi

R. Trapezius

R. Deltoid

R. Pectoralis Major

L. Latisimus Dorsi

L. Trapezius

L. Deltoid

L. Pectoralis Major

Fig. 4. Tearing up paper with both hands.

Fig. 4. Tearing papers with both hands. It can be seen that the EMG activity is recorded in axial and proximal muscles only on the affected side and there is no activity on the unaffected side, even though tearing of papers is done by both the hands. This may be a feature worth noting in the hemiplegic patient. Whether or not this excessive activity in the axial and proximal muscles on the affected side of a hemiplegic is a reflection of withdrawal of cortical inhibition and thereby demonstration of free play of the cerebellum, is worth considering.

VISUAL INPUT AND FIRING RATE OF HUMAN MOTOR UNITS IN ISOMETRIC CONTRACTION

Three young adults were made to sit comfortably on chairs with their right arms resting on a couch. Each subject was asked to hold between thumb and fingers a small plastic container used for storing 35-mm film rolls. This lightweight plastic container was chosen in order to get a minimal isometric contraction, so that a single motor unit potential could be elicited from the area covered by a concentric needle electrode inserted in the abductor pollicis brevis muscle. The rate of firing of a motor unit was checked every second for ten consecutive seconds, so that a mean could be calculated later. This experiment was performed with the eyes of subject open as well as blindfolded. In order to compare the influence of various inputs, the rate of motor unit firing was also studied with a blood-pressure cuff applied to

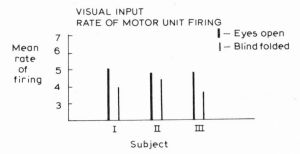

Fig. 5. Visual input and rate of motor unit firing.

the arm (120 mm/Hg) in order to reduce group Ia input. Exteroceptive input from skin receptors was excluded by inserting gauze pieces between the container and finger and thumb. Ears were also plugged in some subjects to obliterate auditory input. In some cases a strap was put around the mouth as a control. Various combinations of different inputs being eliminated or reduced simultaneously were also tried out e.g. eyes blindfolded and ears plugged, eyes closed and cuff pressure etc., and the rate of motor unit firing was studied under these different conditions.

The mean rate of motor unit firing in all trials seemed to vary between three and six per second. Tokizane (1964) has described such motor units with a low rate of firing. The rate of firing in this experiment seems to be slightly lower than that described by Grimby (1968) as shown in Fig. 5 (means are of 10 readings, rate of motor unit firing is per sec). It can be seen that, in all the three subjects, the mean rate of firing of motor units is reduced on blindfolding. In Fig. 6, the table shows mean values in different situations. It is noticed that in comparison to the original eyes-open position,

VISUAL INPUT STUDIES
Learnt activity in 3 normal subjects
rate of motor unit firing in abductor pollicis brevis, mean values

Eyes open	4.9
Eyes open, mouth closed with strap	4.2
Eyes open, cuff pressure 120 mm Hg	4.05
Eyes open, ears closed	4.4
Blindfolded	3.9

Fig. 6. Visual input studies. Learnt activity in 3 normal subjects. Rate of motor unit firing in abductor pollicis brevis, mean values.

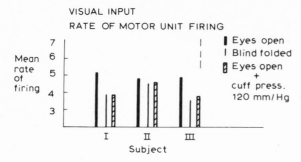

Fig. 7. Visual input rate of motor unit firing.

there is reduction in the rate of firing irrespective of which input is reduced or eliminated (even the control situation of mouth closed with strap shows some reduction). However, the most significant reduction in the mean rate of firing is seen when the subjects are blindfolded (from 4.9/sec to 3.9/sec). Reducing group Ia input also produces a significant drop in the rate of firing (from 4.9/sec to 4.05/sec). It can be argued that 120 mm/Hg cuff pressure does not cut off spindle input completely as the blindfolding does in the case of visual input. Fig. 7 shows the reduction in the mean rate of motor unit firing on blindfolding as against that seen on applying cuff pressure (reducing group Ia input). Fig. 8 demonstrates the same phenomenon with a comparison to ears-closed as well. Fig. 9 shows the comparative reductions in motor unit firing rate when visual and auditory inputs are cut off. Here again the effect of visual input seems to be much more pronounced. Fig. 10 shows the detailed behaviour of the rate of firing of motor units per second for ten consecutive seconds following the elimination of various inputs and in various combinations. It can be seen that elimination of visual input causes

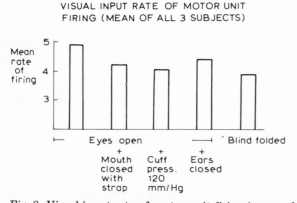

Fig. 8. Visual input rate of motor unit firing (mean of all 3 subjects).

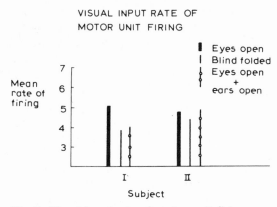

Fig. 9. Visual input rate of motor unit firing.

maximum reduction in the rate of motor unit firing which is further reduced when group Ia input is also obliterated. Maximum reduction, however, is seen when the major inputs like visual, auditory, group Ia, and cutaneous afferents are all cut off simultaneously. This seems not only to confirm the work of several physiologists who have concentrated on the influence of different inputs on the motor neurone pool, but also to validate the reliability of the experiment.

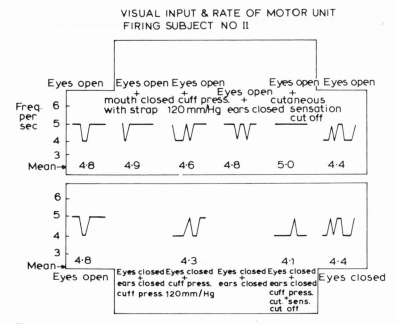

Fig. 10. Visual input and rate of motor unit firing, subject no. II.

Tokizane (1964) in his classification has mentioned motor neurones which fire at a slower rate than 'C'-type units. It seems that, for steady isometric contraction, it is these units which are called upon. Henneman has reported in his animal experiments, and recently verified in man (Hennemann and Shahani, 1974) that the order of recruitment of motor neurones is fixed as far as isometric contractions are concerned, while this order may be more flexible in isotonic contractions. However, these authors do not claim any fixed rate of firing. The reduction in rate of firing of motor units on eliminating or reducing various sensory inputs would suggest that a programme of such a voluntary activity is already present in the central nervous system which may be carried on without sensory inputs. It also seems that sensory inputs are tending to accelerate the rate of firing of motor units. As it is evident from the experiment that the act of holding a lightweight object continued even when inputs are being reduced, the question then arises of the possible effect of the increased rate of firing of motor units on the receipt of sensory inputs. It is difficult to answer this clearly; however, it could be postulated that the increased rate of firing of motor units due to various inputs perhaps keeps the nervous system in a better state of preparation for any need for a change in the learnt programme, although it can also be argued that when a programme of any motor activity has been learnt and stored, the same can be carried out as effectively and perhaps more efficiently without any sensory inputs.

VISUAL INPUT AND MONOSYNAPTIC AND POLYSYNAPTIC REFLEXES

The excitability of the motor neurone pool has also been extensively studied using mono- and polysynaptic reflexes. The 'H' reflex or Hoffmann's reflex is an extremely suitable method of studying the monosynaptic reflex, as in this case, as against the tendon reflex. Not only is gamma spindle bias reduced but it is also possible to give precisely measurable stimuli. Polysynaptic reflexes can be followed up better by studying withdrawal reflexes or flexion reflex. It has been shown that the response of the tibialis anterior muscle on stimulation of the sole of foot gives two components, first and second or early and late, in the same fashion as seen in the blink reflex (Shahani and Young, 1968) when the response is picked up from the orbicularis oculi muscle on stimulation of the supra-orbital nerve on the same side. Both these reflexes were therefore studied in normal and hemiplegic patients (in whom they can be more easily elicited). In hemiplegics there is also the advantage that psychic influences on reflex behaviour and other parameters are reduced, in view of the partial release of control of the lower motor neurone pools from the cortex.

Surface electrodes were used to stimulate the medial popliteal nerve and recording for 'H' reflex was made on or near the threshold stimuli for the

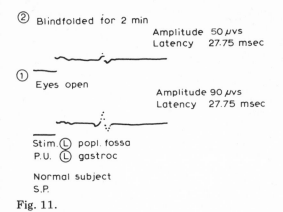

Fig. 11.

gastrocnemius muscle using a concentric needle electrode. Fig. 11 shows reduction in the amplitude of 'H' responses when the responses were averaged by a signal averager on blindfolding the subject for two minutes. Fig. 12 in another subject shows not only reduction in the peak-to-peak voltage on cutting the visual input (blindfolding for two minutes) but also shows slight increases in the latency and duration of the response. However, the slight increase in the duration of response cannot account (by desynchronisation) for the reduction in peak-to-peak voltage. It would seem therefore that, on elimination of visual input, some of the motor units that were contributing to the composite 'H' response failed to respond, perhaps due to increase in their thresholds of excitability or it can be argued that afferent input is now less effective due to either increase in the threshold level of group Ia or due to some other factors desensitizing the neurones presynaptically.

Flexion reflex or withdrawl reflex is a polysynaptic reflex and has two components, early and late. Fig. 13 shows this reflex in an adult (18-years old) with hemiplegia. It is easier to study this reflex in pyramidal lesions than in normal subjects because of the factors already described, and the fact

'H' REFLEX
NORMAL SUBJECT

	l	d	h
200 Volts Eyes open	29·1	9·8	163
200 Volts Blind folded for 2 minutes	29·3	10·4	43·9

Fig. 12. 'H' reflex, normal subject.

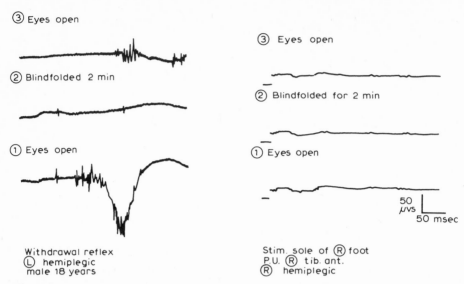

③ Eyes open

② Blindfolded 2 min

① Eyes open

③ Eyes open

② Blindfolded for 2 min

① Eyes open

50
μvs

50 msec

Withdrawal reflex
Ⓛ hemiplegic
male 18 years

Stim. sole of Ⓡ foot
P.U. Ⓡ tib. ant.
Ⓡ hemiplegic

Fig. 13. (Left) Withdrawal reflex in an 18-year-old adult with hemiplegia.

Fig. 14. (Right) The early (1st) component of withdrawal in a hemiplegic patient.

that the threshold stimuli can be of lower intensity. The recording was made from the tibialis anterior muscle by a concentric needle electrode when stimuli were given to the sole of foot (about 2—3 cm below the great toe) with stainless steel needle electrodes. Recordings were made by the raster method. It can be seen that the withdrawal reflex is completely obliterated when visual input is cut. Fig. 14 shows a study of the early (1st) component of withdrawal reflex in another hemiplegic patient, using the same method. Here, however, the technique of averaging has been used. It is clearly seen that there is significant reduction on elimination of visual input.

Fig. 15 shows the influence of visual input on the late component of blink reflex in a normal subject. The supra-orbital nerve was stimulated with surface electrodes and recording was also performed with silver disc electrodes placed on the orbicularis oculi muscle laterally on the lower lid. It is seen that on blindfolding for two minutes (i.e. on eliminating visual input), the latency of the 2nd component is increased, while the duration of the component is decreased. Some reduction in the maximum peak-to-peak voltage is also observed. Similar changes in latency, duration and amplitude of the 2nd component have been reported in the withdrawal reflex in sleep (Shahani, 1968). It is possible to assume that the main factor responsible for these changes seen in sleep may be the elimination of visual input rather than other factors like biochemical changes associated with sleep. However, the behaviour of latency, duration and amplitude of 1st and 2nd components of

BLINK REFLEX
NORMAL SUBJECT

	l l	d l	h l	l 2	d 2	h 2
Eyes blind folded for 2 minutes	— —	— —	— —	44·8	28·1	120·3
Eyes open for 5 minutes	— —	— —	— —	42·1	43·0	145·3

Fig. 15. Blink reflex, normal subject.

withdrawal reflex on elimination of visual input is not that consistent when higher threshold stimuli are used.

This evidence of reduced excitability of the motor neurone pool on elimination of visual input would tend to suggest that visual input is (either directly or through interneurones) exerting a significant influence on motor neurones; whether the influence is exerted through cortico-spinal and cortico-reticulo-spinal tracts or through tecto-spinal and tecto-reticulo-spinal tracts or through some other descending influences is not yet clear.

VISUAL INPUT AND ITS INFLUENCE ON 'M' RESPONSE

Motor-evoked potential or 'M' response (Adrian and Bronk, 1929) was picked up with surface electrodes on stimulating the median nerve in the arm (or at the elbow) using surface electrodes. Stimuli were near threshold level. 'M' response was obtained using a signal averager. On blindfolding subjects for two minutes, a significant reduction in amplitude was invariably seen (Fig. 16).

Fig. 17 shows in a tabulated form that, on cutting visual input, not only is the amplitude of the 'M' response reduced, but latency and duration also show some marginal changes. Fig. 18 shows, in a diagrammatic manner, the reduction in the amplitude of 'M' response on blindfolding. Although reduction in the duration of 'M' response is also seen (Fig. 19) on elimination of visual input the reduction is not so dramatic. Similarly (Fig. 20) only a marginal increase in the latency of 'M' response is found when visual input is cut. This consistent though small increase in latency would suggest that motor units with faster conduction velocities in their axons are more influenced by visual input. The alternative interpretation, that elimination of visual input may also affect other systems, (like the sympathetic and parasympathetic) which bring about some local changes (vaso-motor or temperature) affecting the conduction velocity of axons or increasing the delay at neuromuscular junctions, is less likely to be true as the changes observed in

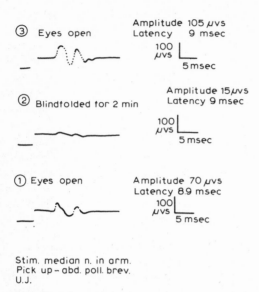

Stim. median n. in arm.
Pick up – abd. poll. brev.
U.J.

Fig. 16. 'M' response from a blindfolded subject.

latency are achieved in a short period (2 minutes) of blindfolding and are also reversible in the same period of time.

These results showing reduction in the amplitude of 'M' response on cutting off of visual input, apart from further reinforcing the significant influence of visual input on the motor neurone pool, also bring into focus a consideration that the excitability of the neuronal pool is also reflected all along the axons. It is remarkable that within a short period of two minutes of blindfolding, the membrane excitability of axons is altered. Whether this establishes change in ionic balance or change in the permeability of mem-

VISUAL INPUT RESPONSE
MEDIAN NERVE

Subject	Eyes open			Blind folded			Eyes open		
	Lat.	Dur.	Ampl.	Lat.	Dur.	Ampl.	Lat.	Dur.	Ampl.
U.J.	8·8	10·6	70	9·0	9·25	15·0	9·0	10·2	10
V.F.	6·0	15·0	5·5	–	–	–	6·0	15·0	6
S.U.	9·5	12·7	20	9·5	11·5	17·5	9·7	11·2	20
S.P	9·7	10·7	20	9·7	8·7	12·5	9·7	8·5	25
I.K.	10·1	10·1	115	12·7	3·7	10·0	10·0	10·7	80

Fig. 17. Visual input response, median nerve.

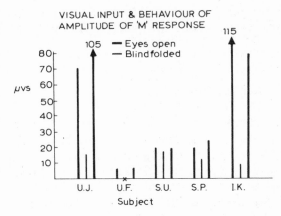

Fig. 18. Visual input and behaviour of amplitude of 'M' response.

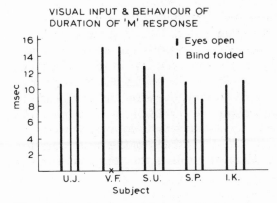

Fig. 19. Visual input and behaviour of duration of 'M' response.

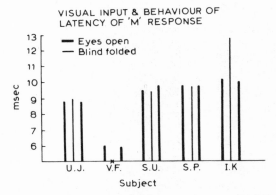

Fig. 20. Visual input behaviour of latency of 'M' response.

brane, or a fast transport of some substance by axonal flow, cannot be said with any confidence at this stage. Yet it opens up many possibilities of research in this area.

VISUAL INPUT AND ITS INFLUENCE ON THE SENSORY SYSTEM

The experiments described earlier demonstrating the significant effect of visual input on such parameters as the 'M' response on threshold stimuli, prompted the author to consider the effect of visual input on the sensory fibres of nerves as well. There are also reports in literature (Fetz, 1968) suggesting the influence of descending tracts on afferent input thresholds. If the visual input were to exert an influence on the alpha pool via cortico-spinal or cortico-reticulo-spinal and tecto-spinal or tecto-reticulo-spinal tracts, it is plausible to assume that it would possibly exert an influence on other afferent inputs, interneurones in the spinal cord playing their own parts.

Orthodromic, sensory-evoked potentials were picked up from the median nerve at the wrist when the digits were stimulated. Fig. 21 shows significant reduction in the amplitude of the sensory-evoked potential when the visual input is cut in one of the subjects. Change is noticed also in the duration of the signal, although latency does not seem to be altered on blindfolding. Fig. 22 shows, in tabular form, the records of latency, duration and amplitude of signals as observed in different subjects in the condition of eyes open and blindfolded. Fig. 23 shows graphically the latency behaviour of the sensory potential, when the visual input is cut off. Fig. 24 shows the mean duration of the sensory potential while Fig. 25 clearly shows that the peak-to-peak

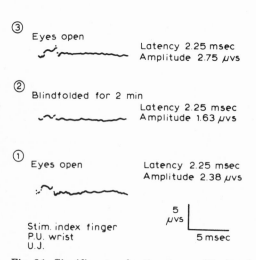

Fig. 21. Significant reduction in amplitude of sensory-evoked potential.

VISUAL INPUT & SENSORY EVOKED POTENTIAL
MEDIAN NERVE

Subj.	Eyes open Lat.	Duration	Amp	Blind folded Lat.	Duration	Amp.	Eyes open Lat.	Duration	Amp.
S.C.	2·75	3·5	3	2·75	3·5	3	2·75	3·13	3·5
U.J.	2·25	5·63	2·38	2·25	5·25	1·63	2·25	5·5	2·75
V.P.	2·25	3·75	5·75	2·13	3·37	5·25	2·0	4·0	5·75
D.D.	2·13	2·12	1·25	2·0	2·13	1·0	1·88	2·37	1·25
MEANS	2·34	3·75	3·09	2·28	3·31	2·72	2·22	3·75	3·31

Fig. 22. Visual input and sensory evoked potential, median nerve.

amplitude of the sensory potential is significantly reduced when visual input is cut, thus clearly establishing that some sensory fibres which were previously contributing to the composite sensory potentials are no longer activated by the same strength of stimuli; their failure to respond can be construed to mean an increase in the threshold of their excitability. This finding, that the peripheral part of the neurone is affected so quickly by a change in the excitability of the main cell, is an interesting discovery which seems to further confirm the similar phenomenon observed when eliciting 'M' responses. Obviously the membrane excitability of axons as well as sensory fibres is very sensitive (in a very short period of time) to all the changes that may be taking place in the parent neurone.

In another experiment, a tungsten micro-electrode (approximately 5 μ tip diameter) was introduced in the median nerve at the wrist of an unanesthetised human subject. As soon as the subject complained of a sensation of numbress and tingling in a specific area of skin (in this case, the lateral aspect

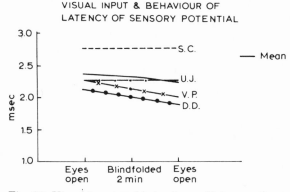

Fig. 23. Visual input and behaviour of latency of sensory potential.

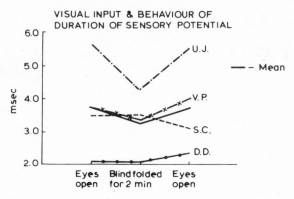

Fig. 24. Visual input and behaviour of duration of sensory potential.

of the distal phalanx of the middle finger), the same area was electrically stimulated and the evoked response was picked up from the monopolar tungsten micro-electrode. The averaged signal was recorded and studied with eyes open and in the blindfolded condition (Fig. 26). It was seen once again that, on blindfolding, the amplitude of the signal was significantly reduced, while the latency was marginally increased. This further reinforces the results gathered when the compound sensory potential of the whole nerve was analysed. In other words, there seems to be clear proof that cutting of visual input so raises the threshold of excitation of the sensory fibres that, with a fixed intensity of sensory input, there is a fall out evident not only in the compound sensory potential (biopolarly recorded) but also in the fascicle potential.

Somatosensory-evoked response from the cortex using surface electrodes

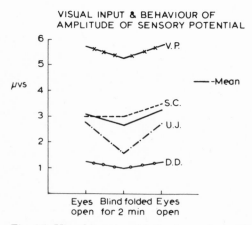

Fig. 25. Visual input and behaviour of amplitude of sensory potential.

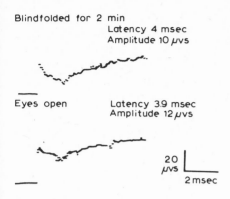

Blindfolded for 2 min
Latency 4 msec
Amplitude 10 μvs

Eyes open   Latency 3.9 msec
Amplitude 12 μvs

20
μvs
2 msec

Stim. midd. finger   G.C.
P.U. med. n. in arm
c̄ microelectrode

Fig. 26.

and signal averaging is a reliable method of studying sensory input and its impact at thalmo-cortical levels. Spinograms present a useful method to study the same phenomenon at the level of roots. In an experiment when SERs and spinograms were analysed in the same subject with eyes open and in the blindfolded condition, significant alteration in the signals was noticed

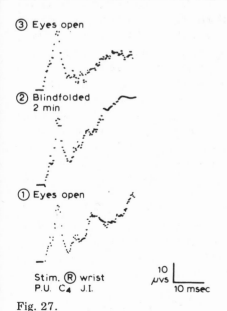

③ Eyes open

② Blindfolded
2 min

① Eyes open

Stim. Ⓡ wrist
P.U. C₄ J.I.

10
μvs
10 msec

Fig. 27.

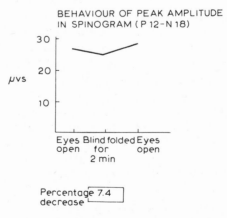

BEHAVIOUR OF PEAK AMPLITUDE
IN SPINOGRAM (P 12-N 18)

30

μvs   20

10

Eyes   Blind folded Eyes
open   for   open
         2 min

Percentage 7.4
decrease

Fig. 28. Behaviour of peak amplitude in spinogram (P12-N18).

both in SERs and spinograms, although no change was seen in latencies or the overall pattern of the signals (Figs. 27 and 28). This is clear proof that visual input seems to affect the sensory input in such a way that at every level, (nerve, spinal root, or thalmo-cortical), there is a significant reduction in amplitude of the potentials, indicating that visual input has an excitatory influence on the threshold levels of various types of sensory inputs. It is known that electrical stimulation of digits may be exciting mainly tactile and other exteroceptive receptors, while it is also believed that the SER occurs mainly as a result of proprioceptive input (Whitehorn, 1969; Giblin, 1969; Halliday, 1963). Similar alterations of SER signals have also been reported in sleep (Allison, 1966). This seems to constitute more proof that mere 'cutting out' of visual input for as short a period as 2 minutes tends to produce results similar to those seen in sleep; similar effects were also demonstrated in the 2nd or late component of withdrawal reflex on blindfolding (Shahani, 1968).

There is now clear evidence that the visual input has a very significant influence on the motor system of man. Considering the experiment in which simple learnt movements were performed by subjects who had a deficit of the pyramidal tract, the excessive activity in proximal muscles of the limbs brings into focus various speculations. Eccles (1971) has asserted that stereotyped movements are largely mediated by the cerebellum. Massion (personal communication) has shown that the cerebellum has maximum influence on the proximal muscles of the limbs, and relatively less on axial muscles and distal muscles in that order. The reduction in the activity of proximal muscles upon blindfolding on performance of the learnt movements in pathophysiological conditions, where cerebellar influence may be functioning with less cortical control, would seem to suggest that the visual input has a direct effect on the cerebellar system (cerebellum and its descending connections). Rubia and Lange (1974) have suggested that visual input may be exerting an influence via the climbing fibres. It would be tempting to involve the red nucleus in this connection, however, there is some gathering evidence that the red nucleus in man tends to be rudimentry and does not play as important a role as in the cat. Wilson et al. (1969) have suggested that Deiters cells projecting to the limbs may be more influenced by inputs other than labyrinthine which have perhaps more to do with motoneurones of neck. We may also have to consider the direct influence of tecto-spinal tracts on the interneuronal pool in spinal cord. Peterson et al. (1971) have suggested that the influence of tectal stimulation on forelimb and hindlimb motoneurones (in cat) may be due to excitation of reticulo-spinal neurones. There are reports that various other types of sensory stimuli like somatosensory (Magni, 1964; Peterson, 1971) and vestibular (Peterson, 1971) are known to influence reticulo-spinal neurones. The reticulo-spinal system thus may be integrating various sensory inputs for their composite influence on motoneurones.

Milner-Brown et al. (1973) have reported that, at low levels of contraction strength, motor-unit recruitment is the major mechanism for increasing force of contraction, but that an increased rate of firing may become a more important mechanism at intermediate to high force levels. Henneman et al. (1974) and Hannertz (1974) have also done some work on the recruitment order of motor units in voluntary contraction. As our experiments involved isometric contraction at minimal levels of tension, the reduction in the rate of firing of motor units on blindfolding did not seem to affect the performance of the voluntary act. From this it is also tempting to deduce that in the performance of learnt activities like holding an object between thumb and fingers, the act can be executed with as much precision with a lower rate of motor unit firing without the visual input. What then could be the functional significance of the increased rate of firing of motor units when visual input is exerting its influence on the central neuronal pool? An answer can be only speculative, that perhaps the increased rate of firing may provide a more suitable state for any need of change in the programme due to any external and internal forces.

Another method of studying the state of excitability of motoneurones and interneurones is by way of reflex studies, both monosynaptic and polysynaptic. Our experiments have shown reduction in excitability on cutting visual input in the case of both these types of reflex. Thus it can be said that motoneurones in the absence of visual input have higher thresholds of excitability. This influence may be exerted upon the motoneurones through various interneurones, but whether through the reticulo-spinal tract, tecto-spinal tract or also direct cortico-spinal fibres cannot be clearly stated with the present state of knowledge. However, it is also possible that visual input has an effect on the threshold levels of other inputs like somatosensory inputs which are applied when we are electrically stimulating the subjects in order to elicit these monosynaptic and polysynaptic reflexes. Fetz (1968) has demonstrated in cats that impulses travelling via pyramidal tracts can also evoke a depolarization of afferent fibres, thereby exerting a presynaptic inhibition on sensory inputs. Our own studies of sensory potentials recorded at various levels — median nerve at wrist, at spinal roots (spinogram), at the level of cerebral cortex (somatosensory-evoked response) — clearly show that cutting down of visual input attenuates all the signals (sensory potentials, SERs etc.). Apart from demonstrating an influence on the threshold of sensory neurones in the spinal cord, it also includes changes at thalmo-cortical projections, as well as signals generated in the post-central gyrus. It also demonstrates that cutaneous as well proprioceptive sensory systems are influenced by the visual input.

The reduction in the peak-to-peak amplitude of 'M' response at near-threshold stimuli when the visual input was eliminated, raises new possibilities of enquiry into the excitability state of the neurone and its axons, in addition to clearly demonstrating the influence of visual input. Within a short period of two minutes of blindfolding the changes were noticed in the threshold of excitation of several axons. If a threshold of excitation of an axon is to be considered in terms of its state of depolarization and hyperpolarization, it is tempting to presume that changes in membrane permeability and ionic balance take place not only at a neuronal level but all along its peripheral appendages. A similar phenomenon in terms of the reduction in the size of sensory potentials further establishes this fact.

In short, visual input has a significant influence on both motor and sensory systems in man. This is proved by studies that have involved voluntary movements by subjects as well as by well known neurophysiological methods of studying stimulus and response (at threshold levels). Whether this influence is mediated through a general integrating system (of various sensory inputs) of reticulo-spinal neurones and/or by other central connections and pathways is not yet clear. Motor as well as sensory neurones in the spinal cord seem to be sensitive to visual input, along with or through appropriate interneurones.

REFERENCES

ADRIAN, E.D. and BRONK, D.W. (1929) The discharge of impulses in motor nerve fibres. Part II. The frequency of discharge in reflex and voluntary contractions. J. Physiol., 67, 119—151.

ALLISON, T., GOFF, W.R. and STERMAN, M.B. (1966) Cerebral somatosensory responses evoked during sleep in the cat. Electroencephalogr. Clin. Neurophysiol., 21, 461—468.

ANDERSON, M.E., YOSHIDA, M. and WILSON, V.J. (1971) Influence of the superior colliculus on cat neck motoneurones. J. Neurophysiol., 34, 898—907.

ANDERSON, M.E., YOSHIDA, M. and WILSON, V.J. (1972) Tectal and tegmental influences on cat forelimb and hindlimb motoneurones. J. Neurophysiol., 35, 462—470.

BURG, D. (1974) Influence of voluntary innervation on human muscle spindle sensitivity. 26th Int. Congr. Physiol. Sci., Satellite Meeting on Motor System: Neurophysiology and Muscle Mechanism, Bombay, India (Abstracts).

ECCLES, J.C. (1971) A re-evaluation of cerebellar function in man. 4th Internatl. Congr. Electromyogr. (abstracts on communications and initial papers), Brussels, p. 167.

ELDRED, E. and HAGBARTH, K.E. (1954) Facilitation and inhibition of gamma efferents by stimulation of certain skin areas. J. Neurophysiol., 17, 59—65.

FETZ, E.E. (1968) Pyramidal tract effects on interneurons in the cat limbo-dorsal horn. J. Neurophysiol., 31, 69—80.

GIBLIN, D.R. (1964) Somatosensory evoked potentials in healthy subjects and in patients with lesions of the nervous system. Ann. N.Y. Acad. Sci., 112, 93—142.

GOFF, W.R., ALLISON, T., SHAPIRO, A. and ROSNER, B.S. (1966) Cerebral somatosensory responses evoked during sleep in man. Electroencephalogr. Clin. Neurophysiol., 21, 1—9.

GRANIT, R. (1955) Receptors and sensory perception. Yale University Press, New Haven, p. 369.

GRANIT, R. and HENATSCH, H.D. (1956) Gamma control of dynamic properties of muscle spindles. J. Neurophysiol., 19, 355—366.

GRILLNER, S. and HONGO, T. (1972) Vestibulo-spinal effects on motoneurones and interneurons in the lumbosacral cord. In (A. Brodal and O. Pompeiano Eds.) Basic Aspects of Central Vestibular Mechanisms. Elsevier Publishing Co., Amsterdam, p. 656.

GRIMBY, L. and HANNERTZ, J. (1968) Recruitment order of motor units on voluntary contraction: changes induced by proprioceptive afferent activity. J. Neurol. Neurosurg. Psychiatry, 31, 565—573.

HALLIDAY, A.M. and WAKEFIELD, G.S. (1963) Cerebral evoked potentials in patients with dissociated sensory loss. J. Neurol. Neurosurg. Psychiatry, 26, 211—219.

HANNERTZ, J. (1974) Discharge properties of motor units in relation to recruitment order in voluntary contraction. Acta Physiol. Scand., 91, 374—384.

HENNEMAN, E., SHAHANI, B.T. and YOUNG, R.R. (1974) Voluntary control of human motor units. 26th Int. Congr. Physiol. Sci., Satellite Meeting on Motor System — Neurophysiology and Muscle Mechanism. Bombay, India (Abstracts).

LUNDBERG, A. (1970) The excitatory control of the Ia inhibitory pathway. In (Anderson, P. and Jansen, J., Eds.) Excitatory Synaptic Mechanisms. Oslo, Universitetsforlaget, pp. 333—340.

LUNDBERG, A. (1972) The significance of segmental spinal mechanisms in motor control. Symposial paper, 4th Internatl. Biophys. Congress, Moscow, pp. 1—13.

MAGNI, F. and WILLIS, W.D. (1964) Subcortical and peripheral control of brain stem reticular neurones. Arch. Ital. Biol. 102, 434—448.

MATTHEWS, P.B.C. (1972) Mammalian Muscle Receptors and their Central Actions. Edward Arnold (Publishers) Ltd., London, p. 630.

MILNER BROWN, H.S., STEIN, R.B. and YEMM, R. (1973) Changes in firing rate of human motor units during linearly changing voluntary contractions. J. Physiol. (Lond.), 230, 371—390.

PETERSON, V.W., ANDERSON, M.E., EILION, M. and WILSON, V.J. (1971) Responses of reticulospinal neurones to stimulation of the superior colliculus. Brain Res., 33, 495—498.

PETERSON, V.W. and FELPEL, L.P. (1971) Excitation and inhibition of reticulo-spinal neurones by vestibular, cortical and cutaneous stimulation. Brain Res., 27, 373—376.

SHAHANI, B. and YOUNG, R.R. (1968) A note on blink reflexes, J. Physiol. (Lond.), 198, 103—104.

SHAHANI, B. (1968) Effects of sleep on human reflexes with a double component. J. Neurol. Neurosurg. Psychiatry, 31, 575—579.

SHAHANI, M. (1973) Visual input and alpha pool in spasticity. J. Postgrad. Med., 19, 139—144.

SHAPOVALOV, A.I., KURCHAVJI, G.G. and STRONGONOVA, M.N. (1956) Synaptic mechanisms of vestibulo-spinal influences on alpha motoneurones. Fiziol. Zh. SSSR (USSR) 52, 1401—1409.

SHERRINGTON, C.S. (1898) Decerebrate rigidity and reflex co-ordination of movement, J. Physiol. (Lond.), 22, 319—332.

STRUPPLER, A. and VELHO, F. (1974) Single flexor reflex afferent recording in man. 26th Int. Congr. Physiol. Sci., Satellite Meeting on Motor System-Neurophysiology and Muscle Mechanism. Bombay, India (Abstracts).

TOKIZANE, T. and SHIMAZU, H. (1964) Functional Differentiation of Human Skeletal Muscle. University of Tokyo Press, pp. 1—62.

VALLBO, A.B. (1970) Slowly adapting muscle receptor in man. Acta Physiol. Scand., 78, 315—333.

WHITEHORN, D., MORSE, R.W. and TOEVE, A.L. (1969) Role of the spino-cervical tract in production of the primary cortical response evoked by forepaw stimulation. Exp. Neurol., 25, 349—364.

WILSON, V.J. and YOSHIDA, M. (1969) Comparison of effects of stimulation of Deiter's nucleus and medial longitudinal fasciculus on neck, forelimb and hindlimb motor neurones. J. Neurophysiol., 32, 743—748.

5

The effects of tonic, isometric contraction on the evoked EMG

Gyan C. AGARWAL and Gerald L. GOTTLIEB

The M-wave is a direct, evoked EMG elicited by electrical stimulation of motor nerve fibers. The amplitude of the response may be measured both by EMG recording from the muscle and by sensing the muscle twitch. Voluntary contraction of the stimulated muscle influences these measures and the effects on the EMG differ from those on the twitch.

INTRODUCTION

When the tibial nerve in the popliteal fossa is electrically stimulated, the first fibers to be excited are the Ia afferents from the spindles of the gastrocnemius-soleus muscles (GSM). About 30—32 msec after the stimulus, a synchronized EMG burst, the Hoffmann reflex (H-wave), is recorded from the GSM (Hoffmann, 1922; Magladery and McDougal, 1950; Paillard, 1955, Gottlieb et al., 1970). As the intensity of stimulation is increased, the H-wave amplitude increases until the threshold of GSM alpha motor fibers in the same mixed tibial nerve is reached. At this point an EMG burst called the M-wave is seen about 8 msec after the stimulus. Further increase in stimulus amplitude results in a monotonic increase in the M-wave until full recruitment of all motor units is achieved. As the M-wave grows the H-wave decreases and by the time the M-wave is maximal the H-wave has vanished. For methodology and further explanation see Táboríková and Sax, 1968, and Hugon, 1973.

The H-wave is influenced by all the spinal and supraspinal mechanisms (such as agonist contraction, antagonist contraction, the Jendrassik manoeuvre, vibration, mental activity, peripheral ischemia) which converge on the alpha motor neurone. (Hoffmann, 1922; Magladery et al., 1950; Paillard, 1955; Hagbarth, 1962; Brunia, 1971; Gottlieb and Agarwal, 1973a,b; Hagbarth, 1973).

The M-wave, being a wholly peripheral phenomenon, is not directly influenced by spinal mechanisms. Peripheral ischemia causes the M-wave latency to become progressively greater and then decay rapidly in amplitude to virtual extinction (Magladery et al., 1950). A marked post-tetanic depression of the M-wave occurs with a tetanic stimulus of frequency greater than 200 Hz and duration greater than 30 sec (Hagbarth, 1962). This depression of the M-wave is accompanied by a small increase in the latency of the response. Vibration and slow muscle stretch do not effect the M-wave (Delwaide, 1971; Mark et al., 1968).

Recently, Shahani (1974) has shown that on threshold stimulation of median nerve in man, the peak-to-peak M-wave amplitude from the abductor pollicis brevis muscle is significantly reduced on blindfolding the subjects. Changes in M-wave are also quite evident in Figure 2D of the paper by Stern et al. (1968). Their experiments were done on Parkinsonian patients.

In this paper we will present some data on the effects of tonic, isometric contraction of agonist and antagonist on the M-wave recorded from the soleus muscle.

EXPERIMENTAL PROCEDURE

Our experiments were performed on four normal male adults ranging in ages from 21 to 36 years. A subject was seated normally in a chair with his right leg extended, the knee slightly flexed, and the foot strapped to a fixed plate with an attached strain gauge bridge for measuring isometric foot torque. The signal from this bridge was also used to provide a visual reference to help the subject maintain a constant initial foot torque (IFT) before stimulation. Differential EMG surface electrodes (1 cm diameter) were placed on the centerline of the lower soleus muscle about 3 cm apart and another pair was placed on the anterior tibial muscle. Cutaneous stimulating electrodes were located posteriorly over the tibial nerve in the popliteal fossa and anteriorly just above the knee. All electrodes were coated with Sanborn Redux Creme.

The electrical stimuli of 1.5 msec duration were applied from a Grass S-8 stimulator through a SIU5 isolation unit. This was triggered at 7–10 sec intervals by a digital computer which recorded both the torque and the EMG. The data were stored on magnetic tape for later analysis. (For details see Gottlieb et al., 1970; Gottlieb and Agarwal, 1971).

RESULTS

With a constant stimulator voltage of M-wave intensity, the foot torque is varied by steady voluntary contraction by the subject. The concommitant variation in the M-wave is shown for two subjects in Fig. 1. In Fig. 2, the subject is relaxed and the same torques applied to the foot plate by the

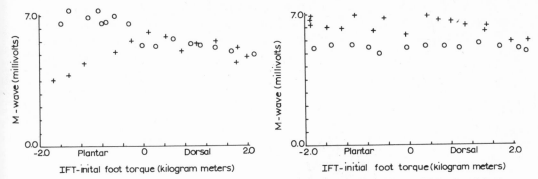

Fig. 1. (Left) Variation in M-wave versus initial foot torque (+ subject, GPO; O subject, GCA).

Fig. 2. (Right) Variation in M-wave versus passive initial foot torque (+ subject, GPO; O subject, GCA).

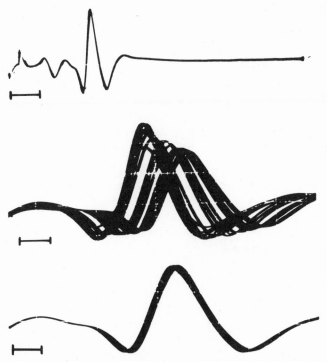

Fig. 3. M-waves during active and passive foot flexion (Subject GCA). (A) Single M-wave with foot relaxed. (B) Series of M-waves (plotted in Fig. 1) during active foot flexion. (C) Series of M-waves (plotted in Fig. 2) during passive foot flexion. Scale: (A) 2 mV and 5 msec, (B) and (C) 2 mV and 1 msec.

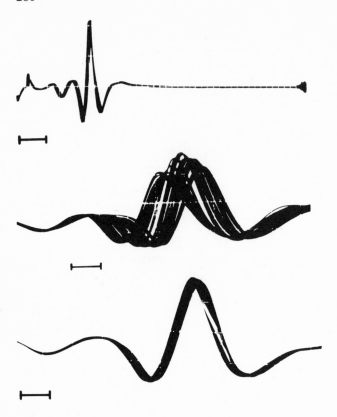

Fig. 4. M-waves during active and passive foot flexion (subject GPO): (A) Single M-wave with foot relaxed. (B) Series of M-waves (plotted in Fig. 1) during active foot flexion. (C) Series of M-waves (plotted in Fig. 2) during passive foot flexion. Scale: (A) 2 mV and 5 msec, (B) and (C) 2 mV and 1 msec.

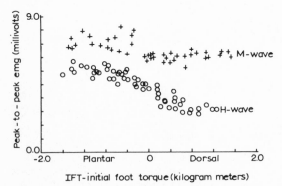

Fig. 5. Variation in H-wave (○) and M-wave (+) with initial foot torque for two experiments at different stimulus intensities.

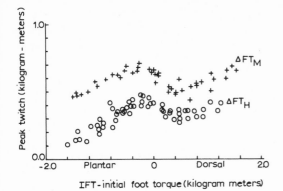

Fig. 6. Variation in twitch for H-wave (○) and M-wave (+) of Fig. 5.

experimenter's hand. Figs 3 and 4 show the actual EMG waveforms of the data in Figs 1 and 2 for both subjects. There is a variation in amplitude of M-wave with IFT and there is a progressive shift in the latency of the peak of the wave, the peak being increasingly more delayed with dorsiflexion and appearing earlier with plantarflexion. There is negligible change in amplitude or phase with passive torques.

Fig. 5 shows the variation in reflex EMG versus IFT for two experiments, one at maximal H-wave stimulation and the other at M-wave intensity suppressing the H-wave. Fig. 6 shows the variation in the twitch amplitudes (ΔFT) with IFT corresponding to these stimuli.

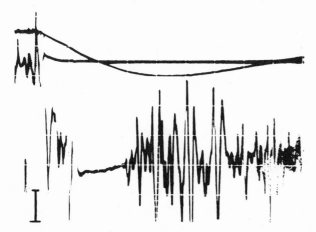

Fig. 7. Reciprocal inhibition of the anterior tibial muscle by a maximal M-wave stimulus delivered to the tibial nerve. Note that the inhibition begins when the H-wave would appear as if it were not blocked by the antidromic component of the stimulus. Upper trace: foot torque 1.2 kg.m./unit; middle trace: GSM EMG 1 mV/unit; bottom trace: ATM EMG 0.05 mV/unit. Time scale 20 msec/unit.

DISCUSSION

In these experiments, the stimulator setting is kept constant throughout a particular run. The assumption made is that the stimulus (in the sense of the number of afferent nerves excited) is constant.

There are two obvious reasons why this assumption might not be valid. The first is that the geometry between the stimulating electrodes and the tibial nerve might change. This is certainly a concern since plantar and dorsi-flexion put different tensions on the tendons crossing the popliteal fossa.

Two considerations dictate against this. The experiments were performed at different degrees of knee flexion and no differences in response were noted other than the normal day to day variations. These variations are a consequence of such diverse factors as electrode placement, skin conductivity and subject fatigue. If geometry at the knee were critical, knee flexion would be expected to be important but it was not. Supramaximal stimuli were used as a precaution against this.

The second question is whether small changes in muscle length and the resulting movement of the recording electrodes might occur between plantar- and dorsi-flexion. Since the foot plate apparatus is not perfectly rigid, some movement is possible. However, flexion of the foot plate by the experimenter's hand produced neither amplitude nor phase changes in the M-wave (see Figs 3 and 4). Muscle shortening due to stretch of muscles' intrinsic series elasticity cannot be excluded, however.

Although the amplitude responses of the two subjects in Fig. 1 do not follow the same pattern, the phase shift is consistant in both. Similar phase shift is also observed for the H-wave. Therefore, this phase shift cannot be the cause of the amplitude changes observed in the M-wave.

The second reason the assumption of constant stimulus is open to question is the fact that for the first 15—25 minutes after stimulation begins the reflex increases in size. If the initial stimulator setting is just below the M-wave threshold, an M-wave will often develop.

The stimulator acts through the SIU5 as a voltage source and one possible explanation for this behavior is that the impedance between the electrodes might decrease as a result of the stimulation. The consequent increase in current flow would then excite more fibers. This is, in fact, a well known phenomenon called the galvanic skin response (Lader and Montagu, 1962) produced by electrical stimulation of the skin.

The problem was resolved by allowing the subject to adapt to the stimulus for 10—15 minutes before beginning an experiment. After that, any residual change was usually too small to notice although, if significant increases did appear, the experiment was aborted.

Since both the stimulus and response are peripheral to the central nervous system, the variation in M-wave is not a function of synaptic mechanisms. Mark et al. (1968) observed no change in M-wave with passive rotation of the ankle joint by 10°. This would indicate that a slight movement of the muscle with respect to the recording electrodes does not appreciably influence the amplitude of the M-wave. What then is responsible for the M-wave variation with IFT?

The change in amplitude is definitely not a consequence of simple summation between the M-wave and voluntary EMG activity. The maximum peak-to-peak amplitude of the EMG measured in these experiments during static voluntary effort is of the order of 80 μV or at least an order of magnitude less than normal M-wave variation. Furthermore, the soleus muscle is inactive during static dorsiflexion when M-wave is reduced. Since the normal firing frequencies of soleus motoneurones is only about 10 pps there is little likelihood of axonal occlusion between the voluntary and reflex inputs.

The peak twitch torque has three distinct phases as seen in Fig. 6. The shape of the response curve is identical for the H-wave and the M-wave.

Starting at the maximum plantar IFT, as IFT decreases twitch increases. This is probably a direct consequence of decreasing incremental gain, with frequency, of the muscle. That is, the twitch caused by a single pulse in a quiescent motor unit is greater than the twitch caused by injecting a single additional pulse into a steady pulse train. In the extreme case, an additional pulse to a maximally tetanized muscle results in no twitch at all. At lower levels of plantar IFT, more motor units are quiescent and each thereby contributes more to the twitch.

There is a second factor leading to a decrease in twitch with increasing IFT. That is the silent period in soleus activity (Granit, 1955) which follows the H-wave (Agarwal and Gottlieb, 1972). This period of silence, lasting about 100—200 msec, is caused by several effects, Renshaw inhibition, Golgi tendon organ inhibition and muscle spindle disfacilitation being among them. This represents an inhibitory 'step input', opposing the excitatory effect of the H-wave (or M-wave).

The silence in soleus activity is total during this period except at very low stimulus levels or very high levels of IFT. Thus, the greater the IFT, the larger is the 'step' of inhibition, its amplitude being the difference between the level of soleus activity prior to the H-wave and the level during the silence. In effect, the reflex twitch is diminished by a transient withdrawal of the voluntary input to the agonist muscle and this would be more significant at higher levels of voluntary effort.

In the region of small plantar IFT to small dorsal IFT, the twitch declines with and to some extent as a consequence of the decreasing EMG. At these low levels of IFT, the changes in incremental gain no longer dominate. However, this decline in twitch does not continue with stronger dorsiflexion and, in the case illustrated, twitch increases to near maximal levels.

We must realize that the foot torque represents the summed effects of two antagonistic muscle groups acting about the ankle joint. Thus, a twitch may represent a transient increase in activity of the soleus and synergistic muscles but may also represent a transient decrease in activity of the anterior tibial muscle and its synergists. During plantarflexion the former mechanism predominates but during dorsiflexion reciprocal inhibition of the anterior tibial muscle as shown in Fig. 7 becomes significant (Gottlieb and Agarwal, 1971; Agarwal and Gottlieb, 1972).

The existence of reciprocal inhibition allows us to understand how the twitch can remain large while the EMG is decreasing. When the twitch is a consequence of this inhibition it represents the difference in anterior tibial activity just prior to and during the transient inhibitory phase. Just as the silent period of an agonist muscle can diminish a twitch, a silent period of an antagonist muscle can enhance it. As long as the inhibition is total, the twitch can be no bigger than the preceding level of activity will allow. Thus, the larger the dorsal IFT, the larger the twitch, as shown in Fig. 6. At larger levels of IFT, the inhibition would presumably no longer be total and the twitch would not increase further.

ACKNOWLEDGEMENT

This work was supported in part by the National Science Foundation.

REFERENCES

AGARWAL, G.C. and GOTTLIEB, G.C. (1972) The muscle silent period and reciprocal inhibition in man. J. Neurol. Neurosurg. Psychiatry, 35, 72—76.

BRUNIA, C.H.M. (1971) The influence of a task on the Achilles tendon and Hoffman reflex. Physiol. Behav., 6, 367—373.

DELWAIDE, P.J. (1971) Etude experimentale de l'hyperreflexie tendineuse en clinique neurologique. Arscia, Bruxelles.

GOTTLIEB, G.L. and AGARWAL, G.C. (1971) Effects of initial conditions on the Hoffmann reflex. J. Neurol. Neurosurg. Psychiatry, 34, 226—230.

GOTTLIEB, G.L. and AGARWAL, G.C. (1973a) Modulation of postural reflexes by voluntary movement. I. Modulation of the active limb. J. Neurol. Neurosurg. Psychiatry, 36, 529—538.

GOTTLIEB, G.L. and AGARWAL, G.C. (1973b) Modulation of postural reflexes by voluntary movement. II. Modulation at an inactive joint. J. Neurol Neurosurg. Psychiatry, 36, 539—546.

GOTTLIEB, G.L., AGARWAL, G.C. and STARK, L. (1970) Interactions between voluntary and postural mechanisms of the human motor system. J. Neurophysiol., 33, 365—381.

GRANIT, R. (1955) Receptors and Sensory Perception. Yale University Press.

HAGBARTH, K.E. (1962) Post-tetanic potentiation of myotatic reflexes in man. J. Neurol. Neurosurg. Psychiatry, 25, 1—10.

HAGBARTH, K.E. (1973) The effect of muscle vibration in normal man and in patients with motor disorders. In (J.E. Desmedt, Ed.) New Developments in Electromyography and Clinical Neurophysiology, Vol. 3, Karger, Basel, pp. 428—443.

HOFFMANN, P. (1922) Untersuchungen über die Eigenreflexe (Sehnreflexe) Menschlicher Muskeln. Springer, Berlin.

HUGON, M. (1973) Methodology of the Hoffmann reflex in man. In (J.E. Desmedt, Ed.) New Developments in Electromyography and Clinical Neurophysiology, Vol. 3, Karger, Basel, pp. 277—293.

LADER, M.H. and MONTAGU, J.D. (1962) The psycho-galvanic reflex: a pharmacological study of the peripheral mechanism. J. Neurol. Neurosurg. Psychiatry, 25, 126—133.

MAGLADERY, J.W. and McDOUGAL, Jr. D.B. (1950) Electrophysiological studies of nerve and reflex activity in normal man. I. Identification of certain reflexes in the electromyogram and the conduction velocity of peripheral nerve fibers. Bull. Johns Hopkins Hosp., 86, 265—290.

MAGLADERY, J.W., McDOUGAL, D.B. and STOLL, J. (1950) Electrophysiological studies of nerve and reflex activity in normal man. II. The effects of peripheral ischemia. Bull. Johns Hopkins Hosp., 86, 291—312.

MARK, R.F., COQUERY, J.M. and PAILLARD, J. (1968) Autogenetic reflex effects of slow or steady stretch of the calf muscles in man. Exp. Brain Res. 6, 130—145.

PAILLARD, J. (1955) Réflexes et régulations d'origine proprioceptive chez l'homme. Librairie Arnette, Paris.

SHAHANI, M. (1974) Visual input and M-response at threshold stimulus. 26th. Internatl. Congr. Physiol. Sci., Satellite Meeting on Motor System: Neurophysiology and Muscle Mechanism, Bombay, India, (abstracts).

STERN, J., MENDELL, J. and CLARK, K. (1968) H-Reflex suppression by thalamic stimulation and drug administration. J. Neurosurg., 29, 393—396.

TÁBORÍKOVÁ, H. and SAX, D.S. (1968) Motoneurone pool and the H-reflex, J. Neurol. Neurosurg. Psychiatry, 31, 354—361.

6

The EMG analysis of certain negative symptoms caused by lesions of the central nervous system*

B.T. SHAHANI and R.R. YOUNG

Though it appears self-evident that the discharge of a patient's spinal motoneurones, and hence his EMG, should be abnormal whenever he is weak because of a disorder affecting the central nervous system (CNS), it has proven remarkably difficult to specify precisely how motor unit behavior in those circumstances differs from normal. It is surprising that the best contemporary EMG laboratories have so little to offer the clinician concerning the objective evaluation of his patients with CNS lesions. Even when one restricts his attention to such patients' purely negative symptoms (e.g., weakness, slowness, akinesia, lack of facility), there is little data to guide one to their EMG characterization. Whereas it is usually possible clinically to recognize and categorize these symptoms according to disease state, site of lesion, and so forth, it is still difficult, or impossible, to do so electromyographically. It remains then for the electromyographer to address himself to the following problem. How (and to what extent) can the abnormal motility in patients with CNS disease (or, for that matter, the normal activity to which the abnormality is contrasted) be described in terms of the performance of single motor units or groups of muscles? This is a brief review of our experience and that to be found in the relatively meager literature bearing upon one aspect of this problem — can the negative symptoms of such patients (including those with what the electromyographer calls 'upper motoneurone lesions') be described in terms of the behavior of small numbers of motor units recorded during a gradual contraction of the affected muscle, and if so, how?

* Supported in part by the Parkinson's Disease Project of the Massachusetts General Hospital and the Allen P. and Josephine B. Green Foundation.

PYRAMIDAL SYNDROMES

The common lesions of the CNS which result in weakness affect, with rare exceptions, both the purely pyramidal and some of the various extra-pyramidal systems. If a hemiparesis or paraparesis results, it is usually referred to as a 'pyramidal syndrome', even though most of the symptoms and signs (particularly the positive ones) result from disorder of non-pyramidal (i.e., 'extra-pyramidal') pathways. For purposes of discussion, we will also use the common term 'pyramidal syndrome', though we wish to make it clear that the causative lesion very rarely is restricted to the true pyramidal system.

Lesions of these CNS systems, dysfunction of which produces hemiparesis or paraparesis, result in weakness by compromising voluntary control over activity of various structures including the final common pathway. EMG documentation of the abnormal activity of spinal or bulbar motoneurones of patients with pyramidal syndromes reveals the following: (1) the number of motor units that can voluntarily be activated or 'recruited' is reduced, and (2) the maximum rate at which they can be activated is also reduced (Hoefer and Putnam, 1940; Sherrer and Metral, 1969; personal observations). Both of these reductions are despite the strongest possible effort on the part of the patient and are to be contrasted with what one records from patients with lesions of the peripheral nervous system. Lesions of the spinal roots or peripheral nerves produce weakness by disconnecting some or all of the spinal motoneurones from their muscles in the periphery. Those uncommon CNS lesions which damage or destroy the spinal motoneurone directly also result in signs of 'lower motor neurone' dysfunction. The result in both instances is also a reduction in the number of motor units that are electromyographically active, though those that remain functionally connected can be activated at a normally rapid rate which depends upon the voluntary effort exerted. Thus, the rate of firing of the few motor units seen in reduced EMG patterns with maximal voluntary effort can give a clue regarding the site of the lesion; if reduced, it suggests an 'upper motor neurone' lesion, whereas if it remains in a normally high frequency range, it usually indicates a 'lower motor neurone' lesion. A normal subject who expends less than maximal effort will also activate fewer motor units but at lower rates than would be seen with greater effort. Fortunately, most patients with malingering or 'hysterical weakness' produce a tremulous, intermittent activation of units, so that one does not always confuse them with patients having structural lesions of the CNS. However, since there is no objective measurement of 'effort', the two EMG signs described above are non-specific — though they are present with so-called upper motoneurone lesions and diverge from normal in proportion to the degree of clinical weakness, they are not absolutely diagnostic of such a lesion. Furthermore, these are the EMG signs associated only with those negative symptoms or motor deficits which are apparent at the beginning of a voluntary movement. This review will not cover the EMG signs of such positive symptoms, or 'release' phenomena, as spasticity, rigidity or tremor, except to mention the confusion they introduce into the study of voluntary control of motor units. In the presence of these positive symptoms, it is possible to activate single units reflexly in response to muscle stretch or cutaneous stimulation. These reflexly recruitable units can usually not be activated voluntarily — in patients with severe or complete paralysis of upper motor neurone type, the units recorded can only be activated reflexly. If, for example, in a patient with a hypotonic 'foot drop', more of the anterior tibial motor units within the recording range of the EMG electrode can be recruited by scratching the sole of the foot than can be voluntarily recruited, the electromyographer or clinician places the lesion within the CNS rostral to the anterior tibial motoneurone pool rather than in the peripheral nervous system. The integrity of the lower motor neurone, in this instance, can be further demonstrated by recording a normal-sized evoked compound muscle action potential (M response) following electrical stimulation of the mixed nerve supplying the weak or paralyzed dorsiflexors of the foot and toes.

Another category of negative symptoms seen with lesions of the CNS is only evident later during the activation of paretic muscles and is loosely termed 'fatigue'. Voluntary activity cannot be sustained for long periods even in those motor units which, with considerable effort, can initially be recruited in such muscles. With muscular activity of comparable strength in normal subjects (that is, with minimal or moderate voluntary effort), single motor units can be seen to be continuously active at rates of 5—10/sec for many minutes (sometimes hours, or even indefinitely). This is particularly true for proximal or axial 'postural muscles', but may be seen also in more distal muscles; data is not at hand to answer the question as to the length of time that motor units can be continuously active, either in normal subjects or in patients with weak muscles. Suffice it to say, most normal tonic units, once recruited, continue to be continuously active for long periods of time. In paretic muscles, some or many units do likewise. Other units, however, are active once or a few times in a short phasic burst at the beginning of contraction. Still others discharge tonically for some seconds before the rate at which they are repetitively active slows gradually to the point that they are 'disrecruited' (cease to discharge). Careful quantitative studies of these phenomena in health as well as disease are yet to be done.

EXTRA-PYRAMIDAL SYNDROMES

Parkinson's disease, the most common 'pure' extrapyramidal syndrome, is the clinical counterpart of dysfunction of nigro-striatal dopaminergic pathways (Hornykiewicz, 1971). There are also other lesions within the CNS, but they are less obvious. Because the symptoms and signs of one patient with

Parkinson's disease (e.g., only unilateral resting tremor) may be so different from those of another (e.g., severe bilateral akinesia without tremor), it is assumed that the biochemical and structural lesions within the nervous system also are multiple and varied. This review will restrict its focus to the chief negative symptom experienced by many, but not all, patients with Parkinson's disease — akinesia. The aspects of normal motility lacking in such patients include: (1) the ability for quick initiation of motion, and (2) facility or dexterity in shifting from one to another of the complicated patterns of contraction (e.g., in muscles of forearm and hand) necessary for the performance of detailed or intricate activities such as writing, buttoning, knitting, etc. These activities and others, such as walking, which normally are perfectly automatic, must, in patients with Parkinson's disease, be consciously thought out step by step. Both of these deficits can be reversed by L-Dopa therapy. The EMG counterpart of the first deficit is slowness in initiation of motor unit activity (prolonged reaction time), but normal numbers of units are usually recruited eventually. They appear to discharge at approximately normal maximal rates, and it is not clear that there is slowness in reaching that rate once a unit becomes active. Certainly, there is usually no apparent immediate failure of tonic contraction of these units. When, with the passage of years, akinesia becomes more severe, 'fatigue' does become prominent — patients may write or speak a few words before the excursion or volume of the motor activity runs down to the point that there is no further output. This fatigue may become so severe that, together with the akinetic difficulty in initiating movements, there is virtual paralysis of voluntary activity. The presence of this sort of paralysis is reflected in the description of Parkinson's disease as paralysis agitans.

The EMG counterpart of the second deficit is even less obvious. Our knowledge of the sequence, timing and relative intensity of activity in each of the muscles involved in any movement (normal or otherwise) is quite limited because of the complexity of the situation and derives from studies of very simple, stereotyped movements, such as a modest amplitude flexion of the elbow (Hallett et al., 1974). We are, therefore, unable to define, in EMG or mechanical terms, the deficits seen in patterns of muscular contraction during complicated movements by patients with extra-pyramidal (or other) lesions.

However, there are a number of observations of the behavior of single motor units and groups of muscles in patients with Parkinson's disease. When rapid phasic movements are attempted (such as tapping the index fingers on a table), the patients initially perform at a maximal rate of 6—8/sec, but this soon changes to the 'resting tremor' frequency of 3—5/sec. Simultaneous EMG recording from a pair of antagonistic muscles (e.g., flexors and extensors of the fingers), shows some interesting features. Initially, there is a tendency to co-contraction with synchronous bursts of EMG activity in these muscles. However, when the tapping rate is reduced to 3—5/sec, the pattern changes into alternating bursts of EMG activity so characteristic of Parkinsonian resting tremor. When this behavior of many units in several muscles during these rather gross movements is compared with the behavior of single motor units during minimal contraction in Parkinson's disease, a striking similarity is noted. Whereas normal subjects can speed up or slow down the rate at which single motor units discharge (within the range of 3—4 or 8—9/sec before other units are recruited), these patients have great difficulty in that respect. The single units that are recruited may initially discharge at a higher frequency of 6—8/sec for a short period of time, but on the whole, there is a tendency to discharge at a rather constant frequency of 3—5/sec. Efforts to speed up the rate recruit other units which, together with the first unit, still discharge at roughly the same frequency and tend to discharge more or less synchronously. Normally, when units are recruited, they discharge without apparent temporal relationship to one another — that is, asynchronously. It is not known which mechanisms are employed so that the spinal motoneurones (within a motoneurone pool) discharge out of phase with one another. In patients with Parkinson's disease, these mechanisms for insuring a non-synchronous discharge are defective, and the early units to be recruited tend to be activated synchronously as a 3—5/sec tremor. The defect which limits the rate, for example, of voluntary flexion and extension of the wrist to 3—5/sec affects the behavior of large numbers of units in these several muscles — though there is as yet no proof, it may be similar to the defect described above in the control of single motor units.

There are other disturbances in the control of single units in Parkinson's disease. After the prolonged reaction time mentioned above, single units can be recruited in isolation by some patients. Though others can certainly recruit motor units (they are not completely paralyzed), and usually normal maximum numbers of units (cf. pyramidal syndrome above), they do not do so normally. There is difficulty in controlling a minimal contraction so as to activate one or several units within the recording sphere of the needle or wire electrode without recruiting so many units as to make it impossible to follow the behavior of a single one in the oscilloscope. Even those Parkinsonians who can activate single units in isolation have difficulty controlling their performance at low levels of effort (cf. 'fixation' at rates of 3—5/sec). With maximum voluntary effort, a great many units become active, the rates approach normal, and the synchronization is usually no longer obvious.

The superimposition, even subclinically, of the positive symptoms of Parkinson's disease, such as the tremor and the tonic background involuntary discharge of units known as rigidity, complicates the EMG analysis of the negative symptoms. For example, some of the single units recorded at 3—5/sec may represent the EMG counterpart of rigidity rather than being the truly voluntary activation of these units. The EMG analysis of most of the other extra-pyramidal syndromes (e.g., dystonia, torticollis, choreoathetosis, hemiballismus, etc.) is even more difficult because they are manifest primarily by positive symptoms. Our preliminary observations indicate that the normal fixed order of recruitment, whereby smaller units are recruited at lower threshold than larger units, may be reversed in some of these conditions.

To return for a moment to the problem of fatigue — as a sustained tonic muscular contraction continues to be maintained, fatigue eventually occurs even in the most normal circumstances. This is manifest as a gradual slowing of the maximal rates of motor unit activity and a 'disrecruitment' of (or progressive cessation of activity in) units, particularly those largest ones which were last to be recruited (Henneman et al., 1965; and see Section II, Ch. 3). This particular type of fatigue is not related to failure of transmission in nerve, muscle fiber, or at the neuromuscular junction, nor to failure of electromechanical coupling or contractile mechanism within the muscle. It is difficult to define precise limits as to when this sort of fatigue occurs, even in normal subjects, because (1) variability in effort from moment to moment makes it difficult to time the onset of the already subtle and poorly discriminated slowing in firing rate and disrecruitment of motor units, and (2) there exist a number of other uncontrollable (or poorly controllable) factors, such as motivation, prior exercise, conditioning, inherited muscle mass and so forth. It is nonetheless true that disease states that produce abnormalities in the central control of motor performance are characteristically associated with fatigue of motor unit function at lower levels of maximum tension or shorter times of sustained contraction than normal. Even so, it is difficult to tell exactly when a movement or sustained posture is beginning to be fatigued, or, during its course, exactly how fatigued it has become. Evaluation of this negative symptom (decrease in motor unit activity) is further complicated in many patients with lesions of the CNS in whom abnormal positive symptoms (such as spasticity, rigidity, choreo-athetosis, tremor) are also present. One reflection of this difficulty is experienced by physical therapists, who are able to grade quite precisely and reproducibly the strength of various muscle contractions in normal subjects and patients with various disorders of the peripheral nerves and muscles. When it comes to quantitative assessment of muscle power in patients with cerebral or spinal lesions, the superaddition of various positive symptoms makes it impossible to quantitate muscle strength accurately.

In summary, the activity of the lower motor neurone or final common pathway (as seen in the behavior of motor units in EMG) does not appear to differ qualitatively from normal when one considers the weakness resulting from such commonplace disorders as cerebrovascular accidents, cerebral tumors, or Parkinson's disease. There appears to be a functional continuum from the subject where the number of motor units and their firing rate is normal to the very weak patient where only a few units can be activated voluntarily, and then only at a low repetition rate. At no point in that continuum can one clearly draw a line separating normal from abnormal. If there were a clearcut, dramatic abnormality in the EMG with certain of the negative symptoms of CNS disease, it would simplify diagnosis (and therefore therapy), as well as the process of clinical (including EMG) and neuropathological correlation by which we have attained much of our knowledge of CNS function.

Careful but non-quantitative EMG analysis of the behavior of single motor units has failed so far to reveal any highly specific quantifiable abnormality in patients with clearcut, easily demonstrable abnormalities of motility caused by CNS lesions. That is, the neurophysiological correlates of classical, clinical 'dysfunctional states' appear to be complex and are not yet reducible to simple, well-defined measurements. Quantitative analyses of the behavioral characteristics of single, low-threshold tonic motor units (Petajan and Philip, 1969), when undertaken in large numbers of patients with well-characterized lesions of the CNS, should be helpful. The concepts of pyramidal weakness, extra-pyramidal akinesia, and 'fatigue' are useful clinically, but even these can be differentiated from normal, or from one another, more easily on the basis of other aspects of the clinical syndrome (i.e., by recognizing a pattern of signs and symptoms), than on the basis of evaluation of the negative symptoms themselves clinically or electromyographically. In a search for the functional units of the motor system, these clinical 'dysfunctional states' have been studied in an effort to gain some insight into what the normal units and their normal function are. Little progress has been made — we have achieved little basic insight by studies of these clinical abnormalities. It is very difficult even to quantify them, e.g., 'how much pyramidal weakness is present now?' To be able to quantitate them would be of immense importance to more certain diagnosis, more accurate prognosis, the evaluation of more effective therapy, and more meaningful insight into CNS function. To be able to define or describe the EMG correlates of these symptoms would not allow us automatically to explain them but would presumably point us toward some understanding of the relevant basic mechanisms.

REFERENCES

HALLETT, M., SHAHANI, B.T. and YOUNG, R.R. (1974) EMG patterns during stereotyped voluntary movements in the human. Proc. Int. Union Physiol. Sci. XXVI. Int. Congr., New Delhi, XI, 184.
HENNEMAN, E., SOMJEN, G. and CARPENTER, D. (1965) Functional significance of cell size in spinal motoneurones. J. Neurophysiol., 28, 560—580.
HOEFER, P.F.A. and PUTNAM, T.J. (1940) Action potentials of muscles in spastic conditions. Arch. Neurol. Psychiat., 43, 1—22.
HORNYKIEWICZ, O. (1971) Neurochemical pathology and pharmacology of brain dopamine and acetylcholine: rational basis for the current drug treatment of Parkinson-

ism. In (F.H. McDowell and C.H. Markham, Eds.) Recent Advances in Parkinson's Disease. F.A. Davis Co., Philadelphia, pp. 34—65.

PETAJAN, J.H. and PHILIP, B.A. (1969) Frequency control of motor unit action potentials. Electroencephalogr. Clin. Neurophysiol., 27, 66—72.

SHERRER, J. and METRAL, S. (1969) Electromyography. In (P.J. Vinken and G.W. Bruyn, Eds.) Handbook of Clinical Neurology, Vol. 1, North-Holland Publishing Co., Amsterdam, pp. 631—649.

7

Asterixis - a disorder of the neural mechanisms underlying sustained muscle contraction *

B.T. SHAHANI and R.R. YOUNG

As described in the foregoing chapter, the EMG analysis of several of the common 'negative symptoms' in clinical neurology is unsatisfactory, and EMG studies have not been particularly helpful with regard to pyramidal weakness, extrapyramidal akinesia, or fatigue with a number of CNS disorders. It is difficult, by means of EMG, either to identify these symptoms of CNS dysfunction or to quantitate the extent to which they are present. There is, however, another common negative symptom (asterixis) which, though it is usually overlooked, has a very characteristic clinical and EMG appearance. Because the deficient EMG activity constituting asterixis is easily recognized, this negative symptom stands in contrast to all the others in which the EMG picture is far from unique or distinctive.

Described initially by Adams and Foley (1953), asterixis refers to a jerky, flapping intermittency of sustained posture. It is characterized by arrhythmic, brief, abrupt lapses, or relaxations, of tonically contracting muscles (Fig. 1). These lapses may occur as often as several times a second or as infrequently as one per minute or longer. The EMG counterparts to these relaxations are periods of complete electrical silence (35—200 msec) (Fig. 2) during which sustained posture is overcome by gravity. Then, when the motor units begin to be activated again in normal numbers and at as rapid a rate as prior to the pause ('complete interference pattern'), the body part is jerked back to the formerly maintained posture (often with an overshoot depending on the circumstances). The latter, restorative movement is more rapid (and therefore, jerky) than the gravity-induced initial movement which occurred during the EMG pause (Fig. 1). The subject has no control over these pauses, is astonished to find that they have happened, and complains that his arm, for example, is jerking involuntarily. If the pauses occur very

* Supported in part by the Parkinson's Disease Project of the Massachusetts General Hospital and the Allen P. and Josephine B. Green Foundation.

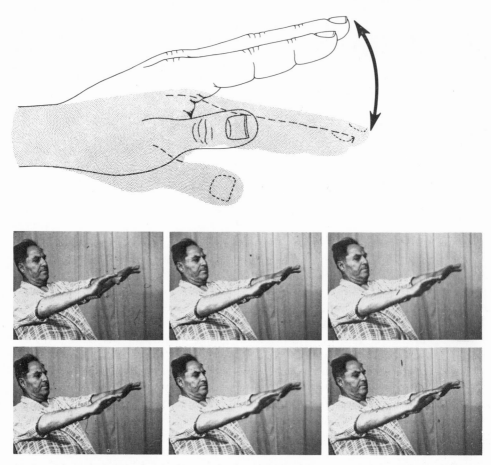

Fig. 1. (A) This illustrates the changes in posture of the voluntarily dorsiflexed hand seen with asterixis. During the cessation of EMG activity in muscles responsible for dorsiflexion of the wrist, gravity pulls the hand into the position denoted by the stippling. When the EMG resumes, the hand is quickly dorsiflexed again. (B) The sequence described in (A) is depicted by the sequential photographs of the patient's right hand. Note that the posture of the patient otherwise, including the rest of the right upper extremity, does not change during this sequence. There is approximately 85 msec between frames, and the sequence proceeds horizontally, beginning with the upper left and ending with the lower right frame.

frequently, the jerking becomes almost rhythmical, and the abnormal movement can be mistaken for a tremor. The pauses occur synchronously throughout the muscles of one limb, but there is little correlation in the timing of the lapses in both arms, for example. There is no change in the EEG associated with these movements. The termination of EMG activity and its reinstitution are instantaneous — the motor unit activity is switched off

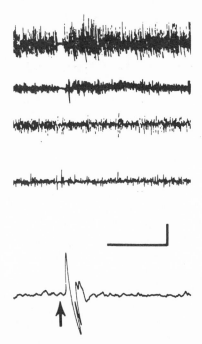

Fig. 2. The upper 4 lines are surface EMG activity recorded from a patient's wrist extensors, wrist flexors, triceps, and biceps muscles, respectively. The bottom tracing is an accelerometric record of movement in that hand. Note the typical brief cessation of EMG activity associated with asterixis (above the arrow) and the biphasic acceleration of the hand which follows. These are the EMG and accelerometer counterparts of the clinically evident 'flap' or 'jerk.' Calibrations are 1 sec and 50 μV.

and then on again without any obvious change, such as reduction in numbers or rates of motor unit firing just prior to or following the pause. These brief pauses with quick, jerky movements are, of course, not seen when a muscle or limb is absolutely at rest (i.e., no background EMG activity). Even when there is background EMG activity against which they could be seen, the pauses and lapses of posture are difficult to recognize during the ballistic phase of the actual movement (i.e., during phasic aspects of muscle contraction). They are readily apparent, often within a matter of seconds, after the sustained posture has been reached (i.e., during the tonic, isometric phase of muscle contraction). They are seen during the tonic phase of (1) conscious voluntary movements (such as dorsiflexing the wrist), (2) involuntary, postural contractions (such as supporting the trunk on an arm while leaning backwards in the sitting position), and (3) reflex muscle contractions (such as the grasp reflex).

Our hypothesis is that these lapses reflect an abnormality of the neural mechanisms underlying sustained muscular contraction. It is tempting to suggest that this abnormality involves those CNS circuits subserving tonic (as opposed to phasic) muscle contraction. Certainly that would describe, dichotomously, the situations in which one does and does not see the lapses clinically (vide supra). We prefer to use the term 'sustained' contraction rather than the more specific terms "tonic" or "phasic" because, in such patients, we have recorded brief periods of silence even during the alternating 3—4/sec bursts of EMG activity in wrist flexors and extensors associated with voluntary tapping of the fingers. Many more careful observations are required of the presence or absence of asterixis in various situations of movement, posture, etc., to allow a maximally precise description of the circumstances of motility in which asterixis is most prominent. The tonic—phasic dichotomy, a simple though useful one, may not reflect adequately the strategies employed by the CNS. In any case, these lapses of EMG activity certainly interrupt what would normally be a well-sustained (brief or prolonged) contraction — as such, asterixis provides a readily quantifiable EMG (and clinical) sign of an abnormality within what is, theoretically at least, a restricted CNS system. Unfortunately, the anatomical and neurochemical details of this system — a disorder of which causes asterixis — have not been worked out yet. There are, however, a number of very tantalizing leads. These flaps, or lapses of posture, are seen in normal people as they fall asleep in an upright position (i.e., without prior relaxation of postural muscle contraction). The muscles of the neck — principally extensors, but at other times (depending on position of head) flexors, are involved so the head nods and is quickly jerked upright. If upper limb muscles are tonically active (holding a paper or a book), they are also involved with the typical jerks of asterixis when the normal subject dozes off. Under slightly less normal circumstances, we have seen several patients without apparent CNS lesions who developed prolonged, typical, bilateral asterixis while receiving anticonvulsants (Young and Shahani, 1973). Other metabolic or biochemical abnormalities can (as noted below), by way of the circulation, affect the CNS to produce bilateral asterixis without a corresponding structural change in the CNS. A series of patients with focal CNS lesions demonstrates contra-lateral asterixis only while receiving the anticonvulsant diphenylhydantoin (Young and Shahani, 1973). The anatomical lesions, as demonstrated in these patients, unfortunately are not restricted to one CNS structure or another. However, there was no clear weakness of the arm, no sensory loss, and no 'cerebellar signs' in these patients. Other patients, as they recover from a hemiparesis, suffer from asterixis even without diphenylhydantoin; small, very focal CNS lesions can also produce asterixis. Patients with Parkinson's Disease and other movement disorders characteristically demonstrate contra-lateral asterixis during stereotaxic neurosurgical procedures as the lesions in the VL thalamus are gradually enlarged. Neurosurgeons then terminate the procedure, having made what they consider the maximal lesion possible without permanent pyramidal tract dysfunction. The production of asterixis by a thalamotomy at the point where damage is beginning to extend to the internal capsule (and/or other structures) suggests that very slight weakness may relate in some way, to asterixis. That may also be the case with the patients who have focal CNS lesions -- though when the leg contra-lateral to the lesion was quite weak, the contra-lateral arm always appeared normally strong, or nearly so. Unfortunately, we are unable to be certain of the presence or absence of slight weakness and, therefore, cannot make a correlation with asterixis. Tyler and Leavitt (1965) have described asterixis in patients with profound sensory loss, but this has not been our experience. Certainly the clinical setting in which asterixis is most common does not include demonstrable sensory loss or weakness. Generalized, bilateral asterixis is not uncommon when patients in a general hospital are examined, afflicting, as it does, approximately 10% of such patients at any one time (Leavitt and Tyler, 1964). It is particularly prominent in patients with one of several metabolic abnormalities: (1) hepatic failure (or porto-caval shunting of blood from the G.I. tract into the systemic circulation without its having passed through the liver, even if the latter is normal) where various amines and ammonia itself are increased in the blood; (2) chronic pulmonary disease with elevated blood pCO_2, and (3) chronic renal disease with increased retention of urea, creatinine, and other metabolic products. Such patients all manifest reduced levels of alertness, confusion, and stupor, if not actual coma or semi-coma. This has been considered to reflect a generalized CNS defect or defects (Tyler and Leavitt, 1965) — its association with asterixis has resulted in the latter fragment of the whole clinical picture of hepatic encephalopathy, for example, being overlooked as the result of a possible focal deficit (focal in the sense of either an anatomical focus or a disturbance in one pharmacologically discrete system).

It has been suggested that the multiple clinical signs of these apparently unrelated metabolic disorders arise from abnormalities produced in CNS function by changes in neurochemical transmitter substances (Fischer, 1974). For example, various amines (e.g., octopamine) and their amino acid precursors circulate in elevated quantities in patients with liver disease (Fischer and James, 1971). They may enter the CNS, where they release the normal endogenous neurotransmitters and can be taken up by catecholaminergic neurones, in which octopamine, for example, would serve as a 'false transmitter'. That is, the synaptic vesicles would contain both the false and true transmitter substances in varying proportion. An impulse arriving in that axon terminal would release both and, since the false transmitter would not have the normal post-synaptic action, the effect of that presynaptic impulse on the post-synaptic cell would be subnormal. Unfortunately, we have no knowledge of which transmitter substances are involved in the production of asterixis. The role of diphenylhydantoin in the evocation of this syndrome in patients, when it is given in the presence of certain contralateral focal lesions (Young and Shahani, 1973), is a fairly specific one and, if we knew the CNS actions of diphenylhydantoin in detail, might pinpoint the neural mechanism responsible. Unfortunately, diphenylhydantoin has many CNS actions, including augmentation of cerebellar Purkinje cell discharge rate (Halpern and Julian, 1972) and a recently described effect on dopamine metabolism (Mendez et al., 1975).

We assume that the neural mechanism which is episodically dysfunctional during asterixis is one concerned with the maintenance of sustained muscular contraction — which may be described as tonic, isometric contraction, concerned perhaps more with posture than movement. In patients with asterixis, there appears to be less disorder of projected or ballistic movements, their initiation, changes in posture, or the phasic muscle contractions underlying them. The realization that asterixis is an easily recognizable, quantifiable sign of a rather specific neural dysfunction is exciting. It is now clearly dissociable from stupor and other complex and diffuse CNS symptoms. Once its anatomical, physiological, and pharmaco-biochemical substrate is more clearly understood, the presence of asterixis can be used to infer something about the pathophysiology of the disease process under study. We should also have insight into an important functional subunit within the motor system, the situations in which it is malfunctioning, the disabilities produced, and perhaps a clearer picture of the role that that particular building block plays in the whole scheme of the neural control of muscular activity.

REFERENCES

ADAMS, R.D. and FOLEY, J. (1953) Neurological disorder associated with liver disease. In (H.H. Merritt and C.C. Hare, Eds.) Metabolic and Toxic Diseases of the Nervous System, Res. Publ. Assoc. Res. Nerv. Ment. Dis., 32, 198—231.
FISCHER, J.E. (1974) False neurotransmitters and hepatic coma. In (F. Plum, Ed.) Brain Dysfunction in Metabolic Disorders, Res. Publ. Assoc. Nerv. Ment. Dis., 53, 53—73.
FISCHER, J.E. and JAMES, J.H. (1971) Mechanism of action of L-DOPA in hepatic coma. Surg. Forum, 22, 347—349.
HALPERN, L.M. and JULIAN, R.M. (1972) Augmentation of cerebellar Purkinje cell discharge rate after diphenylhydantoin. Epilepsia, 13, 377—385.
LEAVITT, S. and TYLER, H.R. (1964) Studies in asterixis. Arch. Neurol., 10, 360—368.
MENDEZ, J.S., COTZIAS, G.C., MENA, I. and PAPAVASILION, P.S. (1975) Diphenylhydantoin: blocking of levodopa effects. Arch. Neurol., 32, 44—46.
TYLER, H.R. and LEAVITT, S. (1965) Asterixis. J. Chron. Dis., 18, 409—411.
YOUNG, R.R. and SHAHANI, B.T. (1973) Anticonvulsant asterixis. Electroencephalogr. Clin. Neurophysiol., 34, 760a.

8

A review of physiological and pharmacological studies of human tremor*

B.T. SHAHANI and R.R. YOUNG

Tremor, which may be defined as more or less regular rhythmic oscillation of a part of the body around a fixed point, can be demonstrated in the outstretched hands of all normal persons. This type of tremor is termed 'physiological' and does not usually produce symptoms except under stressful conditions, when it becomes exaggerated and then is commonly attributed to nervousness. Tremor, however, can also be a manifestation of a variety of neurological disorders. Since recent studies have shown that certain types of tremors can be controlled by specific drug therapy, it is important that methods be evolved which would help the clinician in the proper diagnosis and management of this movement disorder. In a detailed physiological study on a large number of normal, healthy, control subjects and patients with various neurological disorders, we have found that it is possible to identify different types of tremor on the basis of rate, rhythm, pattern of EMG activity in a pair of antagonistic muscles, accelerometric recordings and effect of attempted voluntary effort and fine discrete movements on these various parameters. Although none of these factors alone is specific for one type of tremor, a combination of the study of various physiological parameters and the therapeutic response to specific pharmacological agents can be extremely useful in the differential diagnosis and treatment of tremors. This review is a brief description of our clinical, physiological and pharmacological evaluation of tremor in a number of patients with a variety of neurological disorders.

ACTION TREMORS

Action tremors are present only when a limb is actively maintained in a certain position or during the course of a voluntary movement. This type of

* Supported in part by the Parkinson's Disease Project of the Massachusetts General Hospital and the Allen P. and Josephine B. Green Foundation.

tremor disappears when the limb is relaxed and is not greatly exaggerated as the limb nears the target of a movement.

Physiological tremor

   As mentioned above, physiological tremor can be demonstrated in all normal individuals. It is an action tremor seen in outstretched hands and has a frequency of 8—12/sec. Simultaneous EMG recordings from a pair of antagonistic muscles (e.g., extensors and flexors of wrist) may show continuous activity (interference pattern) (Fig. 1A) or bursts of EMG activity occurring synchronously in these muscles. Under stressful conditions, there is an increase in the tremor amplitude with its rate remaining constant. In addition, there is then a tendency for EMG bursts to become more discrete, perhaps due to greater synchronization of the activity of motor units. Isoproterenol, a beta-adrenergic stimulating agent, given intravenously produces similar effects in the amplitude of the tremor and the pattern of EMG activity in the antagonistic muscles. However, when introduced intra-arterially into the brachial artery, isoproterenol produces enhancement of the tremor only in the perfused arm, a finding which has brought attention to the existence of peripheral tremorogenic beta-adrenergic receptors in the limb itself (Marsden et al., 1967; Young et al., 1974). The isoproterenol-enhanced tremor can be

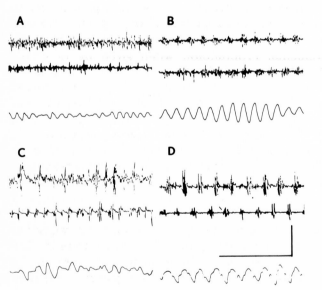

Fig. 1. EMG and accelerometer recordings from patients with (A) physiological, (B) essential, (C) neuropathic, and (D) Parkinsonian resting tremor. Calibrations are 1 sec. and 100 μV or 1 g.

blocked by propranolol given intra-arterially, intravenously, or by previous chronic oral administration, though the underlying physiological tremor appears to be unaffected.

The physiological tremor does not produce symptoms and therefore needs no treatment. Whether or not tremors seen in various metabolic disorders (e.g. thyrotoxic tremor) are exaggerated physiological tremors remains to be proven. Certainly, the metabolic tremors respond to treatment of the underlying disorder, but in addition, beta-adrenergic blocking agents acutely reduce the tremor of thyrotoxicosis, for example.

Essential tremor

When an action tremor becomes symptomatic and appears as the only neurologic abnormality in a patient, it is termed 'essential' tremor. When the essential tremor occurs in several members of the same family, it is called 'familial' (usually dominantly inherited) and, when seen only in old age, 'senile'. Electrophysiological analysis of this tremor usually shows both discrete bursts of EMG activity occurring synchronously in the pair of antagonistic muscles and smooth, regular sinusoidal accelerometric recordings (Fig. 1B). The rate of this tremor tends to be slower than physiological tremor and varies from 4—8/sec. In a few patients with essential tremor (approximately 5%), EMG bursts may alternate in the antagonistic muscles — although the significance of this finding is not clear at the present time, it is possible that this small group may include those patients who go on to develop a full-blown Parkinson's syndrome at a later date. Essential tremors are not present at rest and become enhanced when subjects are asked to perform fine discrete movements. Propranolol, when given by mouth in divided daily doses of 60 to 240 mg, can effectively suppress the amplitude of essential tremor and its senile and familial variants (Winkler and Young, 1974). Similarly, a cocktail containing ethanol (e.g., equivalent to 45 cc of 80-proof Vodka) taken by mouth can abolish it (Growdon et al., 1975) although the tremor may get worse after the effect of alcohol has worn off. When propranolol or alcohol are injected intra-arterially in pharmacologically active concentrations, they fail to produce a significant decrease in the amplitude of the essential tremor — a finding which suggests that therapeutic effects of these two pharmacological agents are not due to blockage of peripheral beta-adrenergic tremorogenic receptors (Young et al., 1974). All the experimental evidence at the present time points toward a central, rather than peripheral, mechanism for the production of essential tremor. The therapeutic effect of propranolol, like that of ethanol, should, therefore, be due to its effect on structures within the central nervous system rather than on peripheral tremorogenic receptors.

Neuropathic tremor

A type of action tremor may be seen in a small group of patients with acquired, chronic, relapsing — remitting, steroid-sensitive polyneuropathies (Adams et al., 1972). It is most prominent in distal parts of limbs and becomes exaggerated when patients are asked to perform certain discrete tasks. It is more marked during one phase of the disease, when the neuropathy is severe, only to disappear completely after the steroid-induced improvement in the underlying illness has taken place. EMG recordings from antagonistic muscles show bursts of EMG activity which vary from second to second from being synchronous to alternating (Fig. 1C). Accelerometric recordings show an irregular tracing. The rate of this tremor usually varies from 6—8/sec. Propranolol by mouth has no therapeutic effect on this kind of action tremor. Most of these patients respond well to steroid therapy with improvement in their neuropathy and amelioration of tremor.

The neuropathic tremor described above must be differentiated from the familial tremor seen in certain kinships with Charcot—Marie—Tooth Disease. It is suggested by some authors (Yudell et al., 1965) that combination of these two disorders in the same patient constitute the syndrome described by Roussey and Levy. Analysis of this tremor (when it occurs in combination) in our laboratory has shown that it has all the physiological and pharmacological characteristics of essential tremor described above. In contrast to neuropathic tremor, this latter type should be treated with propranolol given orally in divided doses (Shahani et al., 1973).

TREMORS AT REST

This type of tremor is present when the limbs are more or less in repose. The most common example in this category is the 'tremor at rest' seen in most patients with Parkinson's Disease.

Parkinson tremors

Although the majority of patients (approximately 75%) with Parkinson's Disease have typical tremor at rest, there are a significant number who have an 'action tremor' which may co-exist (40%) or occur independently of the resting tremor of Parkinsonism (Schwab and Young, 1971).

Electrophysiological features of the typical Parkinson tremor at rest are shown in Fig. 1D. The bursts of EMG activity alternate in the pair of antagonistic muscles (in contrast to synchronous EMG activity seen in most action tremors). The rate ranges from 3—7/sec, and this type of tremor is usually suppressed, at least for a brief period, by voluntary activity. At times, with voluntary activity, the tremor may change its character to a faster frequency tremor (8—12/sec) with synchronous bursts of EMG activity in the antago-nistic muscles — a physiological tremor (Lance et al., 1963). There are, however, a large number of patients with Parkinson's disease who have symp-tomatic action tremor with all features of the essential tremor described above. Another, smaller group of patients with Parkinson's disease have a 'myoclonic' tremor as defined below, either with L-Dopa (Klawans et al., 1975) or without it (Growdon et al., 1975b).

The most useful pharmacological agent in the treatment of the Parkinson tremor at rest appears to be ethopropazine or, sometimes, L-Dopa. The essential tremor, when present, may worsen with L-Dopa therapy and should be treated with oral propranolol.

MISCELLANEOUS MOVEMENT DISORDERS WHICH MAY MIMIC TREMOR

Cerebellar tremor

Cerebellar ataxia (tremor), also called 'intention tremor' or 'ataxic trem-or', should be differentiated from other types of tremor. Unlike action trem-ors, which are present in the outstretched hands, cerebellar ataxia can usual-ly be brought about only by a willed movement which requires precision. The ataxia is most marked during the terminal part of the movement near the target, when the limb oscillates in different directions. This is in contrast to action tremors, which also may have increased 'terminal oscillations', though they are usually in one plane. Moreover, the rate of the increased terminal oscillations seen with action tremor is essentially the same as that of the underlying tremor, whereas a much slower (2—3/sec) rate and much coarser terminal oscillations are seen with cerebellar ataxia. Finally, there is no effect of beta-adrenergic blocking agents on the cerebellar tremor, and ethanol may, in fact, make it worse. Some improvement in the limb ataxia is noted by attaching weights to distal parts of the extremity and thereby increasing the sensory feedback to the CNS (Hewer et al., 1972). Recording of EMG activity from the antagonistic muscles has not shown any character-istic patterns for this type of movement disorder.

Myoclonic tremor

Myoclonus is the term applied to irregular, quick, lightning-like move-ments of the limb seen in a variety of medical and neurological disorders. With 'negative myoclonus', sustained voluntary activity is interrupted by brief pauses resulting in quick, jerky movements so characteristic of myoclo-nus (see previous chapter). 'Positive myoclonus', on the other hand, also produces quick movements, but in this instance, they are a result of sponta-neous activity ranging from a single motor unit discharge to bursts of EMG activity, occurring at random or synchronously in various muscles of the same limb. When the jerky movements, produced either by negative or positive myoclonus, occur frequently, they give the appearance of a tremor though analysis of the responsible EMG activity can easily differentiate them from other types of tremor.

L-5-Hydroxytryptophan (L-5-HTP) has been shown to be very effective in the therapy of post-hypoxic intention myoclonus (Van Woert and Sethy, 1975) but, in our experience, does not alleviate all forms of myoclonus. Baclofen has also proved useful in the treatment of this and other forms of action myoclonus — its side effects are much less troublesome than those produced by L-5-HTP even when the latter is given together with the peripheral L-aromatic amino acid decarboxylase inhibitor, α-methyldopahydrazine.

Hysterical tremor

It is not surprising that hysterical tremor can simulate the other types of tremors described above in view of the fact that the variety of EMG patterns described, including a single unit discharge at an interval of several seconds (seen in some myoclonic syndromes), can be reproduced by normal, healthy individuals. There are certain clinical features, however, which may help the clinician in the diagnosis of hysterical tremor. This type of tremor is usually restricted to one limb and does not respond to the specific drug therapy for the tremor it mimicks. The management of this tremor depends on the treatment of the underlying psychiatric ailment.

REFERENCES

ADAMS, R.D., SHAHANI, B.T. and YOUNG, R.R. (1972) Tremor in association with polyneuropathy. Trans. Am. Neurol. Assoc., 97, 44—48.
GROWDON, J.H., SHAHANI, B.T. and YOUNG, R.R. (1975a) The effect of alcohol on essential tremor. Neurology, 25, 259– 262.
GROWDON, J.H., YOUNG, R.R. and SHAHANI, B.T. (1975b) The differential diagnosis of tremor in Parkinson's disease. Trans. Am. Neurol. Assoc., 100, in press.
HEWER, R.L., COOPER, R. and MORGAN, M.H. (1972) An investigation into the value of treating intention tremor by weighting the affected limb. Brain, 95, 579—590.
KLAWANS, H.L., GOETZ, C. and BERGEN, D. (1975) Levodopa-induced myoclonus. Arch. Neurol., 32, 331—334.
LANCE, J.W., SCHWAB, R.S. and PETERSON, E.A. (1963) Action tremor and the cogwheel phenomenon in Parkinson's disease. Brain, 86, 95—110.
MARSDEN, C.D., FOLEY, T.H., OWEN, D.A.L. and McALLISTER, R.G. (1967) Peripheral β-adrenergic receptors concerned with tremor. Clin. Sci., 33, 53—65.
SCHWAB, R.S. and YOUNG, R.R. (1971) Non-resting tremor in Parkinson's disease. Trans. Am. Neurol. Assoc., 96, 305—307.
SHAHANI, B.T., YOUNG, R.R. and ADAMS, R.D. (1973) The tremor in Roussy—Levy syndrome. Neurology, 23, 425—426.

VAN WOERT, M.H. and SETHY, V.H. (1975) Therapy of intention myoclonus with L-5-hydroxytryptophan and a peripheral decarboxylase inhibitor, MK486. Neurology, 25, 135—140.

WINKLER, G.F. and YOUNG, R.R. (1974) The efficacy of chronic propranolol therapy in action tremors of the familial, senile or essential varieties. New Engl. J. Med., 290, 984—988.

YOUNG, R.R., SHAHANI, B.T. and GROWDON, J.H. (1974) Beta-adrenergic mechanisms in essential tremor. Trans. Am. Neurol. Assoc., 99, 25—27.

YUDELL, A., DYCK, P.J. and LAMBERT, E.H. (1965) A kinship with the Roussy—Levy syndrome. Arch. Neurol., 13, 432—440.

Organization of learnt movements

1. Prefrontal unit activity of under-trained monkeys in delayed-response tasks
   by K. Kubota and S. Kojima 317

2. Triggered and guided components of visual reaching. Their dissociation in split-brain studies
   by J. Paillard and D. Beaubaton 333

3. Movement and associated postural adjustment
   by H. Regis, E. Trouche and J. Massion 349

4. A proposal for study of a state description of the motor control system
   by L.D. Partridge 363

Prefrontal unit activity of under-trained monkeys in delayed-response tasks

Kisou KUBOTA and Shozo KOJIMA

In order to examine the neuronal activity related to the correct performance of a delayed-response task, single unit activity of the dorso-lateral
prefrontal cortex was studied in monkeys which were not well trained and
performed the task with a lower success rate than in a previous investigation
(Kubota et al., 1974).

In 4 under-trained monkeys a total of 112 prefrontal units showed activity
correlating to events of delayed-response tasks in which the sequence included inter-trial interval, visual cue, delay and response. Ninety-four units
were activated during cue and response phases. With an increase of error trials
in longer delay intervals, the increase in the discharge rate of visuokinetic
units during cue, delay and response phases of correct trials became less
frequent. Eighteen visuokinetic units were studied in detail. In about 40% of
these units examined, the increase of the discharge rate in one or more phases
of error trials was significantly reduced, compared with the rate in correct
trials. In 20% of the units, an increase of the discharge rate occurred during
the error trials. In 40% of the units no difference was found between the
discharge rates of correct and error trials.

Results support the view that visuokinetic activity is essential for eliciting
the correct performance in this delayed-response task.

As shown by lesion and cooling studies (Fuster and Alexander, 1970; cf.
Teuber, 1972), the dorso-lateral prefrontal cortex of the Rhesus monkey is
implicated in the performance of delayed-response type tasks (delayed response and delayed alternation) in which monkeys are required to remember
the location of a presented cue, (e.g., left or right cue) or self-produced
behavior (e.g., left or right lever depression) occurring a short time before.
These facts lead to an operational proposition, as originally proposed by
Jacobsen (1935), that this part of prefrontal cortex is involved in spatial
short-term memory processes. The search for a neural correlate of spatial
short-term memory, possibly involved in the execution of delayed-response
tasks, has been attempted in several laboratories, analyzing single unit activity or the mass DC potentials of the dorso-lateral frontal cortex, while monkeys are performing the task. While a satisfactory answer is as yet unavail-

able, possible candidates have been suggested. Fuster (1973) studied prefrontal units in a delayed-response procedure and, for wide areas of the prefrontal cortex, found a higher discharge rate of unit activity during the delay period than in the control inter-trial interval period. This activity was coupled with an increase or decrease of the rate of discharge in the preceding cue presentation period (B and C-type units). Since this activity during delay and cue periods did not differ between left and right choices, Fuster concluded that the activation during the delay is providing the basis for the correct execution of the task. Kubota et al. (1974) studied units in the dorso-lateral area during a delayed-response task with two visual cues (left and right). The majority of units related to the task were activated during cue, delay and response periods (visuokinetic unit). Between left and right choices a fraction of visuokinetic units showed a differential increase of the discharge rate or an antagonistic change (increase on one side and decrease on the other side) in cue and delay periods. A suggestion was made that the differential activity in the cue and delay phases are essential in choosing the correct location of the reward in the delayed-response task and hence may be related to a spatial mnemonic function. Similar differential activity of prefrontal units during visual delayed-response is also briefly reported by Niki (1974).

If the unit activities of this cortical area, such as visuokinetic, are indeed involved in processes of the spatial short-term memory, it may be expected that discharge patterns are different between correct and error responses during performance of delayed-response paradigm. Sufficient information concerning the relation of neuronal activity to error responses is as yet unavailable, since previous single-unit studies were obtained from over-trained monkeys and report anecdotic observations during error performances in which error performance was related to a reduced activity in the delay phase (Fuster, 1973). Further, Abplanalp and Mirsky (1973) showed in delayed-alternation tasks that the high amplitude EEG waves of the prefrontal cortex appear at an intermediate performance level (75%) but not at low (50%) or high (90—100%) performance levels. Stamm and Rosen (1969, 1972) showed that, during delayed-response tasks, a slight steady potential shift (a mnemonic potential shift) in the dorso-lateral prefrontal cortex could be correlated to the performance level; the higher the DC shift, the more correct the performance. These studies of the EEG potentials, together with occasional observations of unit activities in delayed-response tasks, may indicate that the unit activities associated with correct performance be distinguished from those of error performance.

In the present study experimental subjects were monkeys that had been trained to perform a delayed-response task at the shortest delay time (0.2 sec) with 100% success rate but had not been exposed to a task of several seconds delay. During experiments, they performed 1-sec delay tasks initially at a chance level and gradually improved their performance scores but did not attain 90% success rate even at the final stages of the experiments. The relationships of prefrontal unit activities between correct and error trials were studied. A preliminary report was made in the 50th Meeting of the Japan Physiological Society held in June 1974 at Sapporo, Japan.

METHODS

Four Rhesus monkeys were used. Experimental set-ups and recording techniques were exactly the same as previously reported for the delayed-response task (Kubota et al., 1974) except that the monkeys were naive, under-trained for the task.

The monkey in a primate chair faced a panel on which were located two tungsten filament bulbs, 6.5 cm apart, positioned slightly above the monkey's eye level. (cf. Fig. 1 of Kubota et al., 1974). Five cm below each lamp was placed a lever, protruding toward the monkey. This assembly of lamps and levers was set on the right hand side of the panel so that, with his right hand, the animal could reach either one of the levers. The third lever (hold key) was set 12 cm below the assembly and 15 cm nearer to the monkey from a panel, in order to place the hand in a certain spatial position. Monkeys had to press this lever to start the task. Initially they were trained for 1 or 2 months until they invariably performed the delayed-response task at the shortest delay time (0.2 sec, minimal-delay task). In a typical sequence, the monkey at first depressed the hold key with his right hand to start an inter-trial interval period. After depressing the key for 3 sec, one of the cue lamps, either left or right, was lit for 1 sec (no-go signal, cue period). Thereafter, the lamp was turned off and a delay period of 0.2 sec started. After this delay period, both left and right lamps were simultaneously turned on, signalling the reward availability (go signal, response period). When the monkey pressed the lever located just below the lamp lit during the cue period, the lamps were turned off, and 0.1—0.3 ml of an artificial orange juice was delivered to his mouth (correct trial). On the other hand, depression of the lever above the lamp that was not lit during the preceding cue period, resulted in turning-off the lamps without reward (error trial). Releasing the lever and returning his hand to the holding key position again led to a new trial. Sequential controls of the stimuli and responses were accomplished by a minicomputer (PDP-12A) (for programs, see Kubota, 1974). In a single day's experiment monkeys performed 400—1000 trials.

Surgery. After completion of the training, surgery for unit recording was performed under phencyclidine hydrochloride anesthesia (1.5 mg/kg). A cylinder (20 mm in diameter) was implanted in the skull over the dorso-lateral prefrontal cortex. Bolts and nuts for restraining the monkey's head were also implanted. After about one week's rest, unit recording was started with tungsten micro-electrodes.

RECORDINGS AND DATA REDUCTION

Unit activity related to events of the delayed-response task was examined while the monkey was performing the minimal task (0.2-sec delay). If changes in the discharge rate were found during cue and/or response periods, the delay period was prolonged, usually to 0.5—3 sec, rarely up to 12—24 sec. Therefore, monkeys received training with 'longer' delay times only when relevant unit activities were being recorded. During recording sessions of 1.5—4 weeks learning scores at 1-sec delay time were improved gradually from 50% to 90%. Daily progressions of the success rates at different delay times are illustrated in Fig. 1 as cumulative curves of 3 monkeys. Cumulative numbers of trials at each delay time in sec and the percentage rate of correct trials out of total trials in a single day's session are plotted in the ordinate against the days of recordings in the abscissa. The day when a related unit activity was recorded for the first time is shown as the first day. After 300—500 trials of 1-sec delay for 10—25 days, no monkeys attained a 100% performance level. After recordings of 2 weeks, one monkey (no. 17) attained an 80% level at 1-sec delay, but the success rate at 3-sec delay fluctuated widely from 50 to 100% and at 6-sec delay it was slightly above chance level. Another monkey (no. 18) reached, after 10 days training, 80% performance level at 1 sec. The rate at 3 sec was 65% on the 11th day. In a third monkey (no. 16) the levels at 1- and 3-sec delays at the later phase of recordings were slightly above chance level. To a fourth monkey (no. 19, not illustrated), a somewhat different delayed-response task was assigned in which, on responding to the go signal, the monkey had to continue to press the hold key for an initial 0.3—0.5 sec. In other words, this monkey was pre-trained with 0.5—0.7-sec delay instead of 0.2-sec delay. Compared to the other 3 monkeys, the success rate of this monkey at 1-sec delay rose quickly with fewer trials, reaching a plateau of 90—100% after 3 days of recordings, but the rate at 3-sec delay fluctuated between 50 and 100%. This modified task was intended to see whether there were any changes in the discharge which could be related to the lever depression and which were separable from changes caused by the visual stimuli. Since the results of the fourth monkey did not yield new findings, they were not separated from those of the other 3 monkeys.

Single-unit activity and five event marks (left and right lamp signals, hold-

Fig. 1. Daily changes of trial numbers and success rates at different delay times (0.5, 1, 3, and 6 sec) in three under-trained monkeys. Three pairs of curves from one monkey obtained at different delay times are arranged vertically. Ordinate: cumulative trial numbers (●——●——●) and daily correct rates in % (●- - -●- - -●). Abscissa: days after the delayed task with delay of more than 0.5 sec was started. L or R denotes the side of the brain from which unit recordings were done. There is an interval of more than a week when the recording side of the brain was changed.

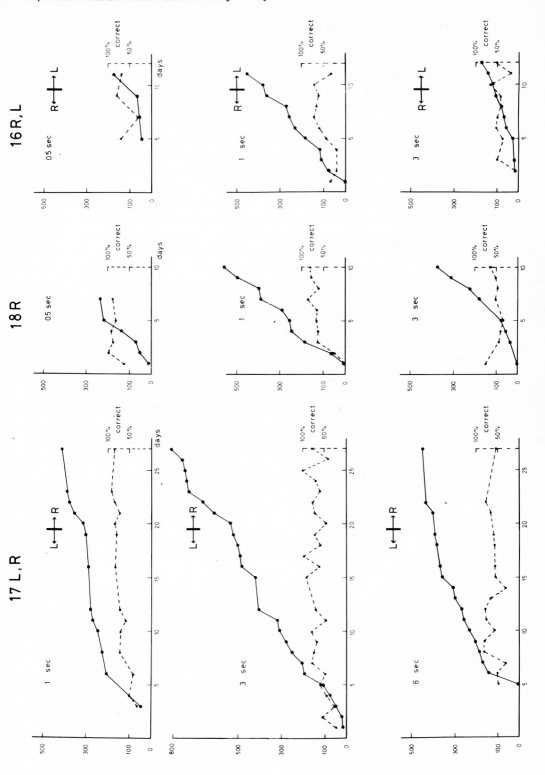

key depression, left and right lever depression) were recorded on tape with a 7-channel tape recorder. Using the PDP-12A, these analog data were digitized and stored on the disk. Unit activity was fed into AD converter inputs of PDP-12A. Sample rates were variable, and were usually 20 msec per bin. Except for a small number of units whose activity was not isolated, all averaging and numerical calculations were performed from the digitized data of the disk, separately for left (L) and right (R) trials and also separately for correct (O) and error (X) trials. Unit activity which was difficult to isolate by a window discriminator was recorded on Kodak Direct Print paper and spike numbers were counted if possible. Later calculations were performed by a computer. Computations were obtained in four groups, representing left—correct (LO), left—error (LX), right—correct (RO) and right—error trials (RX). Averaged data were shown on the computer display (512 × 512 bins), spike discharges being represented as dots (cf. Fig. 2). Displayed data were photographed routinely by Kodak Polaroid Camera (C-5).

For quantitative analysis in each single unit, spike numbers per sec (represented by spikes/sec) were calculated at different phases of the trials, such as I (time from 2 sec prior to the cue to 1 sec prior to the cue onset), C (cue period, 1 sec), D (delay period) and R (response time from go-signal onset to hold-key release). Time values were represented by multiples of 12.5 msec. For statistical treatments trials with reaction times longer than 0.7 sec were excluded. Significant increase or decrease of the rates at different phases, compared with I values were tested statistically (t-test). Any significance between two corresponding values out of the 4 groups was also detected by use of the t-test. All procedures were performed by programs written in FOCAL-12 or assembler languages.

After completion of the experiments the brain was perfused by Ringer solution followed by 10% formalin. Serial sections of the penetrated area were made and stained by the Nissl method.

RESULTS

General

In four monkeys, single-unit recordings in the behaving state were started as soon as the monkey learned securely to press the correct lever at the minimal-delay (0.2 sec) task. Units were searched for by lowering the microelectrode step by step, while the monkey was performing this task in which a left or right no-go visual cue was presented for one sec and, after 0.2-sec delay, left and right lamp signals were presented simultaneously with the go signal. A monkey was permitted to release his hand from the hold-key position and to proceed to depress the lever only during the go phase.

If the discharge rate of a given unit changed in association with events of the task, the activity was recorded on tape for more than 10 trials at this minimal delay time. Subsequently, while continuing tape recordings, the delay time was prolonged to 0.5, 1, 2, 3, or up to 24 sec, with frequent returns to a 0.2-sec delay. At longer delays these under-trained monkeys pressed the correct lever with a lower rate of success (cf. Fig. 1).

During 187 penetrations of 4 monkeys in the peri-principal area, mostly locating in the caudal half-portion of the lateral bank of the principal sulcus, 112 units showed a correlation to the task with minimal and longer delays. In these, increases or decreases of the discharge rates were judged rather roughly by observing changes of the averaged response of peri-stimulus time histograms (cf. Kubota et al., 1974). Most of these units (94 units) were activated both at initial cue and go phases with or without increases during lever depression. In 8 units depression occurred during cue and/or go phases. Further, in 8 units increase occurred only during lever depression and in 3 a transient increase with the shortest latency period occurred during cue and go phases. In 65 units data of a sufficient number of trials were collected to yield statistical analysis in both minimal and longer delays. Since units other than those activated during cue and go phases were not influenced by an increase of the error trials, further descriptions of the activity of minority groups were not made in this study. The units to be described are considered as representing the visuokinetic units in the naive state (Kubota et al., 1974) because these units behaved similarly during cue and go phases, and other kinds of units which were considered to be significantly involved in delayed response were not found.

Exact locations of the electrode recordings were unable to be determined in 2 monkeys because of partial damage to the dura and cortex. But it was ascertained that all units to be described were located in the caudal half of the bank of the principal sulcus, never away from the 6–8 mm of the sulcus, where visuokinetic units were found in a previous paper (Kubota et al., 1974).

Responses at minimal delay

Discharge patterns at the minimal delay task were studied in 94 units. During inter-trial interval time most recorded units had a background activity up to 20 spikes/sec. They were rather irregular. Compared to the rate in the preceding inter-trial interval, 35 units showed a significant increase or decrease during cue phases ($P < 0.05$, t-test). Out of these units, 14 were activated significantly by either of the cues, 9 units only by the left cue and 10 units only by the right cue. Two units were depressed by one of the cues (left). In 2 other units there were combinations of increase on one side and decrease on the other side. If, in these units, the rates were compared between left and right cue phases, 12 units showed a side difference, 6 units exhibiting a higher rate in the left cue and the other 6 in the right cue.

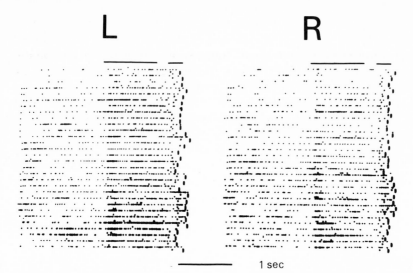

1 sec

Fig. 2. Dot displays of responses of a single prefrontal unit during performance of the minimal delayed response (30 left and 30 right trials, 100% correct). Left (L) or right (R) visual lamp signal was presented according to a Gellerman's series but trials were illustrated separately in temporal sequence according to left or right cue. Longer lines above dots represent times of the lamp signal and shorter lines times of go phase when two left and right lamps were presented. Spike numbers were counted every 20 msec. Occasional dots above dotted line indicate that two spikes appeared in one 20-msec bin. Dots seen below dotted spike trains at go phase represent the timing when the monkey released his hand from the hold key. Vertical bars at the right ends of dots represent the timing of the lever depression. Time calibration was represented at the center bottom (1 sec = 50 bins).

Raster patterns of Fig. 2 illustrate examples of the discharges of a single unit at a minimal delay task. During the inter-trial interval there was an irregular spontaneous activity (mean ± S.D., 10 ± 13 spikes/sec). During cue lights, as shown by the longer lines above dots, the unit was activated by no less than 100 msec light and activation continued as long as the light was on. On the average, the rate was about 32 spikes/sec in the left and 25 spikes/sec in the right. During go phases, as shown by the shorter lines above dots, the rate of increase was not remarkable. From the go-signal onset till hold-key release (as indicated by a large dot below a train of smaller dots for spikes) the average rate was 25 spikes/sec in the left and 15 spikes/sec in the right. At timings from hold-key release to lever-press (vertical bars at the right end of dot trains indicate the moment of lever depression), the rates were slightly higher than in the preceding inter-trial interval. Timings from go-signal onset to hold-key release were, on average, 123 msec for the left and 136 msec for the right. Further, it took about 160 msec from hold-key release to lever-presses on either side.

Out of 35 units with a significant increase at cue phases, 22 units showed a significant increase at go phase of left and/or right trials and 13 units did not. Further, 7 units with no significant increase at either of the cue phases showed an increase at the go phase. Finally, compared to the increase at the cue phase, increase at the go phase was significantly larger in 12 units and significantly smaller in 3 units. Thus, in the naive state activations were observed in both cue and response phases as in the over-trained state. The decrease in the unit activity during the go phase in contrast to increase in activity during the cue phase was not observed in visuokinetic units in the previous study (Kubota et al., 1974). Although this fact seems of interest in considering possible mechanisms of the formation of delayed response behavior, the number of sampled units (3 units) was regarded as being too small to permit further discussion.

Unit responses at lower success rates

An attempt was made to find a difference in the discharge rate in longer delay trials which had more errors. Examples of responses at different delay times of a single unit are illustrated in Fig. 3, as paired peri-stimulus time histograms. Responses to left (L) and right (R) cues are averaged at 0.2, 0.5, 1.0 and 3.0-sec delay times. The longer the delay, the lower the success rate. In the control inter-trial interval there was an activity at 10–20 spikes/sec at minimal delay. The unit was gradually activated by the left cue and reached about 40 spikes/sec in its later phase. The increase continued during the go phase, significantly, though less remarkable. A gradual change was not clear with respect to the right cue, but the total number of spikes at the cue was greater than that in the control and the increase was significant ($P < 0.05$). A significant increase was also observed in the go phase, immediately before the hold-key release. When the delay was 0.5 sec (80%), increase by the cue was seen on both sides, but only the left side increase was significant ($P < 0.05$). During delay increases are not seen on both sides, a significant increase occurred during the right go-phase. At 1-sec delay (62%) an increase was seen on left cue trials, whether or not the response was correct, and on right cue trials, a weak increase was seen in cue and go phases. Significant increase was only observed during left cue phase of correct trials (LO). At 3-sec delay (56%) no significant increase was seen at any phase, although a slight increase was seen during left cue of correct trials (LO). Further, no significant differences between correct and error trials of any delay times were seen in either side except for rates during delay at 3-sec delay trials. From the results in Fig. 3 it is seen that, with a decrease of the success rates of the trials, a significant increase of the discharge rate during cue and go periods becomes less striking, both in correct and incorrect trials.

A tendency, observed in a unit illustrated in Fig. 3, that less activation during cue and go phases in longer delay tasks, was also seen in the responses

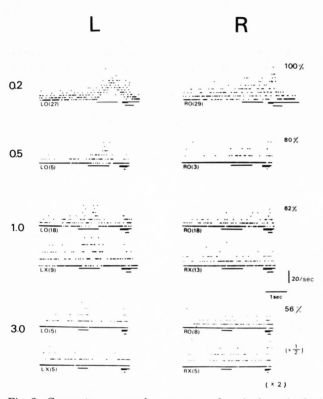

Fig. 3. Computer-averaged responses of a single unit during left (L) and right (R) cue trials in the delayed response at different delay times (0.2, 0.5, 1.0 and 3.0 sec.) LO, LX, RO and RX at the bottom left of each response represent, respectively, left cue—correct press, left cue—error press, right cue—correct press and right cue—error press. Numbers at bottom left in parentheses represent average trial numbers. Short bars below the response in the middle of each figure represent the cue stimuli of 1 sec. Continuous thick and thin lines at the right bottom in each response represent the go phase. The beginnings and ends of the shortest lines represent times with shortest and longest times of lever depression, respectively. All other lever depressions occurred during times shown by a short line. Another short line below the thick—thin line indicates timings during which the hold key was released. Amplitude calibrations for 0.2, 0.5 and 1.0-sec delay trials are represented at the right between 1.0 and 3.0 delay trials. In 3.0-sec trials the time calibration is 2 sec and amplitude 10 Hz (1 bin = 40 msec).

of other units. As shown in a tabulated form in Table 1, computations of 12 units were performed from a series of trials with different delay times separately for left and right trials. In each unit responses were categorized into one of 4 stages according to success rates (I, 100—95%; II, 85—70%; III, 70—55% and IV, 55—0%).

At each stage mean values were computed at different phases from correct responses of the task (I, inter-trial interval; C, cue; D, delay and R, go

TABLE 1

Responses of 12 selected units in different performance levels. Averaged rates (spikes/sec) of 4 phases of the delayed-response (I, C, D, and R) were categorized into 4 stages according to the success rate, that is, I (100—95, minimal delay time), II (85—70), III (70—55) and IV (55—0%). ↑ or ↓ indicates a statistical difference ($P < 0.05$, t-test) from values in the control values. V or Λ is attached if a significance was found between paired values ($P < 0.05$). The side of initial visual cue is given by L or R after the unit code number. Numbers in parentheses show number of trials of the same side of I—IV stages.

| | | | | I | | | | II | | | | III | | | | IV | | |
			I	C	D	R	I	C	D	R	I	C	D	R	I	C	D	R
1	19R, 7-1A	L	(26,10,13,-)	0.2	10 ↑		0.8	0	0.6↑	0.4↑	0.6	0	0.6↑	0.8↑	0.9↑				
		R	(29,12,13,-)	0.2	2̂5 ↑		3̂.6↑	0.1	0.9↑	4.5↑	3.1↑	0	0.8↑	1.5↑	0.7				
2	18 R,10-5A	L	(15, 7, 6, 4)	0.5	0.1↓		6.3↑	0	0.3	10.0↑	3.5↑	0.2	0	2.7	2.3	0	0.8	2.0↑	2.5
		R	(18, 9, 4, 2)	0.1	2̂.4↑		5.2↑	0	2̂.7↑	10.1↑	2.3	0.5	0	0.5	0.7	0	0.5	1.4	4.9
3	18 R,10-3	L	(9, 9, -,4)	1.2	2.2		0.8	1.9	5.1↑	13.2↑	4.8					2.3	1.5	5.6	3.4
		R	(10,12, -,5)	0.2	1.4↑		3.2	2.6	6.8↑	7.8	4.8↑					1.0	1.4	1.6	1.9
4	16 R,25-1A	L	(28, 5,13,5)	1.5	9.8↑		5.7↑	1.8	14.6↑	3.6	2.1	1.4	5.5↑	0.7	1.1	1.5	6.8	0.5	7.4
		R	(26, 3,13,8)	1.3	3.9↑		3.9	1.4	5.3	1.3	8.2↑	0.9	1̂.2	1.5	4.1	0.6	2.6	0.9	8.4
5	18 R,13-6	L	(20, -,11, 7)	1.0	10.1↑		32.6↑					0.2	9.0↑	7.0↑	10.7	1.6	22.9↑	14.0↑	20.2↑
		R	(20, -,10, 4)	2.0	8.2↑		35.1↑					2.7	4̂.1	4̂.2	14.4↑	2.8	8̂.7	7̂.2	23.9
6	18 R, 9-1A	L	(28, 7,12,5)	1.9	3.1↑		0.4↓	2.1	6.2↑	3.6	3.4	2.3	2.2	0.5↓	1.7	1.6	3.5	0.3	0
		R	(29, 8,14, 7)	2̂5	1̂.2↓		0.1↓	2.3	3̂.0	2.0	1.1	1.7	1.5	2.0	0.6	2.6	0.3↓	0.6↓	1.5
7	18 R,17-1	L	(8, - 6,4)	1.9	7.1↑		14.1					3.0	4.8	5.2	17.8	2.8	16.3	9.4↑	35.8↑
		R	(7, - 7,6)	2.4	5.1		17.2					2.7	7.1↑	8.0↑	13.9↑	3.0	8.6↑	6.5↑	23.6↑
8	18 R,10-4	L	(24,10, 5,9)	3.0	4.4↑		24.5↑	2.1	4.2	13.4↑	11.8↑	0.8	2.9	4.5↑	5.1	0.4	1.1	5.7↑	6.3↑
		R	(24, 9, 7,7)	2.4	4.7↑		15.0↑	2.8	3.4	10.4↑	12.2↑	1.6	2.5	4.6↑	7.4↑	0.3	0.7	1.9↑	2.4
9	18 R,24-1	L	(27,16, 9, 3)	4.3	9.9↑		14.5↑	4.9	6.8	3.4	11.1↑	7.5	4.7	2.7	29.5↑	5.8	12.3	6.6	18.8↑
		R	(27,19, 6, 5)	4.0	9.3↑		18.1↑	5.8	12.0↑	6.9	16.5↑	9.6	13.2	4.3	32.0↑	9.9	12.4	5.4	21.8
10	18 R,18-1	L	(12, 3,-,5)	5.8	6.8		9.7↑	6.0	5.8	9.5	8.7↑					6.2	9.6↑	8.6	11.5↑
		R	(13, 5, -, 4)	5.8	8.5↑		14.9	4.8	11.8↑	10.9	10.9↑					9.1	15.7	10.4	8.9
11	17 L,13-4	L	(3, 3, 5,2)	14.2	14.3		35.1↑	6.7	25.7↑	21.9↑	43.1↑	21.3	31.2	29.0	38.5↑	16.7	21.5	20.7	18.2
		R	(4, 5, 3,4)	18.6	3̂3.0↑		42.7↑	3.5	11̂.2↑	8̂.9↑	22.3↑	18.7	2̂5.7	29.8↑	37.5↑	17.1	23.3	28.3↑	9.5
12	18 R,15-1	L	(20, 7, 9,-)	20.3	37.1 ↑		61.7↑	31.9	42.1↑	38.6	53.1↑	18.6	37.6↑	24.4	47.1↑				
		R	(18, 8, 8,-)	19.4	31.9↑		58.7↑	26.3	41.0↑	40.9↑	49.8↑	19.4	39.7↑	29.5↑	50.7↑				
	Means			4.7	8.8		17.2	5.7	11.1	11.8	14.2	5.5	9.9	7.8	15.5	3.9	9.6	7.3	12.4
				4.9	9.3		18.1	5.0	9.8	10.4	13.1	5.8	9.6	8.6	16.2	4.6	7.4	6.4	10.7
	Numbers of ↑			-	18		16	-	13	10	13	-	7	8	10	-	3	6	6
	↓			-	2		2	-	0	0	0	-	0	1	0	-	1	1	0
	>or<			-	5		2	-	3	3	1	-	3	1	0	-	1	2	0

phases). If significant changes of the rate in a given phase from the inter-trial interval values are found ($P < 0.05$), asterisks (↑ or ↓) were attached to mean values. At stages I and II in most units, a significant increase was observed at least in one of the cue and go phases. At stages III and IV significant increases became less frequent. The ratio of occurrence of significant increase per unit at the cue time decreased gradually from 0.75 (I), through 0.65 (II) and 0.35 (III), to 0.15 (IV). The occurrence of a significant increase at the delay time also decreased with decrease of success rates from 0.5 (II), through 0.4 (III), to 0.3 (IV). Thus, at any phase of the task, with decrease of the success rate, the frequency of significant increase decreased. As for the discharge rates, at the inter-trial of lower success rates there were no instances of significant changes. This reduction of changes of the significant rate increase in III and IV stages may be argued to be due to the fact that trial numbers for data collection in stages III and IV are of the same order as those in stages I and II, therefore with decrease of the success rate, trials of correct choice decreased and trials of incorrect choice increased. As seen in parenthesis in Table 1, the numbers of correct trials decreased with increase of error trials, but the above-mentioned tendency cannot be solely attributable to the lack of sufficient trial numbers for the statistical test, because, even if the trial numbers at cue were the same between two stages, less increase was observed in trials with less success rate. Simultaneously, instances in which there was a significant difference between left and right trials at $P = 0.05$ also decreased gradually at any phase of the task from stage I though II and III, to IV, as shown at the bottom of Table 1.

In order to see if there were any differences between the discharge rates of correct and error trials, calculated values of 18 units, obtained at different delay times, were combined. In each unit from corresponding values of different delay times new representative values (averages with S.D.s) were calculated in 4 different groups, that is, left cue—correct (LO), left cue—error (LX), right cue—correct (RO) and right cue—error trials (RX), and yielded values are tabulated in Table 2. Significant increase in cue, delay and go phases were observed both in correct and error trials, though the frequency of significant increases is 30% less in cue, delay and go phases of error trials. Since these units showed a variety of changes, changes of the average rates of 6 units were illustrated in Fig. 4 in graphic form. Fig. 4A illustrates an example in which significant rate differences were not found during any phases of the task (no. 3 of Table 2). Whether the cue was left or right and whether the response was correct or incorrect, the unit was activated by the cue (1.0—2.5 spikes/sec). The rate during delay further increased to 5.6—6.7 spikes/sec and during go phase it fell to 0—1.5 spikes/sec. In Fig. 4D (no. 13 of Table 2), in contrast to the unit in 4A, a side difference was found between left and right trials (LO = LX vs. RO = RX) but no difference was found between correct and error trials. The unit was activated when the right cue was presented whether it was correct or not. There was a slight activation by the left cue during delay and go phases. A unit illustrated in Fig. 4B (no. 9 of Table 2) showed differences between correct and error trials. In LO trials the rate increased by the cue from 2 to 4 spikes/sec, during delay the rate was the highest (10.8 spikes/sec) and at go phase it became slightly

TABLE 2

Comparisons of averaged discharge rates of 18 selected units between correct and error trials (I, III; C, cue; D, delay; R, response). Means and S.D.s were calculated separately in left correct, left incorrect, right correct and right incorrect groups. Values referring to the left cue are shown on the left side (L) and those to the right are on the right (R). In each unit values of correct responses are in the upper line (O) and values of incorrect responses in lower line (X). If, in each group, a significant increase or decrease was found compared to the rate in the values in inter-trial interval (I), then ↑ or ↓ is attached. If a significant difference was found between correct and error trials to left or right cues, > or < was attached. Numbers in parentheses below the unit code number represent times of the delay sampled. Total number of trials sampled and % correct score are also shown in (n).

No	UNIT	%	(n) L	I (L)	C (L)	D (L)	R (L)	(n) R	I (R)	C (R)	D (R)	R (R)	
1	19R, 7-1A (2,3)	71	23	0 ±0	06±05?↑	06±100↑	08±115↑	25	0 ±020	09±105↑	30±415↑	19±250↑	O
			20					20	0 ±0	13±150↑	20±182↑	06±083↑	X
2	18R,10-5 (05,1,15,3)	57	25	0 ±020	04±103	65±522↑	23±330↑	23	01±028	21±256↑	65±682↑	23±349↑	O
			20	01±030	03±078	51±426↑	12±307	16	0 ±0	12±165↑	25±379↑	12±273	X
3	16R,19-1 (05,1)	60	6	03±034	25±096↑	62±290↑	10±183	6	01±013	10±183	65±308↑	15±204	O
			5	01±012	20±167	56±242↑	10±200	3	0 ±0	10±082	67±340↑	0	X
4	16R,24-1 (1,3)	56	6	10±101	10±075	17±159	49±683	8	05±07?	30±269↑	15±196	65±536↑	O
			4	16±064	10±123	03±056↓	09±152	7	08±073	17±088	13±195	31±514	X
5	17L,40-1 (05,2,3,6,9)	70	16	07±069	26±154↑	25±150↑	45±315↑	23	09±0?1	20±176↑	11±135	47±373↑	O
			12	09±102	26±240↑	11±093	31±240↑	5	09±028	18±271	11±061	37±265	X
6	18R,10-4 (1,2,4)	67	24	12±120	28±248↑	87±530↑	83±698↑	23	17±176	23±217	60±469↑	78±744↑	O
			13	19±166	14±130	69±439↑	70±304↑	18	14±157	19±231	47±421↑	83±578↑	X
7	16R,25-1A (1,15,2,3,4,6)	50	37	18±185	84±863↑	14±184	36±684	33	13±130	31±388↑	12±167	69±1050↑	O
			34	19±138	57±536↑	11±136↓	24±397	36	21±179	23±263	21±208	42±557↑	X
8	18R,13-6 (3,5)	80	18	07±105	144±905↑	97±485↑	144±1419↑	14	27±425	54±439	50±291	171±875↑	O
			14	18±268	90±625↑	55±270↑	158±972↑	11	14±161	57±601↑	60±308↑	189±705↑	X
9	18R,10-3 (1,2)	59	13	20±200	40±341	108±494↑	44±382	17	21±225	52±449↑	60±386↑	39±513	O
			6	12±107	29±246	69±497↑	25±307	15	05±081	28±279	27±238↑	10±116	X
10	18R, 9-1A (1,3,12,15)	56	37	22±212	35±284	14±187	23±242	37	22±160	16±201	15±169	12±158↓	O
			25	27±221	29±270	18±178	30±292	33	25±400	11±158	15±183	13±201	X
11	17L,13-5 (1,4)	52	5	19±14?	54±196↑	208±736↑	237±1107↑	6	27±155	60±129↑	158±687↑	209±1661↑	O
			7	46±340	84±118↑	175±740↑	195±385↑	3	60±179	33±471	105±680	119±889	X
12	18R,17-1 (1,3)	59	10	29±226	94±857↑	69±358↑	250±1281↑	13	29±211	78±432↑	73±247↑	184±754↑	O
			6	35±206	157±427↑	72±346	240±1163↑	10	21±122	83±400↑	96±406↑	200±759↑	X
13	18R,18-1 (1,3)	57	8	61±256	82±276	90±283	104±274↑	9	67±415	135±569↑	107±489	100±324	O
			7	83±400	77±134	89±234	114±382	6	51±217	135±213↑	107±306	111±277↑	X
14	18R,24-1 (1,3,2,4)	69	37	70±674	68±554	39±771	192±1162↑	38	72±767	124±851↑	58±407	218±1279↑	O
			17	95±1004	119±950	65±400	253±1310↑	17	103±1044	158±1533	45±446	232±1492↑	X
15	16R,25-2 (1,2,3,4,6)	50	13	105±541	341±715↑	83±548	253±1388↑	16	94±356	183±429↑	51±380↓	216±1448↑	O
			27	101±464	356±820↑	94±434	292±1844↑	2	62±015	160±0 ↑	85±400	365±1150	X
16	16R,13-2 (5,1)	61	10	102±29?	192±571↑	199±493↑	692±2320↑	10	108±232	163±640↑	302±593↑	771±3463↑	O
			13					13	90±391	145±485↑	239±696↑	441±2778↑	X
17	17L,13-4 (2,3)	56	7	200±705	284±534↑	266±905	327±1042↑	7	178±443	243±406↑	290±443↑	215±1505	O
			8	55±453	221±65?↑	208±1284↑	250±1311↑	3	157±384	157±419	273±1216	182±672	X
18	18R,15-1 (3,6,9)	75	19	233±993	379±1094↑	294±107?	486±1171↑	19	230±772	414±1224↑	331±1029↑	470±1564↑	O
			2	310±1100	485±153	46?±166	500±0	11	247±611	425±1166↑	325±1060	524±903↑	X

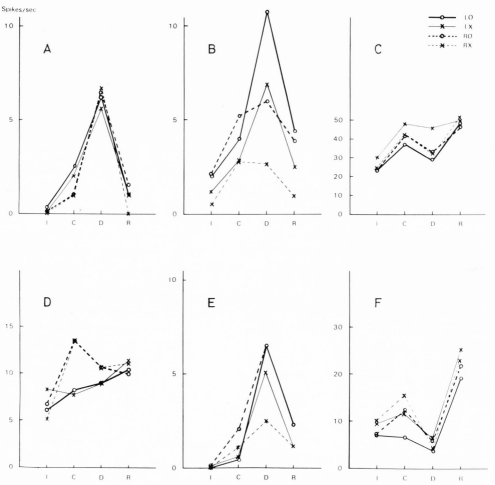

Fig. 4. Comparisons of the averaged rates of under-trained states between correct and error trials of different phases of the delayed response. From A to F, six different examples of units. Ordinate, discharge rate (spikes/sec). I, C, D and R of the abscissa represent, respectively: inter-trial interval, cue, delay and response phases. O: correct trials, X: error trials. Thick lines represent correct trials and thin lines error trials. Real lines represent left-side trials and broken lines right-side trials.

higher than the control value. In RO trials the rate increased similarly during cue and delay phases, though the rate in delay is low. In trials with errors of both left and right sides (LX and RX), corresponding rates were lower than the respective values of any phases of correct trials. In both left and right trials, curves looked as if those of correct trials were moved downwards, parallel to those of error trials. In RX trials rates in inter-trial intervals, delay and go phases were significantly lower than those of RO trials. In Fig. 4E (no. 2 of Table 2) an example with differences between LO and RO cue phases and no differences in rates of inter-trial intervals, shows differences between correct and error trials. Except for left cue phase, rates at error trials were lower, though not significantly, than the respective rates of correct trials. Examples of the increase with error trials are illustrated in Fig. 4C (no. 18 of Table 2) and F (no. 14 of Table 2). A unit in Fig. 4C showed similar rate changes in LO, RO and RX trials. The rates at cue of any trial were about twice those of the control and the rates at delay were between control and cue time, except for LX trials in which the rates during the inter-trial interval and delay were as high as those during cue. Rates in cue and delays in LX trials were higher than those in LO trials. Finally, in a unit illustrated in Fig. 4F, respective rates in cue phases with error trials were higher than respective rates with correct trials. And rates at delay were lower than inter-trial interval values in any trials.

In Table 2 significantly low rates in error trials occurred 8 times (in inter-trial interval, twice; in cue, once; and in delay, 5 times) and significantly high rates occurred 6 times (in inter-trial interval, twice; in cue, twice; and in delay, twice). In units with significantly differential rates in the cue phase between left and right correct trials (L > R, 5 units: R < L, 3 units), differential relations seen between LO and RO trials were retained between LX and RX trials in 5 units, were lost in 4 units and were never reversed. From data shown in Table 2 and Fig. 4 it may be said that in error trials of delayed response about 40% of units showed a reduction in discharge rates in one or more phases of the task and in 20% of these an increase of the rate was observed. In the remaining 40% there was no clear change.

DISCUSSION

Prefrontal unit activity was studied in the performance of the two-choice, visual delayed response of under-trained monkeys. The change of the discharge patterns was examined with respect to success rates of the task and the differences between the discharge patterns of error trials and correct trials were also studied. With an increase of delay times from 0.2 sec to more than 3 sec, the success rate decreased from 100% to chance level. Corresponding to the lowered success rate, an increase of the discharge rate at cue, delay and/or response phases in correct trials was less frequent. The lowered activation of the prefrontal units in choosing the correct response may be interpreted as reflecting that the monkey becomes less attentive to the cue signal and performs the task incorrectly.

Rate changes were compared between correct and error trials, averaged rates could be lower or higher in error than in correct trials. In half of the selected units a decreasing tendency was observed in at least one of the phases of the task, including the inter-trial interval, while an increase was seen less frequently. Possible mechanisms for the changes were hard to infer from these results, because factors influencing the discharge rate in response to the visual space are unknown. Whether the visually activated units have a visual field, as seen in units in the frontal eye field is to be studied (Mohler et al., 1973). Thus, decrease and increase of the rates in error trials reflect unknown characteristics of the prefrontal unit activity. However, two factors seem important. Firstly, decreased activation, seen only in delay periods in error trials, suggests that the visuokinetic units are not capable of discharging properly for the correct selection of the reward. Secondly, decrease of activity is seen in the inter-trial interval, suggesting that the visuokinetic unit is not so much activated in the under-trained state as in the over-trained state. The lack of higher activity may be coupled to the lower success rate in the task.

Lowered activation of the visuokinetic unit may be produced if the background activity in the control becomes lower, as seen in error trials. This will lead to lowered activity in the delay phases, and may be related to the monkey paying less attention to the coming cue stimulus or to finishing the correct lever-press. It is conceivable that, with an improvement of the task performance, the prefrontal unit would be more activated by the cue and therefore more activated during the delay.

REFERENCES

ABPLANALP, J.M. and MIRSKY, A.F. (1973) Electroencephalographic correlates of delayed-alternation and visual discrimination learning in rhesus monkeys. J. Comp. Physiol. Psychol., 85, 123—131.
FUSTER, J.M. (1973) Unit activity in prefrontal cortex during delayed-response performance: Neuronal correlates of transient memory. J. Neurophysiol., 36, 61—78.
FUSTER, J.M. and ALEXANDER, G.E. (1970) Delayed response deficit by cryogenic depression of frontal cortex. Brain Res., 20, 85—90.
JACOBSEN, C.F. (1935) Functions of the frontal association area in primates. Arch. Neurol. Psychiatr., 33, 558—569.
KUBOTA, K. (1974) A neurophysiological approch to study functions of the prefrontal cortex. Seitai no Kagaku, 25, 196—207. (In Japanese).
KUBOTA, K., IWAMOTO, T. and SUZUKI, H. (1974) Visuokinetic activities of primate prefrontal neurons during delayed-response performance. J. Neurophysiol., 37, 1197—1212.
MOHLER, C.W., GOLDBERG, M.E. and WURTZ, R.H. (1973) Visual receptive fields of frontal eye field neurons. Brain Res., 61, 385—389.
NIKI, H. (1974) Differential activity of prefrontal units during right and left delayed-response trials. Brain Res., 70, 346—349.
STAMM, J.S. and ROSEN, S.C. (1969) Electrical stimulation and steady potential shifts in prefrontal cortex during delayed response performance by monkeys. Acta Biol. Exp., 29, 385—399.
STAMM, J.S. and ROSEN, S.C. (1972) Cortical steady potential shifts and anodal polarization during delayed response performance. Acta Neurobiol. Exp., 32, 193—209.
TEUBER, H.-L. (1972) Unity and diversity of frontal lobe functions. Acta Neurobiol. Exp., 32, 615—656.

2

Triggered and guided components of visual reaching. Their dissociation in split-brain studies

J. PAILLARD and D. BEAUBATON

The organization of visual reaching may involve two different components: the triggering of a motor programme for the ballistic transport of the hand toward the target and the final guiding of the movement to ensure the correct placement of the hand on the target. Both aspects were studied on baboons in contra-lateral and ipsi-lateral eye—hand coordination after interhemispheric disconnnection and section of the optic chiasma.

(1) Anticipatory programmes (feedforward) are concerned with the spatial calibration of information required to organize the ballistic movement of the hand. Visual information is the decisive factor but memorized tactile cues may also play a role in connection with proprioceptive information. This type of programme can be triggered in both contra-lateral and ipsi-lateral conditions, with the postural setting of the hand and fingers in relation to the visual identification of the target. This is maintained in the contra-lateral but lost in the ipsi-lateral condition.

(2) Corrective movements (feedback) can be visually guided close to the target by control of the proximal or of the distal musculature. Neither of these controls are preserved in the ipsi-lateral condition. Alternatively, the movements may be guided by tactile cues, which occur as soon as the hand has contacted the target. The corrective adjustments remain unimpaired in both conditions. The anatomo-physiological implications of these results are discussed.

INTRODUCTION

The transportation of the hand to grasp an object or point at a visual target depends on an ordered sequence of functional operations intervening at various stages in the organization of such an action: initiation, programming, execution and adjustment. In this behavioural sequence, visual information plays an important part, but other sensory cues (tactile and proprioceptive) may intervene at different stages in the elaboration of the movement. The origin of visuomotor action must be sought in the operation of detection. At this level visual information, processed as an alerting signal, triggers the saccadic reaction of foveal grasp and the automatic recentering of the head in the direction of the target. Simultaneously, the arousal of attention determines the choice and final ordering of the processing operations. It is then possible to extract from a complex array of information the characteristics of the object that is fixated, and define the qualities (shape, colour, consistency, size, weight, etc.) on the basis of which it is categorised. The object that is identified, however, must also be localised; and it is the spatial coding of visual information which allows the motor programme, with its parameters of adjustment in direction and distance, to steer the hand to the vicinity of the target. The final adjustment is achieved through corrective visual feedback and the cutaneous re-afferents derived from contact with the target. The organization of such a performance may involve, in the first instance, the elaboration of a motor programme, or its selection from a pre-established repertoire. The triggering and execution of the programme may depend on an open-loop operation that does not require retroactive correction. The ballistic trajectory of the hand towards a target, or an object to be grasped, relies to a considerable extent on this type of operation. In contrast, the final positioning of the hand and of the fingers, using visual cues, and the adjustment of the fingers to the shape of the object using cutaneous information, depend on a closed-loop operation. In this case, the motor act is dependent on feedback that enables the programme to be adjusted according to the peripheral conditions of its execution and the precision required to reach the spatial objective.

Within this frame of reference, we have studied problems of visuomotor coordination, in commissurotomised monkeys pointing at a visual target. The 'split-brain' preparation, by sectioning the optic chiasm and the telencephalic commissures, restricts visual information — at least in principle — to one hemisphere. The problem then is to control the capacity of the 'seeing' hemisphere to trigger and guide the movement of the contra-lateral or ipsi-lateral limb during visuomotor performance. Animal studies consistently report that commissurotomy has no effect on the visual guidance of the contra-lateral limb. In contrast, there are notable divergencies regarding the limb ipsi-lateral to the seeing hemisphere: some authors emphasize the importance of dyspraxias following the suppression of inter-hemispheric connections (Downer, 1959; Gazzaniga, 1963; Lund et al., 1970) others describe the motor deficits as transitory and slight, if not totally absent (Myers et al., 1962; Black and Myers, 1965; Hamilton, 1967).

There have been many attempts (Gazzaniga, 1970) to interpret these contradictions which may stem from two main groups of factors. The first concerns the nature of the afferents or re-afferents accessible to the involved hemisphere: their modifications and limitations are imposed by the experimenter or by the experimental paradigm. The second is linked to the definition of the motor act as a response of the subject which involves distal or proximal muscle groups, depending on the complexity of the movement, and ranges from simple, digital pointing to sequences of very elaborate manipulations. Finally, discrepancies may result from differences not only in procedure but also in the criteria used to categorize and quantify the response. Evaluation of the performance may vary according to how one describes the trajectory of a movement, the precision of the point of contact, the coordination of digital movements, and the chronometric aspects of the sequence. In the series of experiments, the task consisted of pointing to a visual target. This type of response can be analysed in terms of the different kinds of sensory information that intervene at the afferent level and, on the efferent side, the different ways of mobilising and organizing motor commands.

METHODS

These investigations were carried out on baboons (*Papio papio*) divided into three groups: split-brain subjects with a section of the inter-hemispheric commissures (corpus callosum and anterior commissure), control subjects

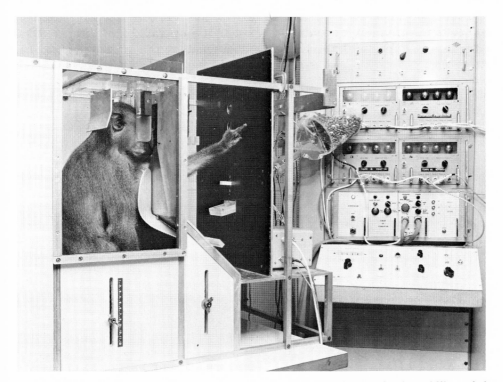

Fig. 1. Experimental apparatus: After distribution of the stimulus in the midline of the panel (Exp. 1) or illumination of a lateral target (Exp. 2—3), the monkey is responding by releasing the lever and pointing at the target.

(with a section of the optic chiasma only) and normal (unoperated) subjects. Throughout the experimental session, the animal is freely moving in a specially-designed cage (Trevarthen, 1972) placed in a soundproof room (Fig. 1). The subject is trained to put his head in a mask fixed on the anterior wall of the cage, which ensures fairly normal posture in relation to the work panel. This mask is fitted with spectacle frames which can be occluded or provided with polarised filters. A system of sliding panels constrains the animal to use only one arm for the response. The work panel, placed vertically 25 cm in front of the cage, contains on the lower section a lever and a cup where food reinforcement is delivered. The monkey determines, by pressing on the lever, the beginning of the trial and thus the inter-trial intervals. Moreover, the lever press standardises the initial position of the active limb.

Experiment 1: Localisation of visual signals in the commissurotomised monkey

Shape discrimination learning in commissurotomised animals is confined to the trained hemisphere (Myers, 1956). This lack of interocular transfer evidences the role, confirmed in numerous experiments involving electrophysiological techniques or lesion studies, of the geniculo—striate system and primary visual cortex in the analysis of the shape and quality of signals. On the other hand, there is ample support for the hypothesis that subcortical structures intervene in the visual processing of spatial information (Held, 1968; Ingle, 1968; Schneider, 1968; Trevarthen, 1968). Thus, although section of the neo-cortical commissures prevents the transmission of information that is cortically processed from one hemisphere to another, it is in theory possible that information provided by mesencephalic structures can be bilaterally distributed. In other words, if shape discrimination learning cannot be transferred from one hemisphere to the other in split-brain animals, we may nevertheless envisage the possibility of inter-hemispheric transfer of positional cues in these animals.

In this first experiment (Beaubaton et al., 1970), four commissurotomised monkeys and two normal animals were trained to point at one of two targets on the left or on the right of a central panel where the discriminanda were displayed. These signals involve shape discriminations (one of the two figures, 0 or 8, appearing in the middle of the screen) or discrimination of positions (the cue given by the presentation of the stimulus at either the top or the bottom of the screen). A correct pointing response to the target at either the left or right of the central panel constitutes the criterion of discrimination for both shape and positional cues.

The results (Table 1) confirmed in split-brain animals the complete absence of inter-hemispheric transfer of form discrimination: when the hand and eye contra-lateral to those used in training are tested, the subjects cannot respond correctly; new training is required for the contra-lateral combination,

TABLE 1

Experiment 1: Inter-hemispheric transfer of form or position discrimination. The symbol "+" indicates, at the end of learning sessions, more than 90% of correct responses and for transfer testing a high-level transfer of training. "O" signifies absence of transfer, the animal failing to solve the task within the testing session.

	Visuomotor coordination	Form discrimination		Position discrimination	
		Split-brain	Normal	Split-brain	Normal
Primary training	Contra-lateral	+	+	+	+
Transfer testing	Ipsi-lateral (trained hand)			+	
Transfer testing	Contra-lateral (untrained hand)	0	+	0	+
Transfer testing	Ipsi-lateral (untrained hand)			0	

of which the duration is comparable to that needed for the initial period of acquisition. Regarding the discrimination of position, inter-ocular transfer is observed immediately: from the first testing session the subjects reach a high level of performance (more than 90% correct responses). In contrast, there is a complete absence of inter-manual transfer in these animals. The normal monkeys show complete transfer in both situations. In so far as the presence or absence of inter-hemispheric transfer permits inferences about the degree of participation of cortical and subcortical structures, respectively, these results confirm the cortical support of operations in shape discrimination learning and suggest the intervention of subcortical structures in the functions of localisation. Moreover, they show that the control of the ipsi-lateral limb in the split-brain monkey can be directly invoked by spatial cues, provided that the trained hand is tested. There is, therefore, inter-ocular but not inter-manual transfer of the performance.

Experiment 2: Hemispheric distribution of visual information and precision of pointing

The results of the previous experiment seem to contradict the proposition, often made implicitly, that the distribution of visual information is restricted to the so-called seeing hemisphere. It is clear that the hemisphere not directly tested receives information about the position of the discriminanda. It remains to be discovered whether this type of information contributes to the correct adjustment of the trajectory of movement, and if this same hemisphere can compensate for the deficit by using visual cues not related to the target or by taking into consideration other sensory afferents. In conditions of monocular training, there may be an asymmetrical division of attention. The effects of this functional asymmetry between the two hemispheres, demonstrated by Trevarthen (1968), have been discussed in relation to visuo-motor performance (Gazzaniga, 1970; Lund et al., 1970; Keating, 1973). The use of polaroid filters by Trevarthen in such experiments enables the restriction of specific visual information to one eye while retaining the possibility of binocular vision of the experimental environment. The problem then arises as to whether this technique, which in some conditions may effect the hemispheric distribution of attention, can influence the precision of performance in a visuomotor task according to whether or not the subject has binocular vision of the experimental environment.

The following experiment (Beaubaton and Chapuis, 1974) using polaroid lens, was carried out to test this hypothesis. The performance of two split-brain monkeys and one control subject (section of the chiasma) was examined in a task of manual pointing at a visual target. The precision of responses for both contra-lateral and ipsi-lateral eye—hand combinations was measured in conditions of monocular vision of the environment 9 (the occlusion of an eye by a mask throughout the experimental session) or binocular vision of the field (the use of polaroid filters). In both cases, the selective distribution of the signal to one eye only was ensured.

The results (Table 2) showed a global decrease of correct responses in the commissurotomised monkeys when the active limb is seen by one eye only, whereas this phenomenon was not observed in the control subject. Moreover, the split-brain animals showed a deficit with the ipsi-lateral eye—hand combination and monocular vision. The fact that this deficit was very slight, if not suppressed, with binocular vision suggests that it is the ipsi-lateral combination which mainly benefits in this condition.

The deterioration of performance by the split-brain animals using the ipsi-lateral command and monocular vision can be interpreted in terms of a difficulty in operating, at the end of the trajectory, a visuomotor correction of the positional errors of the limb in relation to the target (Paillard and Beaubaton, 1975). In contrast, the quality of responses in animals using the same ipsi-lateral device but with binocular vision of the environment, suggests that, in this particular case, the hemisphere which does not receive visual information in relation to the target and its position, nevertheless has access to afferents provided by other sensory modalities. This could concern tactual information provided by the active hand from contact with the target and visual afferents concerning the position of this hand in relation to the body and the spatial frame of reference provided by the work panel. The seeing hemisphere can then trigger the programme of ballistic transport of the ipsi-lateral limb but the terminal adjustment then depends on the contra-lateral hemisphere which can, in certain cases, compensate for the deficit

TABLE 2

Experiments 2 and 3: Data observed in split-brain and chiasma-sectioned monkeys performing a pointing task. Percentages of correct responses are compared with χ^2 tests. Values of χ^2 are followed by * when they reach a $P = 0.05$ probability threshold.

	Split-brain subjects			Chiasma-sectioned subjects		
	Contra-lateral	(χ^2)	Ipsi-lateral	Contra-lateral	(χ^2)	Ipsi-lateral
Exp. 2 Binocular visual field	93.0	(0.24)	88.2	96.4	(5.62)	87.2
(χ^2)	(12.69*)		(43.94*)	(2.32)		(1.42)
Monocular visual field	74.3	(19.26*)	43.8	91.2	(0.07)	92.3
Exp. 3 With tactual information	73.8	(9.5)	52.8	78.9	(1.5)	85.6
(χ^2)	(19.9*)		(30.2*)	(1.4)		(1.2)
Without tactual information	44.4	(19.4*)	15.9	82.5	(0.2)	79.7

due to the commissurotomy by the coordination of visual, tactile and proprioceptive cues.

*Experiment 3: The use of tactile cues in visual guidance of the ipsi-lateral
limb*

The hypothesis has been put forward that tactile cues may be exploited
when visual information is not available to guide the movement of the limb
in its final phase.

These cutaneous cues are in fact directly integrated by the cortex contra-
lateral to the active hand; and they are then capable of guiding the positioning of the digits by direct cortico-spinal pathways. This possibility may explain some aspects of the contradictions expressed in previous work regarding the importance of motor deficits in ipsi-lateral eye—hand control after
commissurotomy.

The possibility of this tactile compensation, observed by Brinkman and
Kuypers (1972, 1973) in a grasping task, can be examined in our pointing
experiment (Beaubaton and Chapuis, 1975). Accordingly, the precision of
pointing was measured in two split-brain subjects and a control subject. The
performance of the contra-lateral and ipsi-lateral eye—hand combinations
was compared in two conditions, with and without tactile information about
the visual target, both conditions being realized by raising or lowering the
metal target in relation to the panel. The results (Table 2) showed a significant deterioration of performance when cutaneous re-afferents from the
target were suppressed in the split-brain monkeys. This phenomenon, which
was observed even with the contra-lateral command, may be attributed to
the conditions of training which may have reinforced the importance of
tactile cues. This lack of precision is in marked contrast to the high level of
performance of the control subjects in all the experimental conditions.

Further analysis is required to specify the role of tactile cues in the
placing of the hand in comparison with their role in association with vision
of the limb and proprioceptive information about the position of the limb at
the moment of terminal contact. Other experiments in our laboratory (Paillard and Brouchon, 1974) have shown that this information can contribute
to the spatial calibration of the terminal position of the moving limb. This
calibrated information can then be used again for the programming of subsequent movement and thus account for the improvement in precision of
performance. Tactile cues are not the only ones which may be exploited for
this process. The correct reponses shown in the absence of cutaneous reaffer-
ences with the ipsi-lateral combination may be due to the use of information
concerning the quality of the immediately preceding response provided, for
instance, by the distribution, or the absence, of reinforcement.

DISCUSSION

The interpretation of the experimental results requires a clear distinction between two components of the reaching performance: (1) the choice and triggering of an appropriate motor programme for the ballistic transport of the band toward the target — the so-callled open-loop aspect of the performance and (2) the final correction of the trajectory to ensure the correct placement of the hand on the target — the closed-loop phase of the operation (Table 3). Ocular movements illustrate the same functional distinction, that is, between a saccadic component triggered by extra-foveal stimulation and an error-correcting mechanism contributing to the foveal capture and tracking of the target.

A similar distinction was made by Hein and Held (1967) in studies about the ontogenetic development of the visual placing reaction of the kitten. These authors contrasted two operations: the visually elicited extension of the forelimb which appears as soon as the kitten is able to see and the visual guidance of the limb (for the correct positioning of the paws on the supporting surface) which necessitates an early exposure of the moving limb. The evidence from studies of pointing performance may be interpreted analogously: the deterioration recorded when one eye controls the ipsi-lateral hand may be attributable to a specific impairment of the mechanisms of final adjustment whereas the ballistic movement, which is visually triggered, can be correctly performed.

The first phase of the triggering mechanisms may require the use of positional cues concerning the location of the visual target; these positional cues are available for the control of the ipsi-lateral hand in split-brain animals (Table 3). It therefore seems unlikely that the geniculo-striate pathways and their cortical projections make a contribution since ballistic reaching to a visual target is preserved in monkeys after complete destruction of cortical visual areas (Humphrey and Weiskrantz, 1967; Humphrey, 1970). Experimental evidence in support of two visual systems leads one to emphasize the role of tectal structures for localisation in contrast with the shape-analysing function of the geniculo-striate system. If the contribution of subcortical structures to the organization of limb movement remains to be specified and can only be hypothetical at this stage of analysis, the problem of the spatial coding of visual cues to trigger the response has to be clarified. Gazzaniga (1966, 1969), in his 'cross-cueing' hypothesis, stressed the role of proprioceptive re-afferents, from the position of the eye and the head, in the spatial coding of visual information. These afferents, which are bilaterally distributed, are available for both hemispheres in split-brain animals and may therefore contribute to the triggering of limb movement in ipsi-lateral control through the contra-lateral hemisphere. Brinkman and Kuypers (1973) however, have questioned this point of view and demonstrated the possibility of visuomotor performance with the ipsi-lateral command, after destruction of

TABLE 3

Organization of visuomotor coordination in split-brain monkeys

Regulatory processes	Functional operations	Stages of movement	Sensory cues	Motor control	Ipsi-lateral visuomotor control
Anticipatory programmes (Feedforward)	localization	ballistic transport	visual (tactile) (proprioceptive)	proximal	fair
	identification	postural setting of the hand	visual	distal	impaired
Retroactive corrections (Feedback)	adjustment	terminal correction	visual	proximal	impaired
		fingers guiding	visual	distal	impaired
		fingers guiding	tactile	distal	fair

the contra-lateral sensory motor area. Nevertheless, as Gazzaniga (1969, 1970) has shown, the steering of the hand by the ipsi-lateral eye in callosotomised monkeys is greatly impaired after rigid fixing of the head in relation to the body. Further demonstrations of the supplementary role of cervical articular receptors in eye—head coordination after labyrinthectomy (Dichgans et al., 1973) as well as the striking motor disorder resulting from rhizotomy of the cervical dorsal roots (Cohen, 1961) evidence the special role played by information about the position of the head in calibrating the trajectory of the limb to reach a target in space (Paillard, 1971, 1974).

The contribution of proximal joints and then of the proximal musculature in setting the direction of the ballistic movement of the limb must also be emphasized. This is consistent with studies (Kuypers, 1964; Lawrence and Kuypers, 1968a,b; Brinkman and Kuypers 1972, 1973) demonstrating the restriction of motor control of the ipsi-lateral limb to the proximal musculature by way of the ventromedial cortico-spinal descending pathways. If the ballistic component of the reaching performance presupposes that the proximal musculature is significantly involved in every instance, it would be predicted that the open-loop reaching for a visual target — whether the contralateral or ipsi-lateral hemisphere is involved — should be comparable, that is to say, equally imprecise in localisation, provided that error-correcting mechanisms were excluded; this effect has been demonstrated by Hamilton (1967). By contrast, closed-loop reaching performance is differentially affected with the ipsi-lateral as compared with the contra-lateral pairing of eye and hand, as shown in previous studies (Downer, 1959) and also by the results of our own pointing task.

From the anatomo-physiological point of view, the connections between visual cortex and motor system have to be considered. Myers et al. (1962) discussed the question as to whether visual information was distributed to sensory motor areas directly through cortico—cortical association pathways or alternately through a subcortical loop down to mesencephalic structures. The possibility of direct control of brainstem motor centres by visual cortex has also been raised (Teuber, 1970). It is known that the visual guidance of movement can be severely impaired by brainstem lesions (Sprague and Meikle, 1965; Sprague, 1966) as well as by caudate lesions (Gybels et al., 1964). Although the integrative role of brainstem structures in sensory motor coordination has been stressed (Lashley, 1924; Penfield, 1954), it seems likely that cortico—subcortical connections are critically involved in the control of visuomotor mechanisms. These interactions which have been demonstrated in anatomical (Altman and Carpenter, 1961) and behavioural (Voneida, 1970) studies, may well contribute to the preservation of the unity of perceptual processes which is shown in the visuomotor performance of callosotomised subjects (Trevarthen and Sperry, 1973).

Finally, we would like to emphasize a somewhat neglected component of the anticipatory mechanisms involved in the reaching movement, namely those dealing with the postural setting of the hand and fingers in relation to the visual identification of the characteristics of the target. This postural setting of the grip depends on the perceived size, shape and weight of the object. This grip-posture may be modified or even absent in split-brain subjects (Downer, 1959; Gazzaniga, 1963; Lund et al., 1970; Brinkman and Kuypers, 1973). As soon as contact is established, the grip is adjusted by means of tactile information which then plays a predominant role in the guidance of digital exploration for the adjustment of grasp. A major handicap in the ipsi-lateral condition may be inability to set the hand and fingers in an appropriate posture, although the perceptual identification of the features of the object may be correctly achieved by the seeing hemisphere (Table 3). This could explain, at least in part, the impairment of finger positioning observed by Brinkman and Kuypers (1973) in the ipsi-lateral condition and attributed by them to the loss of visual guidance of distal musculature. The posture of the hand and digits, when gripping an object, is not in fact 'guided' by direct visual control of finger movement because it can also be observed in the open-loop condition without vision of the hand.

Regarding the second group of processes regulating visuomotor performance in closed-loop conditions, two main sources of feedback can be considered. First, the corrective mechanisms using visual feedback at the end of the trajectory in order to adjust the correct placement of the hand. As we have stressed previously, it is likely that visual information serves mainly to position the hand in steering the proximal musculature and possibly, although to a lesser extent, the fingers. This ability is clearly impaired, even in open-loop reaching, in our callosotomised animals using the ipsi-lateral eye—hand combination. Recent reports of Keating (1973) point in the same direction: this author observed a clear impairment of distal motor control in ipsi-lateral reaching. This inefficacy of visual correction of hand position in the vicinity of the target could be considered in the light of the mechanisms involved in visual tracking and, more specifically, visuomanual tracking of a moving target. There are conflicting studies in the literature: reports of unimpaired performance by split-brain monkeys in visuomotor tracking tasks (Myers et al., 1962; Black and Myers, 1965) compared with the ipsi-lateral deficits noted by other workers (Gazzaniga, 1966; Lehman, 1968). These discrepancies may stem from the failure to distinguish clearly between the use of visual information as spatial cues for triggering movement in open-loop conditions, and as error-signals in a feedback loop.

Moreover, the predictability of the movement of a moving target may be sufficient to account for partial success in tracking tasks in all conditions, and especially with the ipsi-lateral condition in which this mechanism of prediction could compensate for the lack of processing of visual feedback. Further, although the movement of the proximal musculature can be controlled by either hemisphere, only the contra-lateral hemisphere can control the distal musculature, as Brinkman and Kuypers (1972, 1973) have emphasized. These authors rightly suggest that, as soon as the hand comes into contact with the target, the tactile information that is available to the contra-lateral motor area of the non-seeing hemisphere may account for the good manipulative performance of split-brain animals, using the ipsi-lateral eye—hand combination. Our experiments on the effect of suppressing tactile cues in pointing tasks confirm this supposition. Tactile cues are therefore likely to be the main source of information for the positioning of the hand and fingers in relation to a visual target. The role of direct, visual feedback from the position of the distal segments of the limb is therefore minimized and may be supplemented by an anticipatory setting of the grip, that is absent in the steering of the ipsi-lateral hand by the seeing hemisphere.

REFERENCES

ALTMAN, J. and CARPENTER, M.B. (1961) Fiber projections of the superior colliculus in the cat. J. comp. Neurol., 116, 157—178.
BEAUBATON, D., NYSENBAUM-REQUIN, S. and PAILLARD, J. (1970) Etude du transfert interhémisphérique de l'analyse de la forme ou de la position du signal chez le singe à cerveau dédoublé. J. Physiol. (Paris), 62, 343.
BEAUBATON, D. and CHAPUIS, N. (1974) Rôle des informations tactiles dans la précision du pointage chez le singe split-brain. Neuropsychologie, 12, 151—155.
BEAUBATON, D. and CHAPUIS, N. (1975) Champ visuel monoculaire ou binoculaire et précision du pointage chez le singe split-brain. Neuropsychologie, (in press).
BLACK, P. and MYERS, R.E. (1965) A neurological investigation of eye-hand control in the chimpanzee. In (Ettlinger E.G., Ed.): Function of the Corpus Callosum, Little, Brown and Co., Boston, pp. 47—59.
BRINKMAN, J. and KUYPERS, H.G.J.M. (1972) Split-brain monkeys: central control of ipsilateral and contralateral arm, hand and finger movements. Science, 176, 536—539.
BRINKMAN, J. and KUYPERS, H.G.J.M. (1973) Cerebral control of contralateral and ipsilateral arm, hand and finger movements in the split-brain rhesus monkey. Brain, 96, 653—674.
COHEN, L.A. (1961) Role of eye and neck proprioceptive mechanisms in body orientation and motor coordination. J. Neurophysiol., 24, 1—11.
DICHGANS, J., BIZZI, E., MORASSO, P. and TAGLIASCO, V. (1973) Mechanisms underlying recovery of eye head coordination following bilateral labyrinthectomy in monkeys. Exp. Brain Res., 18, 548—569.
DOWNER, J.L. de C. (1959) Changes in visually guided behavior following mid sagittal division of optic chiasma and corpus callosum in monkeys (Macaca mulatta). Brain, 82, 251—259.
GAZZANIGA, M.S. (1963) Effects of commissurotomy on a preoperatively learned visual discrimination. Exp. Neurol., 8, 14—19.
GAZZANIGA, M.S. (1965) Interhemispheric cueing system remaining after section of neocortical commissures in monkeys. Exp. Neurol., 16, 28—35.
GAZZANIGA, M.S. (1969) Cross-cueing mechanisms and ipsilateral eye-hand control in split-brain monkeys. Exp. Neurol., 23, 11—17.
GAZZANIGA, M.S. (1970) The Bisected Brain. Appleton Century Crofts, N.Y., 172 p.

GYBELS, J., MEULDERS, M., CALLENS, M. and COLLE, J. (1964) Lésions chroniques du noyau caudé chez le Chat. J. Physiol. (Paris), 56, 372—373.

HAMILTON, C.R. (1967) Effects of brain bisection on eye-hand coordination in monkeys wearing prisms. J. Comp. Physiol. Psychol., 64, 434—443.

HEIN, A. and HELD, R. (1967) Dissociation of the visual placing response into elicited and guided components. Science, 158, 390—392.

HELD, R. (1968) Dissociation of visual functions by deprivation and rearrangement. Psychol. Forsch., 31, 1—4, 338—348.

HUMPHREY, N.K. (1970) What the frog's eye tells the monkeys brain. Brain Behav. Evol., 3, 324—337.

HUMPHREY, N.K. and WEISKRANTZ, L. (1967) Vision in monkeys after removal of the striate cortex. Nature, 215, 595—597.

INGLE, D. (168) Two visual mechanisms underlying the behavior of fish. Psychol. Forsch., 31, 1—4, 1—51.

KEATING, E.G. (1973) Loss of visual control of the forelimb after interruption of cortical pathway. Exp. Neurol., 41, 635—648.

KUYPERS, H.G.J.M. (1964) The descending pathways to the spinal cord, their anatomy and function. Progr. Brain Res., 11, 178—202.

LASHLEY, K.S. (1924) Studies of cerebral function in learning: V. The retention of motor habits after destruction of the so-called motor areas in primates. Arch. Neurol. Psychiat., 12, 249—273.

LAWRENCE, D.G. and KUYPERS, H.G.J.M. (1968a) The functional organization of the motor system in the monkey. I. The effects of bilateral pyramidal lesions. Brain, 91, 1—14.

LAWRENCE, D.G. and KUYPERS, H.G.J.M. (1968b) The functional organization of the motor system in the monkey. II. The effect of lesions of the descending brainstem pathways. Brain, 91, 15—36.

LEHMAN, R.A.W. (1968) Motor coordination and hand preference after lesions of the visual pathway and corpus callosum. Brain, 91, 525—538.

LUND, J.S., DOWNER, J.L. de C. and LUMLEY, J.S.P. (1970) Visual control of limb movement following section of optic chiasma and corpus callosum in the monkey. Cortex, 6, 323—346.

MYERS, R.E. (1956) Function of corpus callosum in interocular transfer. Brain, 79, 358.

MYERS, R.E., SPERRY, R.W. and McCURDY, N. (1962) Neural mechanisms in visual guidance of limb movements. Arch. Neurol. (Chicago), 7, 195—202.

PAILLARD, J. (1971) Les déterminants moteurs de l'organisation de l'espace. Cah. Psychol., 14, 261—316.

PAILLARD, J. (1974) Le traitement des données spatiales. In De l'espace corporel à l'Espace Ecologique Symp. Assoc. Psychol. Sci. langue française (Bruxelles, 1972). Paris P.U.F., pp. 7—54.

PAILLARD, J. and BEAUBATON, D. (1975) Problèmes posés par le contrôle visuel de la motricité proximale et distale après disconnexion hémisphérique chez le singe. In (Schott B., Michel F. and Boucher M., Eds.) Les syndrome de disconnexion calleuse chez l'homme.

PAILLARD, J. and BROUCHON, M. (1974) A proprioceptive contribution to the spatial encoding of position cues for ballistic movements. Brain Res., 71, 273—284.

PENFIELD, W. (1954) Mechanisms of voluntary movement. Brain, 71, 1—17.

SCHNEIDER, G.E. (1968) Contrasting visuomotor functions of tectum and cortex in the golden hamster. Psychol. Forsch., 31, 1—4, 51—62.

SPRAGUE, J.M. (1966) Interaction of cortex and superior colliculus in mediation of visually guided behavior in the cat. Science, 153, 3743, 1544—1547.

SPRAGUE, J.M. and MEIKLE, T.H. (1965) The role of the superior colliculus in visually guided behavior. Exp. Neurol., 11, 145—146.

TEUBER, H.L. (1970) Subcortical vision: a prologue. Brain Behav. Evol., 3, 1—4, 7—15.

TREVARTHEN, C. (1962) Double visual learning in split-brain monkeys. Science, 136, 258—259.

TREVARTHEN, C. (1968) Two mechanisms of vision in primates. Psychol. Forsch., 31, 1—4, 300—337.

TREVARTHEN, C. (1972) The split-brain technique. In (R.E. Meyers, Ed.) Methods in Psychobiology, Academic Press, London, pp. 251—284.

TREVARTHEN ,C. and SPERRY, R.W. (1973) Perceptual unity of the ambient visual field in human commissurotomy patients. Brain, 96, 3, 547—570.

VONEIDA, T.J. (1970) Behavioral changes following midline section of the mesencephalic tegmentum in the cat and monkey. Brain Behav. Evol., 3, 1—4, 241—260.

3

Movement and associated postural adjustment

H. REGIS, E. TROUCHE and J. MASSION

Forelimb flexion was induced in standing cats by stimulation of the con-tra-lateral motor cortex, of the contra-lateral red nucleus and of the ipsi-later-al superficial radial nerve. Changes in weight supported by each forelimb were measured by strain gauge force transducers.

The decrease in weight associated with the onset of flexion of one forelimb was associated with an increase in weight of the other forelimb. The latency of the increase in weight was longer than or equal to the latency of the onset of the flexion, in the case of cortical or rubral stimulation and equal to or shorter than the latency of the onset of the flexion in the case of superficial radial nerve stimulation.

The amplitude and duration of the changes in weight of both forelimbs were increased when the intensity of the stimulation or the duration of the train were augmented, and the latency of both effects shortened.

Flexion of one forelimb and increase in weight of the other forelimb induced by cortical stimulation were still present after chronic cerebellec-tomy. The same bilateral effects induced by stimulation of the red nucleus were still observed after bilateral chronic ablation of the motor cortex. Ipsi-lateral increase and contra-lateral decrease in weight induced by stimulation of the superficial radial nerve remained unmodified after chronic cerebellec-tomy and after chronic bilateral ablation of the motor cortex.

As a result of the latencies of both effects and of other experimental data it is concluded that the increase in weight of one forelimb associated with flexion of the other forelimb is centrally programmed together with the flexion movement. The site where the postural program associated with movement originates is discussed.

INTRODUCTION

Every movement is performed in a world subjected to the force of gravity. The postural tonus is a permanent contraction of many muscles which coun-teracts the force of gravity and maintains the center of gravity of the body within limits compatible with a good equilibrium of the animal. When a movement of a limb must be made, the distribution of the postural tonus has to be changed in order to shift the animal's weight onto the other limbs and to make the limb free to move. A postural adjustment is also needed during the performance of the movement, in order to prevent the disequilibrium due to the shift of the center of gravity provoked by the movement per se.

Using the dog, Ioffe and Andreyev (1969) described the postural adjustment associated with a conditioned forelimb movement. The weight of the body, which was initially divided between the four limbs, became supported by two diagonally opposite limbs, the contra-lateral forelimb and the ipsi-lateral hindlimb. The same pattern of postural adjustment was observed in the cat, during a placing movement of the forelimb (Massion and Smith, 1974; Regis and Trouche, 1974). In both examples, the movement and associated postural adjustment were closely related in a given motor act. This fact suggests that the central mechanisms involved in the appearance of movement are linked to some extent to the mechanisms producing the postural adjustment.

An indication of the type of link between movement and associated postural adjustment is given by the fact that in some circumstances the postural adjustment may be induced without associated movement; some of the tactile stimulations used to elicit the placing movement with the standing cat (Massion and Smith, 1974), provoked the postural adjustment and failed to induce the placing movement. The same stimulation of the leg applied to cats previously deprived of the cerebellum or of the motor cortex induced only the postural adjustment and not the movement (Regis et al., 1974). It may be concluded that the postural adjustment is usually associated with the movement but may also appear alone as a preparatory mechanism to the projected movement.

The fact that the postural adjustment may be elicited without associated movement does not imply necessarily that the reverse is true and that a movement may appear alone, without any preparatory or associated postural adjustment. In order to investigate this question, the present experimental series was undertaken. A forelimb flexion movement was elicited by direct stimulation of central structures such as the motor cortex and the red nucleus which are on the final command pathway for movement of the limbs (Lawrence and Kuypers, 1968; Wiesendanger, 1969). For comparison, a flexion reflex of the same limb was induced by stimulation of the superficial radial nerve. Two possibilities were envisaged. According to the first, stimulation of the motor cortex or of the red nucleus would initiate the contralateral forelimb movement alone. The postural adjustment would be induced secondarily through the peripheral feedback afferents resulting from the performance of the movement. According to the second possibility, both movement and postural adjustment would be initiated together by the central stimulation, which would trigger directly the postural program needed for the ordered movement. Experimental results were in favor of a central command of both movement and associated postural adjustment.

METHODS

The experiments were performed on 8 adult cats. Among them two animals were chronically de-cerebellated and two other had a bilateral ablation of the pericruciate motor cortex. All were habituated to standing quietly in a restraining hammock with all four feet in contact with a firm supporting surface. The isometric postural pressure exerted by each of the forelimbs was measured by strain gauge force transducers under each limb.

All the animals had electrodes implanted in the motor cortex and/or the red nucleus on one side and on the superficial radial nerve on the other side.

Ten nickel—chrome electrodes insulated except at their tips were implanted inside the motor cortex at a depth of 1.5 mm through narrow trephan holes, and sealed to the skull by dental cement. After recovery from the operation, cortical stimulation was made through pairs of electrodes, and the movement induced was observed. Trains of pulses at 300 c.s., with a duration of 100 msec were commonly used. Only flexion movements of the contra-lateral forelimb were considered.

Stimulation of the red nucleus was performed through a pair of nickel—chrome electrodes, one implanted vertically and the other obliquely. The target zone was the medio-dorsal part of the posterior red nucleus which corresponds to the forelimb area (Pompeiano and Brodal, 1957). Stimulation was used during implantation of the electrodes and the progression was stopped when a clear forelimb flexion was observed. At the end of the

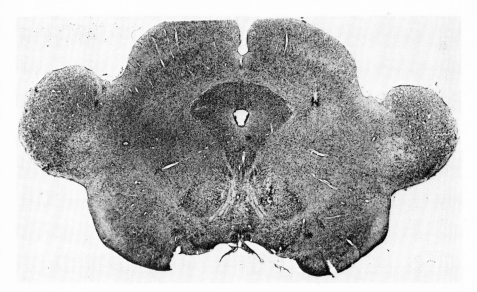

Fig. 1. Histological control of the localization of the tip of one electrode. The tip is located in the dorso-medial part of the caudal half of the right red nucleus (forelimb area).

experimentation, an electrocoagulation was made (50 μA during 15 sec) and an histological control of the position of the tips of the electrodes was systematically performed (Fig. 1). A pair of silver wires was inserted around the superficial radial nerve on the side opposite to the cortical or rubral implantation in a way similar to that described by Pompeiano and Swett (1963). The parameters used for radial nerve stimulation were the same as for cortical or rubral stimulation.

The experimental procedure was as follows: the cat was placed in the hammock in a standing position. The force exerted by each forelimb was measured. The latencies of the changes in weight were measured from the first shock of the stimulating train to a minimal change of 50 g. The intensity of stimulation was adjusted in such a way as to provoke a flexion just sufficient to lift the limb from the supporting tray. Series of ten stimulations with the same parameters were applied. Each experimental session never lasted more than one hour.

RESULTS

Changes of forelimb forces induced by cortical, rubral and radial nerve stimulation

Stimulation of the forelimb area of the motor cortex with a 100 msec train of impulses at 300/sec produced a characteristic change in the forces

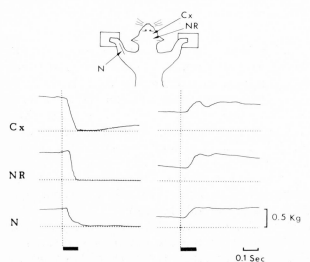

Fig. 2. Changes in forelimb weight induced by stimulation of motor cortex (Cx), red nucleus (NR) and superficial radial nerve (N). On the left, the decrease in forelimb weight is associated with the flexion. The black bar indicates the time and the duration of the repetitive stimulation. On the right, note the increase in weight of the other forelimb.

TABLE 1

Stimulation of cortical forelimb motor area

	Cortical site	Stimulus intensity (volts)	Latency of flexion (msec) (contra-lateral forelimb)	Latency of in-crease in weight (msec) (ipsi-lateral forelimb)
Normal cats				
Grise	a	1.2	35 ±12.2	27.1 ± 8.3
		1.3	27.8 ± 6.9	23.8 ±12.1
Rose	a	2.0	29.1 ± 12.8	58 ± 23.8
		4.0	25.8 ± 11.8·	37 ± 9.4
	b	4.0	70.8 ± 23.3	49.2 ± 6
Tigré	a	3.0	46 ± 8.6	60.7 ± 18
	b	2.0	34.5 ± 6.4	48.1 ± 6
Léonie	a	4.0	58.1 ± 28	44.6 ± 17.2
	b	3.0	66.9 ± 20.5	56 ± 24.5
	c	2.5	30.5 ± 4.3	40 ± 22.2
Decerebellated				
Cerebel 1	a	2.0	28.7 ± 11.2	47.5 ± 20.5
		4.0	29 ± 12	33.6 ± 16.8
Spartacus	a	2.0	59 ± 23	68 ± 28

exerted by each of the forelimbs. There was a decrease in weight of the contra-lateral forelimb, and an increase in weight of the ipsi-lateral forelimb (Fig. 2). The latencies of both effects are summarized in Table 1. It can be seen that some variations occurred between animals, the shortest effect being observed within 25—30 msec. The contra-lateral decrease in weight, which corresponded with the onset of the movement, appeared generally with a latency equal to or a little shorter than the ipsi-lateral increase.

Stimulation of the red nucleus elicited modifications of forces comparable to those induced by cortical stimulation. There was a tendency for the latencies, however, to be somewhat longer in most cases (Fig. 2, Table 2), at least for the increase in weight of the ipsi-lateral forelimb.

Stimulation of the superficial radial nerve induced, as may be expected, an ipsi-lateral decrease of forces which corresponded to the ipsi-lateral forelimb flexion, with a contra-lateral increase in weight. The range of latencies observed for the changes in weight were usually shorter than after cortical or rubral stimulation. In some cases, the contra-lateral increase in weight preceded the ipsi-lateral flexion (Table 3).

TABLE 2

Stimulation of red nucleus

	Stimulus intensity (volts)	Latency of flexion (msec) (contra-lateral forelimb)	Latency of increase in weight (msec) (ipsi-lateral forelimb)
Normal cats			
Rose	2.0	44 ± 13.1	58 ± 10.9
	4.0	23.9 ± 8.6	27.5 ± 5.3
Tigré	4.0	55 ± 19.1	62 ± 6.4
	6.0	40 ± 7	52.5 ± 12.5
Léonie	3.0	36.9 ± 9.8	54 ± 12.2
Bilateral ablation of cortical motor area			
Cécile	0.8	29 ± 18.6	42.8 ± 20.6
Nelly (electrode 1)	2.0	45.3 ± 18.6	51 ± 19.8
Nelly (electrode 2)	2.0	30.9 ± 14.5	32.5 ± 13.2

TABLE 3

Stimulation of superficial radial nerve

	Stimulus intensity (volts)	Latency of flexion (msec) (ipsi-lateral forelimb)	Latency of increase in weight (msec) (contra-lateral fore-limb)
Normal cats			
Grise	0.1	38 ± 5.2	33.3 ± 5.7
	0.15	33.7 ± 7.4	30 ± 5.7
	0.2	30.5 ± 13.8	28.5 ± 12.4
	0.25	25 ± 10.5	24 ± 6.6
Rose	0.5	31.6 ± 10.3	39.2 ± 10.9
	0.6	28.3 ± 15.2	33.3 ± 15.5
Bilateral ablation of cortical motor area			
Cécile	0.8	30 ± 10.9	28 ± 14.3
Nelly	0.8	28.3 ± 4	37.5 ± 7.5
Decerebellate			
Cerebel 1	1.0	35 ± 11.6	41.5 ± 11.9

*Changes of forelimb forces induced by cortical, rubral or peripheral stimula-
tion after motor cortical and cerebellar ablation*

Stimulation of the forelimb cortical area was performed on animals with
chronic cerebellar ablation. Both contra-lateral movement and ipsi-lateral
increase in weight were still observed with the same range of latencies. The
cerebellum and the cerebello-cortical loop were not necessary for the appearance of the responses (Table 1).

Stimulation of the red nucleus was performed in two animals with chronic bilateral motor cortical ablation. The results were comparable to those
observed in intact cats (Table 2). The effects induced by stimulation of the
red nucleus were not secondary to stimulation of brachial fibers passing
through the red nucleus and influencing the motor cortical area through the
ventro-lateral nucleus of the thalamus.

It is interesting to note that both ipsi-lateral flexion and contra-lateral
increase in weight induced after stimulation of the superficial radial nerve
were still noticeable with comparable latencies after motor cortical or cerebellar ablation. Neither effect is relayed through the motor cortex or the
cerebellum.

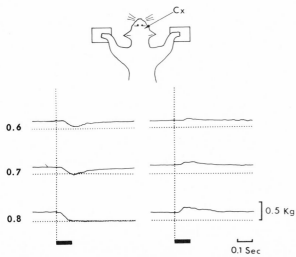

Fig. 3. Influence of the intensity of the stimulation. Same symbols as in Fig. 2. The
intensity values indicated on the left correspond to a relative scale. For an intensity of
0.6, the lifting of the left forelimb is not sufficient to prevent the limb from touching the
tray, as shown by the fact that the trace does not reach the dotted line (zero weight).
Nevertheless, a slight increase of weight of the other forelimb may be noticed. By increasing the intensity, both latencies of contra-lateral decrease in weight and ipsi-lateral increase in weight are shortened whereas the intensity of the reactions increases.

Effect of intensity and train duration

Series of stimulations of progressively increasing intensity were applied to the different target nervous structures in order to see whether both decrease in one forelimb weight and increase in the other forelimb weight appeared with the same intensity of stimulation. The lowest value of the stimulus applied to the motor cortex required for the appearance of the movement was also the threshold value for the increase in weight of the other forelimb (Fig. 3). At threshold values, the latency was longer for both movement of the contra-lateral forelimb and increase in weight of the ipsi-lateral forelimb. Comparable results were obtained for stimulation of the red nucleus and of the superficial radial nerve.

The influence of duration of the train was also investigated. Single shocks applied to the motor cortex or to the red nucleus were ineffective in producing movement of the contra-lateral limb or in evoking an increase in weight of the ipsi-lateral limb. Repetitive stimulation was required, indicating a need for temporal summation. The intensity of contra-lateral movement and ipsi-lateral increase in weight augmented each other when the duration of the train increased (Fig. 4). Variation of train duration also had the same effect on the responses induced by stimulation of the superficial radial nerve.

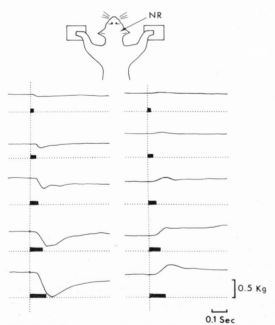

Fig. 4. Influence of the duration of the train. Same symbols as on Fig. 2. Notice the increase of the reactions when the duration of the train is augmented.

Neural versus mechanical origin of the increase in weight of one forelimb associated with a movement of the other forelimb.

When a forelimb movement is induced by cortical stimulation, the ipsi-lateral increase in weight might be explained by neural or by mechanical factors.

To afford a mechanical explanation, for example, the cat could be re-placed by a stool with its four legs resting on the four trays. The sudden lowering of the tray supporting the left forelimb would be accompanied by an increase in weight on the contra-lateral foreleg and the ipsi-lateral hind-legs. The increase in weight would occur synchronously with the sudden lowering of the left foreleg. However, one must bear in mind that the cat does not have a rigid body but is composed of a mixture of rigid parts, the bones, and of viscoelastic elements, the joints and muscles. It may thus be expected that, due to the viscoelasticity of the tissue, the sudden lowering of the tray supporting the left forelimb and the increase in weight of the right forelimb would not be synchronous but that the increase would start with some delay. Actually, the delay was measured with different cats from the onset of the lowering of the tray to a minimal increase in weight of 10 g and was found to be between 15 and 35 msec (Fig. 5). Since after stimulation of the motor cortex, the increase in weight of one limb and the movement of the associated limb may occur synchronously, it is evident that other factors in addition to a solely mechanical process are involved.

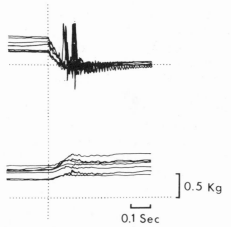

]0.5 Kg

0.1 Sec

Fig. 5. Effect of the sudden lowering of the tray supporting one forelimb on the weight of the other forelimb. The dotted vertical line indicates the onset of the sudden lowering. On the upper trace, the large artefact indicates the moment when the falling tray is mechanically stopped. The lower traces show the corresponding changes in weight of the other forelimb. Notice that the increase in weight appears with some delay with respect to the onset of the lowering.

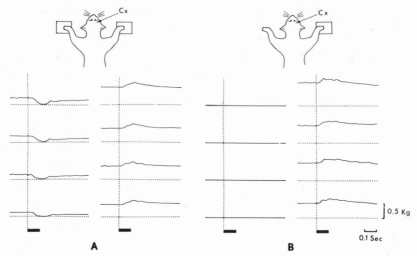

Fig. 6. Contra-lateral flexion elicited when the moving limb is not supported at the time of the stimulation. Stimulation of the right motor area. In A, both forelimbs are supported by a tray at the time of the stimulation and the usual responses are observed. In B, the left forelimb is gently pushed out of the tray and the cortical stimulation is applied in these conditions. Notice that the increase in weight of the right forelimb is still present with the same latencies.

A purely mechanical effect was also excluded by another set of experiments. The left forelimb was gently pushed out of the supporting tray in such a way that prior to cortical stimulation, the body weight was only supported by three limbs. When stimulation of the right motor cortex was applied under these conditions, an increase in weight of the right forelimb was still observed (Fig. 6). The mean latency of the increase in weight was augmented, but latencies as short as those observed with the left forelimb supported by the tray were noticed. The same results were obtained after stimulation of the red nucleus and the superficial radial nerve.

The increase in weight exerted by one forelimb during the movement of the other forelimb may thus be reasonably attributed to a neural mechanism. The question as to whether the increase of force is triggered by the cortical or rubral stimulation or induced through afferents associated with movement will be raised in the discussion.

DISCUSSION

The experiments were undertaken in order to analyze the relations between movement and associated postural adjustment.

Stimulations of motor cortex, red nucleus or superficial radial nerve were performed in order to initiate a forelimb flexion. The same stimulations induced an increase in weight of the other forelimb. This increase in weight could not be interpreted as being the result of a pure mechanical response to the lifting of the limb undergoing the flexion, as already discussed. Neural mechanisms were presumed to be responsible, at least partly, for the increase in weight which resulted from postural adjustment associated with the movement.

The stimulation of motor cortex, red nucleus or superficial radial nerve could be responsible for the postural adjustment in different ways. Firstly, the stimulation could directly induce the flexion movement but not the postural adjustment; the peripheral afferents associated with the performance of the movement would be responsible secondarily for the associated postural adjustment. Secondly, the stimulation could provoke directly and simultaneously the movement and the postural adjustment (see Fig. 7, A and B).

The first hypothesis, according to which the postural adjustment would be initiated by the peripheral afferents associated with the movement, may be disregarded because the latency of the postural adjustment was not systematically longer than that of the movement. However, it might be proposed as an alternative that a contraction of the spindles preceeds the contraction of the flexor muscles and that the postural adjustment would be initiated by the spindle afferents before the onset of the movement. However, the time required for such a servo action would be too long to take account of the latency of the postural adjustment (see Matthews, 1972; Stein, 1974).

It may thus be suggested from the results that the cortical or rubral stimulation commands both the movement and the associated postural adjustment. The recent observations from Gahery and Nieoullon (1974) are still more demonstrative, since these authors observed that the postural adjustment associated with a hindlimb flexion induced by cortical stimulation clearly preceeds the movement by about 10 msec.

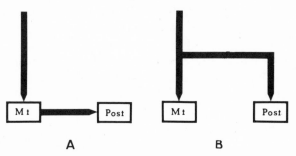

A   B

Fig. 7. Scheme of the possible mechanisms for the postural adjustment associated with movement. In A, peripheral feedback. In B, central command. For further details, see discussion.

It is interesting to emphasize that peripheral cutaneous afferents may be at the origin of the postural adjustment, which may preceed the flexion movement which is therefore centrally programmed. These afferents might be responsible for the onset of the postural adjustment preceeding the placing movement elicited by a tactile stimulation of the forelimb (Massion and Smith, 1974). They might also contribute to the postural adjustment associated with the performance of movement due to the fact that tactile afferents are stimulated by the developing movement.

One ˈay question the mechanism by which the command of the postural adjustment by motor cortex or red nucleus is performed. It is possible that the central command utilizes the spinal circuits responsible for the crossed extensor reflex (Sherrington, 1910). The fact that stimulation of a cutaneous forelimb nerve induces an increase in weight of the other forelimb with a relatively short delay is in favor of this interpretation. The postural adjustment of the hindlimbs (Gahery and Nieoullon, 1974) might be performed through the proprio-spinal pathways discussed by various authors (Rustioni et al., 1971; Miller and Van De Burg, 1973).

The central command of the postural adjustment might also utilize the spinal circuits of locomotion. Actually, the pattern of the postural adjustments which accompany a flexion movement is comparable to the pattern which appears during walking (Shik et al., 1966; Roberts, 1967; Lundberg, 1969; Grillner, 1973; Stuart et al., 1973), although it does not have the same rhythmic character.

The basal ganglia might be another site where the postural adjustment associated with movement could take place. This hypothesis was suggested by, among others, Martin (1967) on the basis of the marked difficulties in postural adjustment which are observed in Parkinsonian patients. More experimental evidence is needed to confirm this last hypothesis.

ACKNOWLEDGEMENTS

The authors wish to thank F. Gambarelli for his very helpful assistance during the performance of the experiments and the analysis of the results. R. Massarino realized the mechanical devices used in this study, and R. Haour was responsible for setting up the electronic equipment. They are warmly acknowledged, as is J. Howard for his help in translating the manuscript into English. This work was supported by contract no. 73-5-107-8 from INSERM.

REFERENCES

GAHERY, Y. and NIEOULLON, A. (1974) Etude des réactions posturales accompagnant des mouvements provoqués par des stimulations corticales chez le chat. J. Physiol. (Paris), 69, 250 A.

GRILLNER, S. (1973) Locomotion in the spinal cat. In (R.B. Stein, K.B. Pearson, R.S. Smith and J.B. Redford. Eds.) Control of Posture and Locomotion, Plenum Press, New York, pp. 515—535.

IOFFE, M.E. and ANDREYEV, A.E. (1969) Inter-extremities coordination in local motor conditioned reactions of dogs. Zh. Vyssh. Nerv. Deyat. Pavlova, 19, 557—565. (In Russian).

LAWRENCE, D.G. and KUYPERS, H.G.J.M. (1968) The functional organization of the motor system in the monkey. I. The effects of bilateral pyramidal lesions. Brain, 91, 1—14.

LUNDBERG, A. (1969) Reflex control of stepping. The Nansen Memorial Lecture. V. Universitetsforlaget, Oslo, pp. 1—42.

MARTIN, J.P. (1967) The Basal Ganglia and Posture, Pitman, London, p. 152.

MASSION, J. and SMITH, A.M. (1974) Ventrolateral thalamic neurons related to posture during a modified placing reaction. Brain Res., 71, 353—359.

MATTHEWS, P.B.C. (1972) Mammalian Muscle Receptors and their Central Actions. Arnold, London, p. 630.

MILLER, S. and VAN DE BURG, J. (1973) The function of long propriospinal pathways in the coordination of quadripedal stepping in the cat. In (R.B. Stein, K.B. Pearson, R.S. Smith and J.B. Redford, Eds.) Control of Posture and Locomotion, Plenum Press, New York, pp. 561—577.

POMPEIANO, O. and BRODAL, A. (1957) Experimental demonstration of a somatotopical origin of rubrospinal fibres in the cat. J. Comp. Neurol., 108, 225—252.

POMPEIANO, O. and SWETT, J.E. (1963) Actions of graded cutaneous and muscular afferent volleys on brain stem units in the decerebrate, cerebellectomized cat. Arch. Ital. Biol., 101, 552—583.

REGIS, H. and TROUCHE, E. (1974) Effet des ablations corticales et cérébelleuses sur la réaction de placement et l'ajustement postural associá. J. Physiol. (Paris), 69, 289A—290A.

REGIS, H., TROUCHE, E. and MASSION, J. (1974) Effect of motor cortical and cerebellar ablation on the postural and kinetic components of a modified placing reaction in the cat. Proc. Internatl. Union Physiol. Sci., 11, 163.

ROBERTS, T.D.M. (1967) Neurophysiology of Postural Mechanisms. Butterworths, London, p. 354.

RUSTIONI, A., KUYPERS, H.G.J.M. and HOLSTEGE, G. (1971) Propriospinal projections from the ventral and lateral funiculi to the motoneurones in the lumbosacral cord of the cat. Brain Res., 34, 255—275.

SHERRINGTON, C.S. (1910) Flexion-reflex of the limb, crossed extension reflex, and reflex stepping and standing. J. Physiol. (Lond.), 40, 28—121.

SHIK, M.L., SEVERIN, F.V. and ORLOVSKY, G.N. (1966) Control of walking and running by means of electrical stimulation of the mid-brain. Biofizica, 11, 756—765. (In Russian).

STEIN, R.B. (1974) Peripheral control of movement. Physiol. Rev., 54, 215—243.

STUART, D.G., WITHNEY, T.P., WETZEL, M.C. and GOSLOW, G.E. (1973) Time constraints for inter-limb co-ordination in the cat during unrestrained locomotion. In (R.B. Stein, K.B. Pearson, R.S. Smith and J.B. Redford, Eds.) Control of Posture and Locomotion, Plenum Press, New York, pp. 537—560.

WIESENDANGER, M. (1969) The pyramidal tract; recent investigations on its morphology and function. Ergebn. Physiol., 61, 73—136.

4

A proposal for study of a state description of the motor control system

Lloyd D. PARTRIDGE*

What I wish to discuss today is quite atypical for a meeting of this type. There are few facts and the possibility of measurement of critical factors is questionable. I do not offer the usual field report of a task accomplished, nor do I discuss a tactical attack on a particular problem; rather I question the strategy of the overall approach to research in motor control physiology.

I risk tampering in an emotionally charged subject where the making of any suggestions is rather pretentious. The proposal, however, is only for a change in research emphasis rather than a major change in direction. It is made with considerable hesitancy, but with the feeling that action is essential because our current course is approaching a point where no further progress in understanding can be made. This threat results from the fact that scientific literature has a finite capacity. A continually accumulating literature will eventually fill any storage capacity, but probably before that the ability to retrieve and to read will limit effective capacity. Who, even today, can keep up with the literature? Using questionable extrapolations of counts in *Index Medicus* I recently estimated that the world literature bearing on motor control is already growing at the rate of 1000 published papers per month. Even if this figure is off by a factor of two, we all know that we miss important material for the lack of reading time. Each year valid work becomes lost. At some point that rate of loss from working knowledge will equal the rate of addition, and progress will then disappear into a stirring process which only exchanges the particular knowledge momentarily appearing on the working surface of the science. This will occur, whether by a programmed deletion of old material or only as the result of accidental attrition by loss within an ever growing total pool. If the goal of our research is to increase understanding rather than just to provide us with entertainment and employment, we have an obligation to make best possible use of whatever capacity remains in our information storage system. Improved

* The author wishes to express his appreciation for research support from the National Institutes of Health while developing these ideas and preparing this manuscript.

usage can probably be accomplished through concerted effort without change in our present approaches. On the other hand, perhaps we can profit even more from a change in research emphasis, guided by experience accumulated in other fields. Such a change I advocate today.

With respect to one potential source of guidance, it is perhaps instructive to compare the progress in understanding of motor control to the progress in understanding of flying machines since Leonardo Da Vinci. Starting without the benefit of Newtonian concepts of mechanics or photographic recording, Da Vinci was able to describe mechanical arrangements involved in reciprocal muscles as well as changes in angle of attack involved in climb and turn maneuvers of flight. He described both structure and operation and exhibited an intuitive analysis that was quite similar in the two systems. In the form of pictorial dimensions, Da Vinci provided, in effect, a set of static descriptions with quantification, which for obvious reasons was less modern for the flying machine than for the anatomical detail. However, the overall understanding of machine flight was roughly comparable in Da Vinci's time to that of human locomotion.

Although airplanes and man have more characteristics in common now than then, the studies of aero-engineering and motor physiology have become quite separated since Da Vinci. The goals, and means of approaching them, differ, and even the forms in which data are recorded are quite different. To design a flying machine, it has been necessary to assemble parts to produce a complex system. Thus, knowledge of the parts has been important only insofar as the knowledge has contributed to predicting behavior of the whole. Denied the design opportunity, the biologist seeking understanding has tended to follow the reductionist path, to study even deeper detail of each already functioning sub-system. A verbal and quantitative description of responses of a component provides an adequate terminal description of that part. When we have described but do not understand the operation of a biological system, we devise new and ingenious means of learning about the still smaller parts. In contrast, for engineering design, only enough data about a part is needed to make a usable prediction of the combined action of many parts. For engineering, however, the data must be in a form capable of manipulative use; synthetic tools are essential and engineers have worked hard to adapt mathematical tools for synthetic use. Much data from engineering measurements are available in compact tables, defined in international standard units. Formal mathematical logic is used routinely. On the other hand, in the area of biological movement we have many descriptions of the results of special tests defined in non-standard terms. Predictive calculation is rarely attempted, but the knowledge of parts has been carried in many cases to the submolecular level. In fact, one might question why a biologist would even want to turn back and predict the performance of a system when the performance of that system had been measured before its parts were studied. In any case, these divergent methods have served us well.

Airplanes fly and who could ask for more literature describing parts of motor control. Nevertheless, while we still have no contracts to design biological systems, can we not perhaps make effective use of some of the tools developed for engineering purposes to improve understanding of biology?

Almost a century ago, when Braune and Fisher described locomotion as a special case of Newtonian mechanics, motor physiology was probably more mathematical and more rigorous than flying machine design, but then machines did not fly. Since then, in order to communicate results of measurement, aero-engineers have standardized measurement and have adopted tightly defined terminology based, to a great extent, on definitions from physics. Results of measurements made in one laboratory are routinely used in other facilities to make critical calculations. In motor control, in contrast, if we have not forgotten the calculations of body mechanics by Braune and Fisher, we have at least not done much to advance them nor to standardize definitions. Neither have we developed a rigorous form of description for most of the other parts of motor control. In most areas we tend to agree that our systems are too complex for mathematical description. It is perhaps significant that, without mathematical rigidity, we experience great difficulty in communicating results from one laboratory to another and also have difficulty recognizing conflict or redundancy between results from different laboratories. For example, one might raise questions about either definitions or conflict of data when material assembled in the *Biology Data Book* describes a particular receptor as showing adaptation but having no dynamic response! Furthermore, when an editor wants to avoid publishing redundancy, can he say that when I stretched a cat's leg and someone else shook a dog's leg, we observed the same thing? He certainly would have little basis in our data to determine whether or not, when a monkey moves a lever, he should pull the experimenter's leg.

Have we not reached the point that more rigid definitions would improve communication? Motor control physiologists might at least determine what is measured by the clinician who says that a particular muscle offers 'weak resistance to passive stretch'. We might even define what units would be appropriate for calibration of his measurement. Does not the very complexity of biological systems add to our need to use in their study both the most sophisticated logical tools available and the most careful definitions we can devise?

In applied mathematics the capability now exists to deal with systems that respond with time-dependent rules, and in a nonlinear manner, to multiple inputs; but we do not do as well with our verbal descriptions of motor systems. Although our treatment usually starts with a reference to the whole complexity of the real system, the analysis finally deals with only a part of the whole, which is even more simplified than a mathematical approximation. Unfortunately, this simplification is usually accomplished without identifying the simplifying assumptions which were made. Should not we invest the time to learn how to better use some of the logic tools of the engineer?

We have a long tradition of adapting tools devised by others to our own needs in motor physiology. The clockwork motor to run a kymograph, the Braun tube to record action potentials, and the digital computer to manage experiments are all cases of profitable theft. Is it any worse for us to turn our larceny from hardware to logic tools? Should we be willing to pay for hardware with grant money, but not willing to buy logic with study time? Yet even if we do buy new logic we can expect, as with the oscilloscope, that there will be quite a bit of adapting work left before it will solve our problems.

One example contrasting a traditional and a more formal description might illustrate advantages and problems. The joint system from shoulder to wrist can be described as involving 11 articulations, with each joint capable of one or more movements called either flexion, extension, hyperextension, rotation, supination, pronation, abduction, adduction or circumduction. In contrast, a human-factor engineer pointed out to me that these joints provide for positioning in seven degrees of freedom while, for example, only six degrees of freedom are needed to orient a cup for drinking. Neither description tells anything about muscle involvement and both lump into a single term the action of more than one articulation, but the description using degrees of freedom tells more concisely about drinking problems than comes through all of the Latin stems. The classical terminology is redundant. Thus flexion, extension, hyperextension, adduction, abduction and circumduction describe with six terms only two degrees of freedom in the wrist. On the other hand, the term circumduction, like a Chinese ideograph, aids fast communication, since it compactly describes a common movement that would require an appreciably longer description in the other form. Nevertheless, the reduction to two degrees of freedom becomes useful for formal analysis of wrist movement. Similar cases of redundant terminology are found throughout the motor control system. Can not we make our thinking more precise by reducing some of this redundancy? I do not mean that use of the terms roll, pitch and yaw would necessarily clarify description of movements in the human shoulder, simple transfer of terms could be insufficient.

If we develop a formal terminology to describe parts of motor control this change alone would make it convenient to apply techniques which engineers now use under the name 'system identification'. This is a formalized version of the usual analytical approach of biology; thus system identification seeks, in a formal way, to learn the characteristics of a system from measured activity of that system. This tool might be most valuable in the hands of an astute physiologist as a means of discovering when his imagination had outdistanced his data. It might be of more value in terms of papers not published than in its contribution to description of biological systems.

While biological research has concentrated on the function of parts of the system, a well-established concept in physiology is that many properties of an intact system cannot be found by study of the separated parts. These properties must then originate in the organization of these parts. To study these properties of a system it is first necessary to learn properties of the parts and then turn back from the usual reductionist part and study the rules of organization and their consequences. In general, motor control physiology has not taken these reverse pathways and consequently has probably by-passed many important issues. Thus, from reflex physiology, synaptic physiology developed; but we have little information as to whether the known properties of synapses are sufficient to account for all of reflex behavior. Whole muscle physiology leads to single fiber physiology and then to fibril physiology, but little is known about how muscle fibers interact to produce those parts of whole muscle response that are not in single fibers. Nerve trunk studies gave way to single fiber studies and progressed to study of single ion action. In this well known exception, the reverse route was explored; observed ion and membrane properties were combined to synthesize an explanation of action potentials. It may be significant that this synthetic process involved a significant application of mathematical logic. It seems reasonable that we now might find the exploration of additional reverse pathways more profitable than continuing emphasis on the reductionist route that already has been so carefully prospected. If this is so it could be worthwhile to look for tools among those already developed by the engineers who have concentrated on synthesis.

As a group we affirmed our trust in the synthetic approach when we came to Bombay by air. Did anyone choose this means of travel because of what the engineers knew about the analysis of sulfur to carbon bonds or thermal effects on bacterial metabolism or activation energy of oxidative reactions or even the mobility of electrons in impure silicon crystals — although these were all constituents in our arrival? Probably of more importance to us was the combination of these and other details to produce safe tyres, non-toxic food, effective propulsion and dependable radios. More likely, we thought in terms of the overall safety record which, in fact, results from the interactions of the whole set of incompletely understood components. Parenthetically, it should be noted that the synthesis which produced the working system was not entirely accomplished by engineers using mathematical manipulation, but was absolutely dependent on the insertion of good intuitive judgments at appropriate stages in the development, a point we should remember if we borrow the engineer's tools.

If we borrow these tools to synthesize predictions of the logical consequences of what we already know about parts of various motor systems, we might expect three kinds of reward. In my experience, the most likely consequence of such a prediction is a failure to fit observed fact. This is no basis for publication, but indicates a deficiency or fault in what was originally presumed. When that defect is found and corrected, the synthesis will finally pay off. In other cases, the synthesis may predict, from the interaction of the parts, system properties that are found in the real system. If one of these properties had not been previously recognized in the whole system, the prediction might make an important addition to our total description. On the other hand, if it were a known, but unexplained, property the synthesis would provide a possible explanation in the rules of the interaction. Thus, synthetic study can contribute to knowledge and understanding of motor control, even though we do not need synthesis for the engineer's purpose. We do have reason to turn back from our reductionist route and try to put together knowledge of parts to aid understanding of systems.

Although motor physiology research has not emphasized the synthetic approach, it already contains a basis for applying synthesis. Motor control research is built on the belief that at any given moment the system will respond to its inputs according to rules, even though we realize that as a result of these inputs the rules for future inputs may be altered. The alteration of rules is also presumed to obey other rules, and it is this totality of these rules which we seek in our research. While these assumptions are not proven, they are implicit in most of our analytic understanding of motor physiology. Insofar as we accept these assumptions of orderly behavior we have the necessary basis for application of a type of synthetic logic which has developed under the label 'state variable'. As used here, this logic is really just a rigidly formal means of manipulating data on the basis of those assumptions. The state of a system is defined in the form of some minimum set of terms representing the present conditions in that system, which are dependent on its history. The future of a deterministic system depends both on its present state and on its future inputs. Engineers have assembled a set of procedures by which mathematical representations of the system's state and presumed rules can be conveniently manipulated to produce a description of the expected temporal behavior of that system. If we express our analysis of system components in a mathematical form, the engineers' tools become readily usable. Although some problems develop in the forms used for this manipulation, multiple inputs, time-changing rules, and nonlinear properties are handled routinely. Thus a form exists for manipulation of information which seems to be suitable for the synthesis of predictions of the logical consequences of interactions between what we believe to be the rules of parts of the motor system.

The state variable methods, however, have no exclusive licence to manipulate this type of data. For any particular system the state can be represented in a variety of different forms. Further, there exist many other logic forms — both verbal and mathematical — that can be used to manipulate information about a system of parts in order to predict that system's behavior. Of course, whatever forms of logic are properly used to manipulate information about a deterministic system the resulting predictions of system properties should all be equivalent. Advantages of a particular logic then appear as either convenience for manipulation or as ease of recognizing error. The state variable methods are well defined, flexible, and are particularly suitable for dealing with separately determined experimental data about parts of a system to predict the properties of their conjoint operation. While the state variable form is not unique in this ability to predict, it is available, tested, and much more constrained than the purely verbal speculations that are often used. Too, the state variable form deals with nonlinear aspects better than some other mathematical techniques, such as frequency response based logic. If we take a synthetic route I commend the state variable tool until better is found.

In summary, I propose that because of the ultimately limited capacity of the literature we must make every effort to conserve this resource. One means of literature conservation lies in an intense effort to reduce ambiguity, redundancy and bulk of added material by working toward more rigorous and more formal description of our results. If mathematical formalisms are used to refine our results before publication, the rate of total literature accumulation can be reduced by reducing error content. A possible second means to conservation involves a shift of emphasis in motor physiology to an increased study of the relatively unexplored topic of properties introduced by interactions between components, at the expense of less effort to extend detailed descriptions of parts. This should not consist of unrestrained speculation, but formal logic, such as the use of 'state variable' descriptions, should be used to test the validity of speculated consequences. This route would not be easy but is perhaps necessary for continuing progress in understanding of motor control.

Subject index

A-alpha fibres, 140, 148
A-bands, 28
A-delta fibres, 140, 149
Acetylcholine (ACH), 121
    synthesis, 83
Achilles' reflex (*see* Reflex)
Action potentials, 15—17, 19—21, 23, 25, 29, 32, 79, 81, 84—86, 366, 367
    polyphasic, 86
Acute spinal animal, 228
Adaptation, 6
Adrenergic, 111
Afferents, 37, 40, 42, 43, 112, 117, 136—138, 141, 143, 173, 175, 182, 201, 229, 247, 252, 274, 334, 360
    fibres, 111, 114, 140, 141, 279
    high threshold, 139
    inflow, 114, 145, 182, 228
    message, 170
    peripheral, 176
    primary, 211, 212, 214, 217, 220, 224, 225
    primary spindle, 99—101, 103, 107, 117, 122, 124, 136, 141—143, 147, 175, 182, 189, 197, 201, 204, 206
    signals, 231
    skin, 261
    system, 229
After effect, 103
    depolarization, 21—23, 29, 51, 53, 54, 60, 279, 280
    potential, 18, 21, 50
Agonist contraction, 283
Akinesia, EMG of, 296, 299, 301
Alcoholic polyneuropathy, 89, 309
Alertness-dependent pacemaker, 240
Alpha, 49, 50, 206
    axons, 121, 123
    drive, 206
    motor fibres and motoneurones, 119, 120, 123, 124, 129, 130, 166, 197, 206, 283

motoneurone axon collaterals, 119, 120, 283
    pool, 261, 274
Amplitude, 270—272, 274, 276, 278, 308, 349
Amyotrophic lateral sclerosis, 86
Androgen-sensitive, 8
Anesthesia, 240, 249, 319
Anion, 23
Anisotropy, 64
Antagonist contraction, 283, 310, 311
Anterior horn cell disorders, 84, 86
Anterior lobe, 247—249
Anticipatory, 333—345
Antidromic, 123, 190, 193, 221, 253
    excitation, 224
    inhibition, 121
    spikes, 218, 219
Antigravity, 7
Articulation, 146, 148
Asterixis, 301, 304—306
Ataxia, cerebellar, 311
ATPase, 5—7
Attention, 334
Auditory input, 265—267
Augmentation, 176
Autogenic inhibition, 119, 123, 124
Autonomic ganglionic blocker, 121
Axial muscle (*see* Muscle)
Axon, 49, 50, 79, 89, 272, 279, 280
    collaterals, 121, 135
    terminals, 214
Axonal, 240
    conduction velocities, 43, 120
    degeneration, 89
    flow and axoplasmic flow, 274
    occlusion, 289

Background discharges, 122
Background excitatory drive, 248
Background noise, 225
Barbiturate, 177, 248

Basal ganglia, 360
Basket cells, 248, 253—255
Behavioural data, 245, 343
Biological movement, 364
Bismuth subnitrate, 28
Bisynaptic arc, 138
Blink reflex *(see also* Reflex)
   137—139, 148, 158, 159, 268, 270
Brainstem, 135, 136, 155, 242, 343
Brainstem reticular formation, 220
Bulbar reticular formation, 140
Busy line phenomenon, 182

Cable theory, 15
Cajal's intermediate nucleus, 216
Calcium ion, 26
Calcium transport, 6
Callostomised, 343, 344
Capacity, 16, 17, 19, 20
   muscle fibres, 15
Castration, 8
Cellular differentiation, 27
Central, 349, 360
   drive, 104
   level, 142
   nervous system, 135, 293—295,
      298—301, 304—306, 309, 311
Cerebellar cortex, 239, 248, 254, 255,
   257
Cerebellar function, 253
Cerebellectomy, 240, 245
Cerebello-cortical loop, 355
Cerebral cortex, 279
Cervical segments, 212
Charcot—Marie—Tooth Disease, 310
Chemical transmitter, 26
Chloride, 22, 23
Cholinergic transmission, 121
Chronic cerebellar ablation, 355
Chronic spinal conditions, 228
Chronically deafferented cerebellum, 255
Climbing fibres (CF), 252—255, 257, 278
   activation, 248, 252, 254
   activity, 247, 253
   afferents, 248
   burst, 247, 248, 250, 252, 254
   collateral activation, 253
   collaterals, 247, 253
   input, 247, 254—256
   Purkinje cell synapse, 253, 257
   response, 248, 249
   stimulation, 254
Clonidine, 177
Clonus, 111, 113, 114

Closed feedback loops, 255, 334, 341,
   343, 344
Code, 242
Collateral reinnervation, 89
Collateral sprouting, 7, 85, 89
Commissures, 335
Commissurotomised, 334, 336, 338, 340
Common pathways, 229
Computer, 16
Concentric needle electrode, 69, 79
Conditioned forelimb movement, 350
Conditioning, 81, 298
   maneuver, 175
   mechanical tooth stimulation, 144
Conduction velocities, 19, 117, 124, 218,
   221, 222, 242, 271
Conjugancy, 242
Constant current pulses, 16
Contractile myofilaments, 26
Contraction, 7, 15, 26, 29, 38, 106, 204
   properties, 6
   speed, 5, 9
   strength, 37, 40, 43, 45
   threshold, 29
   time, 6, 7, 9, 43
Control of movement, 256
Convergence, 254
Convergence movements, 238
Cooling, 59, 317
Correct and error trials, 328, 331
Cortex, 268, 276, 323, 340, 349
Cortical, 197, 264, 318, 337, 341, 352
   control, 278
   stimulation, 349, 351, 352, 357—359
Cortico-cortical, 343
Cortico-spinal, 211—214, 217
   220, 271, 274, 340
Cortico-spinal pathway, 279, 343
Cortico-reticulospinal, 271, 274
Cranial level, 155
Cranial nociceptive reflex, 160
Cross-autogenic inhibition, 142
Crossed polysynaptic connection, 146
Cross-extensor reflex, 360
Cross innervation, 6
Cross transplantation, 6
Cross union of nerves, 6
Cue, 323—325, 331, 332, 341, 344, 345
   and delay phase, 318, 330
   and go phase, 323, 325, 327, 328
   period, 319
   phase, 323, 325, 331
   presentation period, 318
   time, 328

Curare, 83
Cutaneous, 149, 187, 279, 340
  afferents, 226, 227, 267, 334, 340, 360
  mechano-receptors, 138
  origin, 148
  stimulation, 166, 173

Deafferentation, 228
Decerebellated, 351
Decerebrate state, 261
Decerebrated animal, 119, 120, 122, 123,
  140, 146, 156
Decerebrate rigidity, 140
Degenerating fibres, 214
Degeneration techniques, 254
Deiter's nucleus, 212
Delay, 322, 331
Delay and go phase, 330
Delay period, 318—320, 333
Delay phase, 318, 328
Delayed alterations, 318
Delayed response, 317—320, 323,
  325, 331
Delayed time, 318, 320
Denervated axons, 7
Denervated muscles, 7, 9
Denervation, 6, 7
Depolarization, 21, 22, 29, 51, 53, 54, 60,
  279, 280
  presynaptic, 145
  threshold, 82
Depolarized, 29, 50, 56, 57, 59
Depolarized zone, 64, 65
Depolarizing stimulus, 23
Depression, 120, 121, 123, 211, 227, 250,
  284, 323
Descending, 211, 227—229, 274
  fibres, 216
  influences, 271
  inhibitory neurones, 212
  pathway, long, 211, 214, 217, 225
  projections, 214
  regulatory actions, 227
  signals, 211, 225, 228
  spinal cord pathways, 121
  system, 229, 231
Desensitizing, 269
Desynchronization, 50, 51, 55, 57, 59—61,
  63—65, 69
Dielectric walls, 64, 65
Diffusion time, 21
Digastric motoneurones, 143
Digital computer, 366
Diphenylhydantain, 304—306

Dipoles, 17
Discharge,
  changes, 320
  patterns, 331
  rate, 317, 318, 320, 322, 323, 325,
    328, 331, 332,
Disfacilitate, 139, 159, 248, 253, 254,
  289
Disinhibition, 253, 257
Distal limb muscles, 211
Distal motoneurones, 223
Disynaptic, 140, 141, 147, 224, 226
Donder's law, 238
DOPA, 229
Dorsal funiculus, 218
Dorsal horn, 214, 216, 220, 225
Dorso-lateral funiculus, 218—220
Dorso-lateral nuclei, 216
Dorsal root ganglion, 117
Double discharge, 83
Duration, 54, 68, 269—271, 274, 349
Dyspraxia, 334

Eccentric gaze, 240, 244, 245
Efferent drive, 96
Elasticity, 288
Electric axis, 62, 63, 68
Electric centre, 65, 66
Electrical
  activity, 15
  behaviour, 17
  signal, 15
Electrolyte disturbances, 83
Electron microscopy, 16, 26, 27, 29, 30,
  217, 254, 255
Electronic interaction, 21, 23
EMG (electromyography), 51, 69, 74, 79,
  80, 86, 88, 98, 103, 105, 165, 166, 184,
  185, 199, 211, 212, 262, 264, 283, 284,
  287, 289, 290, 293—312
  amplitude, 185
  frequency spectrum, 81
Endplate, 6—8, 50, 51, 54, 60, 64, 68,
  83, 90
  immature motor, 86
Endurance, 5, 6
Enzymic properties, 5
EPSP, 117, 146, 212, 213, 219—221,
  227
Equipotential lines, 64
Equivalent circuit, 17
Error performance, 318
Error trials, 317, 328, 331, 332
Eserine, 121

Evoked
  activity, 252
  potentials, 249
  response, 276
Excitability, 163, 189, 190, 254, 268,
  272, 279
  state, 279
Excitation, 23, 121, 229, 242, 245, 252,
  280
Excitation—contraction coupling, 29
Excitatory, 77, 140, 141, 212, 223, 226,
  252, 278
  effect, 45, 187, 253, 255, 257, 289
  inhibitory interrelationship, 244
  reflex responses, 141, 145
Excited interneurones, 253
Exogenous peroxidase, 30
Extensor, 122, 159, 163, 166, 167, 175,
  176, 212, 227
  cells, 221
  nuclei, 176
  movements, 229
  motoneurones, 77, 127, 130, 166, 223
Extra-pyramidal syndrome, EMG of, 295,
  296, 299, 301

Facilitation, 99, 101, 103, 104, 141, 163—
  167, 176, 177, 192, 197, 206, 226, 229
Facilitatory, 96, 108, 187, 211, 252
  action, 108
  effect, 211
Fascicle potentials, 276
Fatigability, 39, 43, 57—59
  non- 43
Fatigue, EMG of, 295, 296, 298, 301
Fatigue resistance, 5
Feedback, 73—76, 139, 212, 255, 333
  mechanism, 137
Fibre, 17
  pattern, 8
  radius, 16
  surface, 16, 19
Fibrillar striation, 29, 32
Fibrillation potentials, 7
Fibrils, 26
Field potentials, 247, 248, 251, 253
Filaments, 9
Fink—Heimer's technique, 214
Firing frequency, 199, 201
Firing pattern, 79, 89
Flexion movements, 349, 351, 359, 260
Flexion reflex, 268, 269, 350
Flexor, 122, 159, 163, 164, 166, 167,
  175, 176, 212, 221, 229, 357

motoneurones, 77, 127, 166, 211, 223,
  227, 229
nuclei, 176
reflex, 127—131, 197, 199, 204, 206
reflex afferents, 176
spasm, 127, 130
Force, 39—41, 43, 45, 279
Frequency pattern of stimulation, .6, 7
Frontal cortex, 239, 317
Frontal eye fields, 239, 332
F response, 189—194
Fusimotor
  activity, 122, 189
  drive, static, 95, 96, 104, 106, 107, 109
  innervation, 142
  dynamic control, 136
  system, 107, 109, 172

Gamma, 124, 129
  axons, 121
  drive, static, 96, 99, 106—109, 114, 206
  efferents, 95
  motoneurones, 114, 119—123, 197, 212
  motor system, 197
  neurones, 166, 176
  spindle bias, 268
Ganglion spikes, 117
Gating charges, 15
Gaze holding, 244, 245
Generator equivalent, 62
Geniculo-striate system, 336, 341
Glass microelectrodes, 249
Glycerol, 16, 23
Glycogen, 6, 7
Glycolytic, 5
Glycolytic enzymes, 8
GO phase, 323—325
GOLGI, 199
  cells, 248, 253—255
  method, 254
  tendon organ, 37, 124, 142, 143, 187,
  289
Granular cells, 248, 254, 255
Grasp reflex, 303
Group Ia
  afferents, 143, 166, 172, 175, 176,
    186, 192, 229, 283
  input, 189, 265—267, 269
  lingual spindle afferents, 148
  receptors, 200
Group Ib muscle afferents, 143, 226, 227
Group II
  muscle afferents, 177, 197, 206
  cutaneous fibres, 170, 176
Group III cutaneous fibres, 170

Habituation, 129, 138, 245, 351
Hemiplegic patients, 264, 268, 270, 294
Hering's law, 238
Heterogenous muscles, 39
Histochemical motor unit, 85
Histochemistry, 6, 10, 39
Hodgkin—Huxley equations, 15
Hormonal influences, 6, 8, 9
Hormone sensitivity, 8
Hypertrophy, 9
Hypoglossal motoneurones, 145
Hypoglosso-hypoglossal reflexes, 148
Hypoxia, 57, 58
H-reflex, 108, 111, 112, 114, 127—131,
    163, 169, 175, 176, 181—183, 186,
    187, 189, 192, 193, 268, 269, 283,
    287—289

Immobilization, 9
Impedence measurements, 17, 19
Impulse activity, 7
Impulse blocking, 86, 88
Inferior olive, 253
Inherent rhythmicity, 240
Inhibition, 111, 119—124, 140, 156, 159,
    160, 164, 166, 173, 176, 177, 183,
    226, 229, 242, 244, 248, 253, 256,
    264, 289, 290
    direct, 253
    long latency, 140
Inhibitory, 37, 137, 140, 141, 144, 145,
    176, 193, 212, 252, 254, 255, 290
    cerebellar interneurones, 253
    connections, 243
    effects, 253, 256
    interneurones, 247, 248
    post-synaptic potentials (IPSP), 140,
        146, 219, 221, 253
Initial pause, 250
Innervation, 7
Integrative functions, 255, 257
Interneurones, 166, 176, 193, 211, 214,
    218, 221, 224—228, 271, 279, 280
    last order, 226
Interneuronal, 278
    apparatus, 211
    pathway, 231
    systems, 212
    transmissions, 229
Internuclear circuitry, 242
Interpotential time, 81
Inter-saccadic intervals, 238
Inter-trial interval, 318
Interval velocity curve, 81

Intracellular membrane system, 28
Intracellular microelectrode, 17, 19
Intramuscular nerve filaments, 117
Intra-territorial recording, 51
Ionic balance, 272, 280
Ischemia, 83
Isometric contraction, 43, 74, 77, 95, 96,
    98—101, 107, 144, 182, 201, 262, 264,
    268, 274, 284
Isometric postural pressures, 351
Isoproterenol, 308

Jaw jerk, 142
Jendrassik maneuvre, 102, 167, 172, 194,
    200, 283
Jitter, 82, 83, 85, 86, 88, 89
Joint receptors, 199

Kinetric tonic reflexes, 212
Knee jerk, 181
Krause's membrane, 32
Kymograph, 366

Labyrinthectomy, 240, 341
Labyrinthic stimulation, 166
Labyrinthine, 278
Labyrinth receptors, 148
Late components, 231, 270, 278
Latency of response, 139, 269—271, 274,
    276, 278, 284, 287
    long, 137, 140, 141, 148
    short, 137, 140, 141, 144, 147
Lateral, 211, 221
    column, 216
    descending system, 211—214, 216,
        218, 224—227
    funiculus, 216, 217, 219—222
    gaze, 240
    inhibition, 247, 248, 253
    pathways, 223
    jaw movement reflex, 145
    vestibular nucleus, 166
L-DOPA, 122, 123, 296, 311
Leak conductance, 16
Learnt activities, 261, 262, 278
Learnt programme, 268
Length—tension curves, 137
Linear capacity, 16
Linguo-hypoglossol reflex, 146
Lip reflex, 148, 149
Lip tap reflex, 148, 149
Listing's law, 238
Load, 237, 238

Local,
    anesthesia, 83
    cooling, 172
    ischemia, 172
Locomotion, 360, 365
Logic tools, 366
Long loop pathways,186, 187
Lower motoneurone pool, 268, 298
L-5 hydroxytryptophan, 312

Macamylamine, 121
Mass response, 221
Mastication, 148
Mathematical logic, 364
Mean fibre density, 84
Mechanical properties, 39
Mechanical stimulation, 95, 104, 105,
    166, 199
Mechano-receptors, 146
Medial descending system, 211, 212, 216,
    217, 221, 224
Medulary reticular formation, 166
Membrane, 6, 7, 15, 17
    excitability, 272
    permeability, 280
    systems, 26
Memory process, 317
    spatial short term, 317
Mental activity, 283
Metabolism, 5
Microelectrode, 22, 322
Microelectrode recording, 211
Microneurography, 169, 172
Midbrain, 228
Monoaminergic, 229
Monoaminergic descending pathway, 211
Monopolar, 59, 60, 66, 74
Monosynaptic, 74, 77, 117, 137, 141—
    143, 147, 166, 186, 206, 212, 213,
    221, 224, 225, 227, 243, 279
    connections, 211
    descending action, 213
    pathway, 176, 182
    reflexes, 128—130, 148, 156, 169,
        173, 176, 177, 193, 262, 268
    response, 176
Morphology, 25, 211
Mossy fibre (MF), 247, 248, 253, 255—257
Motoneurone
    critical firing levels, 75
    size-principle, 77
Motor
    activity, 9, 237
    axon, 25, 120, 124

control, 139, 146, 160, 197, 343, 363—
    368
cortex, 350, 351, 355—360
cortical ablation, 355
function, 141, 181
innervation, 119
nerve endings, 26
nerve impulse, 6, 25
neurone, 166, 176, 189, 212—214,
    221, 225, 227, 229, 231, 237, 239,
    261, 278, 279, 280, 293
    firing rate, 237
    forelimb, 261, 278
    hindlimb, 261, 278
    hypoglossal, 143, 147, 148
    masseter, 140, 141
    neck, 261
    pool, 190, 193, 261, 268, 271, 272,
        297
performance, 227, 338
physiology, 364—366, 368, 369
programme, 333, 334, 341
syndrome, 179
system, 96, 102, 108, 197, 238, 261,
    262, 278, 280, 343, 365
unit, 6, 25, 26, 38—45, 49—69, 73—90,
    138, 185, 269, 271, 283, 289, 302
    fast, 5, 43
    firing rate, 37, 43, 45, 264—266,
        268, 279, 298, 303
    mechanical properties, 43
    recruitment, 37, 41—45, 73, 279
    slow, 5, 8
Movement, 96, 358
    willed, 102
M-response, 189—191, 262, 271—275, 279,
    283—289, 293
Multi-electrode, 65
Multiple inputs, 365
Muscle, 6, 242
    axial, 278, 295
    cell, 26, 27
    contraction, 26, 74, 96, 107, 108, 298
    cooling, 83,
    fascicle, 199, 206
    fast, 5, 7—9
    fibre, 5, 6, 15—17, 22, 26—32
        38—40, 43, 45, 49, 73, 81, 89, 367
    hyperneurotised, 8
    length, 9, 45, 101, 102, 107, 108, 181,
        288
    pattern, 5, 8, 9
    plasticity, 6
    propagation velocity, 90

relaxation, 97, 99, 100, 106, 107, 201
 shortening, 101, 102, 107, 288
 slow, red, 5, 6, 8, 9
 stretch, 95
 tonic, 7
Myelin sheath, 89
Mysthenia gravis, 83, 85, 89
Mysthenic fatigue, 83
Myoblasts, 27
Myoclonus, 311, 312
Myofibrils, 15, 26, 32
Myoneural junctions, 26
Myopathy, 89, 90
Myosin, 6, 7
Myotatic, 137, 138, 143
 arcs, 163, 176, 193
 masseter reflex, 155
 reflex, 159, 163
Myotonia, 22
Myotonic discharges, 23

Negative
 after potentials, 19
 phase, 53
Nembutalized, 247—249, 252
Nerve fibre, 15
Neural, 6, 9
 coding, 238
 control, 237
 influences, 8
 mechanisms, 301
 organization, 238
Neuromuscular
 blocking, 83
 disturbances, 82, 89
 functions, 83, 271, 298
 synapses, 49
 transmission, 7, 83, 90
Neuronal, 6, 8, 242, 317
 analogue, 239
 discharges, 245
 level, 280
 output, 244
Neurone, 5, 6, 269, 275
 first order, 138
Neuropathies, 86, 89, 90, 310
Neurotrophic, 6, 7, 9
Newtonian mechanics, 365
Nociceptive, 141, 145, 149, 160, 177
Non-linear cable, 16
Non-linear capacitance, 15
Noxious mechanical stimulus, 139
Nucleus Cuneiformis, 228
Nucleus Giganto-cellularis, 220
Nystagmus, 163—166, 244

Occipital lobe, 249
Occluded, occlusion, 121, 177, 192
Ocular motoneurone, 239, 240
Ocular movements, 238, 341
Oculo-facial, 155
Oculomotor
 behaviour, 238
 defects, 243
 organization, 239
 neurones, 243
 system, 238—240, 245
OFF response, 247—253
Oligosynaptic, 144, 225
ON response, 247—251
ON-pause-rebound response, 252
Orbicularis Oculi response, 159
Orbicularis Oris reflex, 148
Orofacial, 155
Orofacial afferent systems, 142
Orofacial sensory information reflex, 147
Oxidation, 5
Oxidative enzyme, 9

Paccini corpuscles, 199
Pacemaker, 245
Pain, 157
Pancuromium, 249
Parkinson's disease, 172, 284, 295—298,
 309—311, 360
Passive electronic spread of potentials, 21
Pattern of signals, 278
Patterned motor activity, 212, 228
Pause, 139, 140, 142, 144, 146, 155—159
Performance, 317, 335, 340, 341, 344,
 359, 360
 level, 318, 320, 337
 scores, 318
Periodontal
 afferents, 145
 mechano-receptor activity, 143, 144
 reflexes, 144, 145
Peripheral, 6, 9
 afferents, 211, 231, 359
 control, 142
 feedback afferent, 350
 ischemia, 283
 nerves, 218, 294
 receptors, 187
Permeability of membrane, 272
Pharmacology, 169, 175, 307, 309, 311
Phasic, 166, 296
 monosynaptic reflexes, 177
 muscle contraction, 43, 304, 306
 response, 97, 99
 stimuli, 163

Phylogenetic development, 256
Placing movement, 350, 360
Polarization, 140, 254
Polyneuropathy, 84, 89
    tremor with, 310
Polysensory information, 256
Polysynaptic, 65, 77, 137, 138, 140, 146,
    166, 177, 186, 219, 221, 223, 225,
    231, 279
    nature, 220
    reflexes, 170, 177, 193, 262, 268, 269
Pontine reticular formation, 243
Positional reflexes, 137
Positive
    feedback loops, 255
    feedback system, 240
    phase, 53, 54
Post-activation, 211
Post-central gyrus, 279
Postsynaptic, 149, 169, 176, 193, 305
    effects, 229
    hyperpolarization, 229
    inhibition, 121, 139, 140, 144, 158,
        159, 255
    responses, 176, 221
Postural, 212, 344, 349
    adjustment, 350, 358—360
    input, 240
    labyrinthine mechanisms, 137
    oculomotor impulse, 240
    programme, 350
    tonus, 349
Posture, 301, 303, 304
Potassium
    accumulation, 23
    current, 16
    ion, 26
Potential, 52, 53, 57—65
    changes, 19
    complexes, 88
    fields, 60
Prefrontal, 317
    cortex, 318, 319
    units, 318, 319, 331, 332
Presynaptic, 6, 193, 229, 269, 305
    inhibition, 176, 177, 182, 189—194,
        279
Procaine, 172
Progressive spinal muscular atrophy, 88
Propagation, longitudinal, 15
Propagation velocity, 17, 19, 20, 81
Propranolol, 309, 310
Proprioceptive, 136, 137, 139, 143, 197,
    279, 333, 340, 341

fibres, long, 136, 139
    input, 278
    lingual reflex, 148
Proprioceptors of neck, 139, 148
Proprio-spinal fibres, slowly conducting,
    216, 218, 221, 223, 360
    interneurones, 229
    neurones, 211, 215, 217—221, 224
    pathways, 217, 222, 224
    volley, 223
"Private" interneurones, 212, 222, 224,
    227
Protective function, 37
Proteins, 6, 9
PSPs, 223, 225, 229, 231
Psychic influences, 268
Purkinje cell, 247, 249, 251—254, 256,
    306
    activity, 253, 255
    axon terminals, 255
    dendritic tree, 253
    discharge, 248
    firing rate, 253
    membrane, 253
    response, 248
    suppression, 257
    synapse, 253, 257
    target cell, 257
Pursuit movements, 238, 239, 245
Pyramidal, 74, 169, 219, 220, 225, 226,
    229, 299, 301
    lesions, 269
    syndrome, 169, 178
    syndromes, EMG of, 293
    tract, 214, 278, 279, 304

Radial nerve, 353—359
Radial resistance, 17
Rebound, 249
Receptor, 37—39, 170, 193, 197
    block, 83
    capsule, 43
Reciprocal, 139, 146, 156, 176, 229
    inhibition, 140, 211, 226, 227, 290
    innervation, 244
    reflex innervation, 141, 155
Reciprocity, 223, 242
Recruitment, 43, 74—77, 79, 89, 201,
    294, 297, 298
Recruitment order, 268, 279, 298
Recurrent
    axon collaterals, 253
    collateral effect, 123, 235
    effects, 247, 255
    inhibitory pathway, 119—124

Red nucleus, 213, 219, 226, 278, 349—360

Reflexes, 97, 137, 140, 155, 157, 287—289, 295
  Achilles', 176
  arc, 89, 182, 201, 206
  behaviour, 119, 120, 268
  deglutition, 147
  function, 261
  hammer tap, 99
  Hoffmann's (*see* H reflex)
  human, 169
  hypoglosso-hypoglossal, 148
  jaw closing, 141
  jaw opening, 140, 141, 143, 144
  lateral jaw movement, 145
  linguo-hypoglossal, 147
  lip, 148, 149
  lip tap, 148, 149
  monosynaptic (*see* Monosynaptic), 144
  myotatic, 141, 159, 163
  patellar, 181
  periodontal, 144, 145
  phasic monosynaptic, 177
  phasic, contraction, 99
  physiology, 367
  positioning, 137
  skin, 137
  spinal, 127, 169, 211, 227, 229
    activity, 211, 226, 227
    reflex arc, 212
  studies, 177, 279
  temporo-mandibular joint, 146
  tendon jerk (*see* Tendon jerk reflex)
  threshold, 169
  tonic neck, 137
  tonic reciprocal, 139
  tonic vibration (*see* Tonic vibration reflex)
  twitch, 289
  withdrawal, 268—270, 278
Regenerated currents, 21
Reinforcement maneuver, 99, 102, 105, 106, 199, 206
Reinnervation potentials, 86
Relaxation phase, 95, 97, 99, 100, 109, 204
Relaxed muscles, 109
Releasing, 211, 228, 295
  action, 229
  signal, 228
Renshaw cells, 119—121
Renshaw inhibition, 289
Repolarization, 21, 60, 81

Resistence, 16, 17, 19—21
Response, 280
Response periods, 320
Reticular formation, 212, 227, 248
Reticular network, 26
Reticulo-spinal, 163, 166, 211, 212, 274, 279, 280
  fibres, 220
  pathway, 224, 226, 227
Retina, 239
Retinal ganglion cell, 237
Retrograde degenerative changes, 216
Reverberations, 245
Rexede's laminae, 214, 216—218, 222
Rhizotomy, 343
Rhythmic alterations, 229
Rightening, 212
Rousy—Levy syndrome, 310
Rubral stimulation, 226, 349, 352, 358
Rubro-spinal, 169, 212, 214, 217, 219, 220, 229
  pathways, 211

Saccadic movement, 238, 239, 244, 334, 341
Sarcomere, 9, 32
  length, 26
Sarcoplasm, 19, 21
Sarcoplasmic reticulum, 26
Scratching, 211, 229
Segmental interneural pathway, 222
Segmental pathway, 166
Self-propagating signals, 21
Semi-circular canal, 164
Sensitization, 138
Sensory, 280, 305, 338
  evoked potential, 262, 274—276, 279, 280
  fibres, 274—276
  inputs, 268, 276—280
  neurones, 280
Servo-action, 359
Short-axon neurones, 217, 218
Shortening phase, 96, 106, 107
Short latency, 220
Silence, 101, 104, 107, 108
Silent period, 142, 145, 289, 290
Single, 96
  fibre EMG, 83, 90
  muscle fibre potentials, 80, 81
Skeletomotor, 96
Skin, 65
  afferents, 197, 206, 265
  stimulation, 199, 201, 204, 206

Sleep, 240, 270, 278
Sodium
   activation, 29
   channels, 19
   conductance, 18
   current, 15, 16
   dependent action potential, 30
   depletion, 21
   ion, 21, 25, 30
   system, 23
Somatosensory evoked response, 276–279
Somatosensory inputs, 279
Spasticity, 111, 112, 114, 127, 130, 169, 186, 194, 295, 298
Spatial, 214, 252, 257, 317, 333, 336, 337, 340, 341, 344
   distribution, 225, 248, 255
   organization, 256
   mnemonic functions, 318
   separation, 214
   short-term memory, 318
Speed, 5, 43
Speed of contraction, 8
Spike discharges, 19, 322
Spinal, 197, 227, 283
   animal, 229
   circuits, 360
   cord, 280
   cord,section, 121, 221
   mechanisms, 228
   motoneurones, 213
   programme, 229
   pathway, 229
   reflex, 127, 169, 211, 226, 227, 229
   reflex arc, 212
   roots, 278, 279, 294
   state, 122
Spindle, 95, 102, 104,–107, 109, 111, 119, 135, 136, 138, 141, 143, 147, 163, 167, 173, 175, 182, 192, 200, 237, 238, 283, 289
   action, 98, 99, 104, 240
   afferents, 96, 97, 103, 106, 108, 123, 142, 147, 197, 199, 206, 261, 359
   drive, 105, 107
   facilitation, 95, 96, 98, 104, 108, 109
   feedback loop, 96
   frequency, 101
   primary, 99–101, 107, 117, 122, 124, 136, 141–143, 147, 175, 182, 189, 197, 201, 204, 206
   secondary, 99, 107, 117, 124, 136, 142, 199, 201, 206

   sensitivity, 96, 97, 187
   tone, 175
   unloading, 96
Spinogram, 277–279
Spino-olive cerebellar pathway, 247
Spino-reticulo cerebellar pathway, 248
Spiral bands, 32
Splanchnic nerve, 247–249, 252
Splanchic stimulation, 249, 251, 253
Split brain, 333–345
Spontaneous activity, 98, 100, 103, 105, 106, 108, 120, 199, 247–249, 311, 324
Spontaneously firing frequency, 100
State variable, 368
Static sensitivity, 201, 206
Steady state, 23
Stellate cells, 248, 253, 254
Stepping, 211, 228, 229
Stereotyped movements, 278
Stimulus, 280
Stretching phases, 106
Stretch, 9, 38, 97–99, 107, 119, 122–124, 136, 137, 173, 178, 199, 200, 204, 284, 288
   receptors, 127, 212
   sinusoidal, 96, 101, 106, 107, 109
   reflex, 111, 112, 114, 136, 137, 181
   sensitive afferents, 123
Striated muscle cells, 26, 28
Striations, 26, 32
Strychnine, 121
Success rate, 320, 331
Succinylcholine block, 83, 175
Sulphate, 23
Summated potentials, 65
Superior colliculi, 242, 261
Suppression, 140, 155, 157, 182, 183, 189, 191–194, 247, 248, 252–255, 310, 345
Supranuclear, 239, 243
   circuitry, 242
   level, 238
   oculomotor, 244
Supraspinal, 186, 211, 212, 228, 283
   signals, 214
Suprathreshold activation, 104
Surface
   currents, 16
   depolarization, 23
   plasma membrane, 27
Symmetric, 53, 59
Sympathetic and parasympathetic, 271
Synapses, 50, 57, 252

Synaptic
  activity, 213, 218
  connections, 214
  depolarization, 206
  inhibition, 111, 112, 114, 211
  inputs, 213, 214, 240, 244
  junctions, 214
  physiology, 367
Synchronized EMG burst, 283
Synchronization, 185, 308
Synchronous, 50, 103, 225, 296, 308—312
  spike components, 84
System identification, 366
System components, 368

Tactile, 333, 338, 340, 345
  afferents, 278, 360
  stimulation, 156, 158, 360
Tannic acid fixation, 27
Tectal stimulation, 278
Tectal and tegmental, 261
Tectospinal tracts, 271, 274, 278, 279
Tectospinal and tectoreticulospinal, 271, 274
Temperature, 57, 58
Temporal, 252
  behaviour, 368
  correlation, 242
  relationship, 80, 297
  summation, 356
Tendon jerk reflex, 108, 111—114, 127—129, 131, 163, 169, 173, 175, 177, 181—189
Tendon tap, 97, 181, 199
Tenotomy, 9
Tensilan, 83, 85
Tension, 9, 40, 43, 75—77, 298
Testosterone, 8
Tetanic stimulation, 21, 284
Tetanized muscle, 289
Tetrodotoxin, 21, 29
Thalamus, 304, 355
Thalamotomy, 305
Thalamic cortical levels, 277, 278
Thalamic cortical projections, 279
Threshold of excitability, 269, 275, 276, 280
Threshold, 269, 271, 275, 276, 278, 280
Thyrotoxicosis, 309
Tone, 147, 163, 166
Tonic, 166, 284, 295, 299, 303
  alpha motoneurones, 120
  excitation, 227
  muscle contraction, 304

neck reflex, 137
reciprocal reflex, 139
stimuli, 163
vibration reflex, 111, 112, 163—166, 177, 181—183, 185, 189, 193
Train duration, 356
Transmembrane potential, 50, 51
Transmitter, 15, 121
Trans-synaptic activation, 221
Tremor, 295—298, 301, 307—311
  action, 309
  cerebellar, 311
  essential, 309, 311
Triphase potential, 68
Trisynaptic arc, 147
Trophic, 7
T-system, 15, 17, 21—23, 26—32
  depolarization, 26
  network, 28
Tubules, 15, 16, 19, 21
Tubular
  currents, 16
  lumen, 16, 17, 19, 21
  potential, 19, 21
  wall, 16, 19, 21—23
Tungston electrodes, 319
Twitch, 95—97, 99—101, 105, 109, 199, 287, 289, 290
Twitch muscles, 29

Unloading, 200, 206

Vascular, 6, 9
Velocities, 57
Velocity recovery function, 81
Ventral, 211
  funiculus, 211, 216, 218, 222—224, 247
  horn, 221, 224, 229
  horn cell, 89
  roots, 121, 123
  root filaments, 73, 120, 123
Ventromedial nuclei, 216
Vestibular, 137, 163, 238, 242
  afferents, 243
  centres, 242
  influences, 166, 244
  inputs, 256
  ocular connexions, 242, 244
Vestibulo-spinal, 163, 211, 212
  tract, 166, 227
Vibration, 111, 112, 123, 124, 181—194, 199, 201, 283, 284
  induced autogenic inhibitory reflexes, 186
  sensitive receptors in muscle, 119

Vibrator, 183, 190, 193
Vibratory inhibition, 173, 177
Vibratory stimulus, 173, 175, 178
Viscoelasticity, 357
Visual, 137, 333—337, 340—345
  cues, 317, 318, 322, 338
  delayed response, 318, 331
  field, 332
  inputs, 256, 261, 262, 266—280
  space, 332
  reaching, 333, 341
  stimuli, 239, 320
  system, 239
Visually activated units, 332
Visuokinetics, 317, 318, 323, 325, 332

Voltage clamp, 16, 29
Voluntary, 197, 201, 206
  activity, 81, 95, 102, 105—109, 199,
    268, 280, 289, 295, 303
  contraction, 42, 45, 78, 80, 89, 96, 97,
    99, 107, 279, 284
  effort, 289, 294, 297, 307
  input, 289
  muscle contraction, 43
  phalangeal movements, 213

Withdrawal reflex, 268—270, 278

Z-lines, 29, 32

Author index

Abplanalp, J.M. 318
Achari, N.K. 141
Adams, R.D. 301, 310
Adatia, A.L. 146, 147
Adrian, E.D. 79, 271
Adrian, R.H. 15, 16, 22, 26, 29, 30
Agarwal, G.C. 183, 289, 290
Agnew, R.F. 212
Ahlgren, J. 144
Albuquereque, E.X. 6
Allison, T. 278
Almers, W. 21
Alnaes, E. 122
Altmon, J. 343
Anastasievic, R. 220
Anden, N.E. 123, 229
Andersen, P. 248, 253
Anderson, D.J. 143
Anderson, M.E. 261
Andrews, C. 166
Appelberg, B. 96
Armstrong, C.M. 15
Ashby, P. 194
Ashworth, B. 176

Bach-Y-Rita, P. 136, 137
Baker, R. 136
Baldissera, F. 226
Barany, M. 5, 6
Barnes, C.D. 192
Basmajian, J.V. 73, 76, 77
Bass, A. 5, 9
Batini, C. 136
Baum, J. 143
Bayav, K.V. 213, 220, 221, 226, 229
Beaubaton, D. 336, 338, 340
Beaurdreau, D.E. 143—145
Bell, C.C. 248, 254
Bennett, H.S. 26
Bergmans, J. 53, 59, 122
Bernhard, C.G. 9, 213

Bessette, R.W. 145
Bessou, B. 206
Bezanilla, F. 21
Bezhenaru, I.S. 222, 227
Bianconi, R. 182, 189
Black, P. 334, 344
Blom, S. 146, 147, 148
Bloedel, J.R. 248, 253—255
Booth, F.W. 9
Bowden, R.E.M. 138, 139
Bowman, J.P. 147, 148
Branstater, M.E. 38, 49, 79
Bratzlavsky, M. 139—142, 144, 146, 148, 155
Breinin, G.N. 136
Bremer, F. 256
Brinkman, J. 340, 341, 343, 344
Brock, L.C. 176
Brown, G.L. 7, 22
Brown, M.C. 49, 120, 123, 124, 182, 189, 201
Brown, T.G. 228
Bruggencate, G. 227
Brune, H.F. 175
Brunia, C.H.N. 283
Bryant, H.S. 23
Buchthal, F. 49, 66
Budakova, N.N. 229
Buller, A.J. 5, 6, 7, 108
Buresova, M. 8, 9
Burg, D. 96, 97, 108, 199, 248, 254, 261
Burger, H.C. 64
Burke, R.E. 5, 6, 38, 79
Burke, D. 114

Cajal, S.R. 135, 142, 147
Carleton, A. 146
Castaigne, P. 178
Chan-Palay, V. 254, 255
Cilimbaris, P.A. 135
Clare, M.H. 108

Close, R.I. 5
Clough, J.F.M. 74
Cody, F.W.J. 142, 144, 145
Coers, C. 49
Cooper, S. 135, 136, 147, 206
Cohen, L.A. 343
Corazza, R. 212
Corbin, K.B. 142, 144, 145, 147
Costantin, L.L. 21, 29, 33
Crowe, A. 96

Dahlback, L.O. 83
De Gail, P. 112, 163, 166, 177, 182, 186
De Kleyn, A. 137
Delwaide, P.J. 112, 163, 166, 172, 173,
    176—178, 182, 189, 193, 261, 284
Desmedt, J.E. 112, 128
Dichgans, J. 343
Dimitrov, G. 55, 60, 65
Dimitrova, N. 55, 59
Dow, R.S. 256
Downer, J.L. 334, 343, 344
Doyle, A.M. 79
Drahota, Z. 5, 6
Dubowitz, V. 5

Eccles, J.C. 119, 121, 169, 214, 225, 249,
    253—255, 257, 278
Edds, M.V. 7
Edstrom, L. 5, 79
Eisenberg, B. 16, 17
Eisenmau, J. 144
Ekbom, K.A. 148
Eklund, G. 163, 164
Ekstedt, J. 79, 80, 83
Eldred, E. 172, 261
Ellaway, P.H. 119—123
Elul, R. 6
Engberg, I. 227
Engel, W.K. 5
Ezerman, E.V. 27

Falk, G. 15, 17
Fetz, E.E. 274, 279
Fischbach, G.D. 9
Fischer, J.E. 305
Fischman, D.A. 8
Ford, F.R. 137
Forssberg, M. 177
Fox, C.A. 254, 255
Freeman, J.A. 256
Freimann, R. 141
Freund, H.J. 79
Freydang, W.H. 21

Fromm, Chr. 122—124
Fumakoshi, M. 144
Fuster, J.N. 317, 318

Gahery, Y. 359, 360
Galeotti, G. 64
Gazzaniga, M.S. 334, 338, 341, 343, 344
Gassel, M.M. 172, 175
Geddes, L.A. 64
Giblin, D.R. 278
Gillies, D. 166, 178, 182, 189, 192, 193
Gokin, A.P. 214
Goldberg, L.J. 140, 141, 144, 146
Goldman, D.E. 181, 182
Goldspink, G. 9
Golgi, C. 255
Gonzalez-Serratos, H. 15
Goodwin, G.M. 142, 172
Gordon, M. 9, 248
Gottlieb, G.L. 182, 183, 283, 284, 290
Granit, R. 96, 107, 119, 120, 137, 177,
    182, 189, 249, 269, 289
Greenfield, B.E. 145
Griffin, C.J. 144
Grillner, S. 43, 120, 122, 123, 166, 167,
    212, 227, 229, 261, 360
Grimby, L. 79, 176, 265
Grodown, J.H. 309, 311
Guth, L. 5, 7
Gutmann, E. 5—9
Gybels, J. 172, 343
Gydikov, A. 52—54, 58—61, 65

Hagbarth, K.E. 96, 106, 112, 172, 182,
    187, 189, 192, 199, 206, 283, 284
Hakelius, L. 86
Hakansson, C.H. 55, 60, 81
Hallett, M. 296
Hall-Craggs, E.C.B. 5
Halliday, A.M. 278
Halpern, L.M. 306
Hamilton, C.R. 334, 342
Hamori, J. 255
Hannam, A.G. 144
Hannertz, J. 45, 279
Hanson, J. 147—149
Hanzlikova, V. 6, 8
Harker, D.W. 136
Harrison, M.T. 248, 254
Harrison, V.F. 73
Herrick, C.Z. 256
Hewer, R.L. 311
Hein, A. 341
Held, R. 336

Henneman, E. 5, 73, 75, 77, 79, 176, 268, 279, 298
Hill, A.V. 15
Hnik, P. 6, 9
Hoefer, P.F.A. 294
Hodgkin, A.L. 15—17, 19, 21, 26
Hoffman, K.P. 108, 140, 141, 283
Holmqvist, V. 121, 123
Hongo, T. 213, 225, 226
Hornykiewicz, O. 295
Hosokawa, H. 135
Houk, J.C. 37—39
Huber, G.C. 135
Hudlicka, O. 9
Hufschmidt, H.J. 142, 143
Hugon, M. 170, 176, 178
Humphrey, N.K. 341
Hunt, C.C. 119, 122, 124, 206
Huxley, A.F. 29

Iggo, A. 130
Illert, M. 220
Ingle, D. 336
Ishibashi, K. 145
Ioffe, M.E. 350
Ito, M. 253, 254

Jacobsen, C.F. 317
Jankowska, E. 227, 229
Jansen, J.K.S. 8, 122
Jasper, H. 53
Jendrassik, E. 102, 108, 109
Jerge, C.R. 141, 142, 144, 145
Jones, R. 6

Kadanoff, D. 138, 139
Kadefors, B. 81
Karlsen, K. 141
Kato, M. 121, 212
Katz, B. 53
Kawamura, Y. 142, 145, 146
Keating, E.G. 338, 344
Keller, O. 136, 140, 145, 148, 149
Kernell, D. 213
Kerr, F.W. 144
Keynes, R.D. 15
Kidokoro, Y. 140, 141, 143, 155, 156
Kimura, J. 138
Kitai, S.T. 139
Klawans, H.L. 311
Klinberg, I.J. 145
Knotsson, E. 172
Kostyuk, P.G. 213, 214, 216, 221, 227
Kostyukova, A.I. 219

Kosarov, D. 58, 61, 66
Kozhanov, M.V. 224
Kubota, K. 317—319, 323, 325
Kugelberg, E. 79, 88, 137, 138, 142, 148
Kuypers, H.G.J.M. 343

Lader, M.H. 288
Lance, J.W. 168, 173, 182, 186, 189, 192, 311
Landau, W.M. 103, 108
Landgren, S. 213
Langhof, H. 247, 248, 252
Laporte, Y. 176
Larramendi, L.M.H. 255
Lashley, K.S. 343
Latham, A. 248, 249, 254
Law, E. 147
Lawrence, D.G. 343, 350
Leanderson, R. 149
Leavitt, S. 305
Lehman, R.A.W. 344
Leksell, L. 119
Lemkey-Johnston, N.J. 254, 255
Lennerstrand, G. 96, 107, 136
Liddell, E.E.T. 49
Lindstrom, L. 81
Lindervold, A. 53
Lindquist, C. 138, 139, 148
Llinas, R. 227, 255
Lloyd, D. 163, 169, 176, 206, 212
Lomo, F. 6
Lorente, De No R. 53, 135
Lowe, A.A. 145
Lubinska, L. 140
Luco, J.V. 7
Lund, J.P. 145, 337
Lund, S. 212, 334, 344
Lundberg, A. 169, 176, 212, 225, 229, 261, 360

Maekawa, K. 256
Magherini, P.D. 192
Magladery, J.W. 138, 163, 283, 284
Magni, F. 278
Mahan, P.E. 145
Mai, J. 129
Mann, W.S. 9
Manni, E. 136
Mark, R.J. 284, 288
Marsden, C.D. 206, 308
Martin, J.P. 360
Maruo, T. 136
Massion, J. 278, 350, 360
Mathews, B.H.C. 119

Matsunami, K. 142
Matthews, P.B.S. 107, 122, 172, 177,
    206, 261, 359
Mayer, R.F. 189
McCouch, G.P. 136
McIntyre, A.K. 142, 143, 206
McPherson, A. 129, 130
Melichma, J. 7
Mendez, J.S. 306
Miledl, R. 6
Miller, F.R. 140, 147
Miller, S. 360
Milner-Brown, H.S. 42, 45, 77, 79, 278
Mohler, C.W. 332
Morimoto, T. 146, 147
Murphy, J.T. 248, 254, 255
Myers, R.E. 334, 336, 343, 344

Nakamura, Y. 142
Natori, R. 33
Ness, A.R. 143
Niki, H. 318
Noth, J. 120
Nyberg-Hansen, R. 214
Nystrom, B. 5

Oscarsson, O. 247, 256
Overend, W. 137

Paillard, J. 108, 163, 175, 283, 338, 340,
    343
Palkovits, M. 254
Pattle, R.E. 64
Peachey, L.D. 15, 16
Pedersen, E. 112, 128, 129
Penders, C.A. 172
Penefield, W. 343
Petajan, J.H. 79, 299
Petersen, I. 53
Peterson, B.W. 278
Pfaffmann, C. 143
Philips, C. 74, 114
Pierrot-Desilligny, E. 175
Plonsey, R. 55, 64
Pogorelaya, N. 216
Pompeino, O. 116, 351, 352
Pomeranz, B. 214
Porter, R. 15, 146, 147
Posselt, U. 146
Prechtl, H.F.R. 148
Preobrazhensky, N.N. 212
Preston, J.B. 213
Proske, U. 124

Ramon Y. Cajal, S. 255
Ramsey, R.W. 9
Regis, H. 350
Reinking, R.M. 37, 39, 40, 43
Renshaw, B. 169
Roberts, T. 360
Rodewald, R. 28
Rosenfalck, P. 64
Rushworth, G. 137, 138, 172
Rubia, F.J. 248, 251, 252, 255, 278
Ruch, S. 64
Rushworth, A. 189
Rustiomi, A. 360

Sakada, S. 139
Salmons, S. 6
Samaha, F.J. 6
Sapengo, E. 64
Sasaki, K. 137
Sauerland, E.K. 143, 148
Schaerer, P. 144
Scheibul, M.W. 253
Schiaffino, S. 5
Schmidt, R.F. 177
Schmitt, A. 147
Schneider, G.E. 15, 336
Schneider, M.F. 17
Schoen, R. 140, 141, 146, 147, 155
Schoultz, T.W. 38
Schwab, R.S. 310
Sears, ML. 136
Sessle, B.J. 144, 145
Shahani, B.T. 138, 139, 148, 268, 270,
    278, 310
Shahani, M. 261, 284
Shapovalov, A.I. 212, 213, 262
Sherrer, J. 294
Sherrington, C.S. 140, 141, 143, 146, 155,
    157, 163, 261, 360
Shik, M.L. 228, 360
Shwaluk, S. 145
Simon, J.N. 128
Simpson, J.I. 257
Skibo, G.G. 216
Slater, C.R. 7
Snider, R.S. 256
Sommer, J. 103, 108
Sprague. J.M. 343
Sroter, F.A. 6, 8
Stalberg, E. 60, 66, 79, 81—83, 85, 88
Stamm, J.S. 318
Stein, J.M. 5
Stein, R.B. 359
Stephens, J.A. 37, 43, 45

Sterling, P. 216
Stern, J. 284
Stewart, W.A. 147, 220
Struppler, A. 108, 172, 199, 206, 261
Stuart, D.G. 37, 38, 360
Sumi, P. 147
Sumino, R. 140, 141
Szenthagothai, J. 142, 143, 214, 254, 255

Takahira, H. 256
Talbott, R.E. 256
Tanaka, T. 138
Tasaki, I. 17
Taylor, A. 142
Teuber, H.L. 317, 343
Thexton, A.J. 140, 141, 155
Thiele, B. 89
Thilander, B. 145
Thorne, J. 189
Tiegs, O.W. 32
Tokizane, T. 79, 265, 268
Tokumaga, A. 137, 138
Trevarthen, C. 336, 338, 343
Torntelj, M. 138
Tyler, H.R. 305

Uemura, K. 213

Vallbo, A.B. 43, 95, 96, 106, 107, 182, 201, 261
Van Woert, M.H. 312
Vasilenko, D.A. 213, 218, 219, 223, 224
Veale, J.L. 128
Veratti, E. 26
Voneida, T.J. 343
Voss, H. 141, 143

Warmolts, J.R. 79
Weddel, G. 7, 146, 147
Whitehorn, D. 278
Wiesendanger, M. 350
Wilson, V.J. 212, 278
Winckler, G.F. 136, 309
Woodbury, I.W. 55

Yamanaka, T. 189
Yemm, R. 140
Young, R.R. 304, 305, 308, 309
Yu, S.K.J. 141
Yudell, A. 310

Zadorozhny, A.G. 226